72

2002

Specialized
Drug Delivery Systems

DRUGS AND THE PHARMACEUTICAL SCIENCES

A Series of Textbooks and Monographs

Edited by

James Swarbrick
School of Pharmacy
University of North Carolina
Chapel Hill, North Carolina

Specialized
Drug Delivery Systems

MANUFACTURING AND PRODUCTION TECHNOLOGY

edited by
Praveen Tyle

Sandoz Pharmaceuticals Corporation
Lincoln, Nebraska

MARCEL DEKKER, INC.   **New York and Basel**

Library of Congress Cataloging-in-Publication Data

Specialized drug delivery systems.

(Drugs and the pharmaceutical sciences ; v. 41)
Includes bibliographical references.
1. Drug delivery systems. 2. Pharmaceutical industry.
I. Tyle, Praveen. II. Series.
RS199.5.S64   1990   615'.19   89-23311
ISBN 0-8247-8190-2

This book is printed on acid-free paper.

MARCEL DEKKER, INC.
270 Madison Avenue, New York, New York   10016

Current printing (last digit):
10 9 8 7 6 5 4 3 2 1

PRINTED IN THE UNITED STATES OF AMERICA

FOREWORD

A revolution of sorts is under way in the pharmaceutical sciences. Not only are recent developments in molecular biology and the treatment of disease having enormous impact, but as a result the whole nature of drug delivery systems is under scrutiny. New biologically active substances such as macromolecules—particularly proteins and polypeptides—will require special care in preparation and handling and need specialized delivery systems to ensure clinically effective drug concentrations in specific sites. These new drug delivery concepts are not easy to create, research, and manufacture, as shown by their long development times and many failures in the process. Much of this work has been sustained by the sheer importance of the needs. There are and will be many obstacles in the way, but these are exciting times and the potential rewards are many.

While much has been said in recent years about these significant changes in the types of therapeutic agents and therapeutic modalities expected in the future, little attention has been directed at their pharmaceutical technology in terms of manufacturing, production, and regulation. There can be large differences between the demands of laboratory and clinical research and those of the manufacturing environment. It is quite natural that concern be directed to these latter aspects of drug delivery system development as we move ever closer to the mass distribution of the products of contemporary pharmaceutical research. This book addresses these needs and therefore takes its place at the forefront of the communication of new pharmaceutical technology.

The editor and authors are to be complimented on their achievement in producing a volume that will not only answer many questions about these emerging technologies but will also provide guidance and stimulation to others in the pharmaceutical industry.

Sylvan G. Frank
College of Pharmacy
Ohio State University
Columbus, Ohio

PREFACE

With the great advances made during the last several decades in our understanding of the pharmacological and toxicological effects of drug action and with our ever-increasing awareness and appreciation of the practical advantages associated with using specialized methods of drug delivery in therapy, it is only natural that the field of drug delivery pharmaceutics has been receiving more and more attention. Additionally, this past decade has witnessed a steep growth in the development of technical capabilities for manipulation of drug release characteristics that are to the advantage of the patient. These advances have brought about the introduction of various specialized drug delivery systems.

Pharmaceutical technology has undergone another tremendous change in the last decade from the standpoint of maturation and implementation of innovative ideas in the process of drug development. This has been coupled with the various intriguing if not fascinating attempts to design and fabricate novel drug delivery systems. Currently, pharmaceutical technologists are heavily involved in the development of site-specific as well as carefully rate-controlled drug delivery systems. In this pursuit, numerous diversified attempts have resulted in a multitude of drug delivery systems that are either under investigation or on the verge of entering the market with full force.

Specialized drug delivery systems represent a means by which a pharmacologically active moiety may be continuously delivered or monitored either systematically or to a target site in an effective, reliable, repeatable, and safe manner. These systems are also capable of delivering the desired concentration of a drug in a fixed, predetermined pattern for a definite time period. Thus, unnecessary side effects are avoided and the delivery of a desired concentration at a precise time is made possible.

Considering the number of recently published papers dealing with specialized drug delivery systems, it is clear that interest in the development of such systems is rapidly increasing. Most of these innovative ideas are presented to the scientific community on a laboratory scale. However, there is no source that presents various aspects and intricacies associated with the development of such specialized drug delivery systems on a production scale. The time has come to recognize problems associated with their manufacturing in a suitable manner that will establish the link between the laboratory and the marketplace of these advances in the pharmaceutical technology. The aim of this work is to partially fill this gap, and I hope it will act as a stimulus and basis for exchanging information that for the most part has remained proprietary till now. The book is organized to first present in Part One selected basic physical pharmacy, pharmacokinetic, biopharmaceutical, technology transfer, and regulatory considerations that influence the manufacture and production technology of specialized drug delivery systems and their performance. Large-scale manufacture and process/production technology of various specialized drug delivery systems is presented in Part Two of the book. These systems include microspheres, nanoparticles, liposomes, hydrogels, transdermal devices, soft gelatin capsules, and aerosol products. Emphasis is placed on the problems associated with the scale-up of these systems. These types of systems allow a wide range of delivery rates.

This book is designed for individuals of diverse backgrounds who are interested in the design, development, manufacture, quality assurance, use and/or optimization of specialized drug delivery systems, and in carrying the product from R&D to the marketplace. Scientists and management involved in the manufacture, process technology, research and development, and troubleshooting and marketing personnel responsible for innovative manufacturing developments in the drug delivery systems and their use in the future should find this book useful.

I am indebted to specialists in several areas of drug delivery who prepared chapters and perserved through several revisions and deadlines. I am also grateful to my wife, Tanu, for her unqualified patience, endurance, and encouragement. Special appreciation is extended to Sue Kendrick of Sandoz Pharmaceuticals Corporation and to Sandra Beberman and Carol Mayhew of Marcel Dekker, Inc., for their expert assistance and encouragement in the preparation of this book. Additionally, I would like to express my thanks to Dr. Sylvan G. Frank for writing the Foreword to this volume. I owe him a considerable debt for his expert knowledge.

Praveen Tyle

CONTENTS

CONTRIBUTORS

Umesh V. Banakar Associate Professor, Department of Pharmaceutics, School of Pharmacy and Allied Health Professions, Creighton University, Omaha, Nebraska

Victor A. Crainich, Jr. President, CDS, Inc., Kettering, Ohio

Stevin H. Gehrke Assistant Professor, Department of Chemical Engineering, University of Cincinnati, Cincinnati, Ohio

W. G. Gorman Group Leader, Department of Pharmaceutical Sciences, Sterling Research Group, Rensselaer, New York

Foo Song Hom Distinguished Research Fellow, Research and Development Center, R. P. Scherer Corporation, Ann Arbor, Michigan

Jörg Kreuter Professor, Institut für Pharmazeutische Technologie, J. W. Goethe-Universität Frankfurt, Frankfurt, Federal Republic of Germany

Ping I. Lee Professor, Faculty of Pharmacy, University of Toronto, Toronto, Ontario, Canada

Andrew Lowery Chief, Technical Staff, Division of Small Manufacturers Assistance, Center for Devices and Radiological Health, Food and Drug Administration, Washington, D. C.

Jürgen Maass Production Manager, Production Department, LTS Lohmann Therapie-Systeme GmbH & Co., KG, Neuwied, Federal Republic of Germany

Francis J. Martin Principal Scientist and Vice President, Liposome Technology, Inc., Menlo Park, California

Karl F. Popp*   Senior Research Pharmacist, Pharmaceutical Sciences, Sterling Research Group, Rensselaer, New York

Wolfgang A. Ritschel   Professor and Chairman, Division of Pharmaceutics and Drug Delivery Systems, University of Cincinnati Medical Center, Cincinnati, Ohio

John F. Stigi   Deputy Director, Division of Small Manufacturers Assistance, Center for Devices and Radiological Health, Food and Drug Administration, Washington, D. C.

S. Esmail Tabibi   Vice President, Research and Development, Medi-Control Corporation, Newton, Massachusetts

Praveen Tyle   Senior Scientist B, Sandoz Research Institute, Sandoz Pharmaceuticals Corporation, Lincoln, Nebraska

Paul K. Wilkinson   Manager, Pharmaceutical Development, Research and Development Center, Mediventure, Inc., Ann Arbor, Michigan

---

*Current affiliation: Director, Product Department, A. C. Stiefel Research Institute, Inc., Oak Hill, New York.

Specialized
Drug Delivery Systems

part one
BASIC CONSIDERATIONS

Chapter 1

INTRODUCTION TO SPECIALIZED DRUG DELIVERY SYSTEMS: FROM LAB RESEARCH TO PRODUCTION

Praveen Tyle

Sandoz Pharmaceuticals Corporation, Lincoln, Nebraska

Wolfgang A. Ritschel

University of Cincinnati Medical Center, Cincinnati, Ohio

Umesh V. Banakar

Creighton University, Omaha, Nebraska

I. INTRODUCTION

"Alchemists they aren't. But a $5-billion-a-year investment in re-
search and development by drug companies in America is generating
a wave of breakthroughs—from tension relievers and cancer ther-
apies to baldness cures and heart-attack medications—and positioning
pharmaceuticals to become the glamour industry of the 1990s" [1].
The wonder drugs currently being developed through the research
pipeline and emerging from the research laboratories continue to show
promise of the pharmaceutical industry's golden touch. Currently,
the drug industry is marching ahead with a financial record that few
businesses can match. Over the last decade alone (1977–1987), it
registered a 10% annual growth rate in sales and 186% gain in after-
tax profits—from $14 billion to $36 billion. More new drug products
are being introduced into the marketplace than at any time in the
past 15 years. Additionally, most of them are, at the least, claimed
to be superior to anything on the market.
  Discovery, testing, and marketing of new chemical entities, the
so-called medicinal agents, is what differentiates the pharmaceutical
industry from many other enterprises. Furthermore, the products

marketed by this industry make a difference in the quality of life
for millions of people. It is now recognized beyond doubt that during the past five years, the pharmaceutical marketplace has been
rapidly changing. This is the result of significant advances in drug
delivery technology registered over the past 25 years. On the other
hand, advances in drug delivery have been spurred by two major
factors: marked decline in rate of appearance of new drug entities
to the medical profession, and acquisition of capabilities in precise
analytical techniques that have permitted the growth of the pharmacokinetics discipline.

Although this growth has been in all disciplines within the pharmaceutical industry, lately this growth has been regulated more
toward the fundamentals germane to the design of drug product.
Numerous reasons can be pinpointed while evaluating the shift of
the interests in drug industry from drug entity to drug product intricacies.

The primary objective of this chapter is to determine the impact
of various factors that have forced the drug industry to direct efforts toward development of modified-release or so-called specialized
drug delivery systems. Additionally, this chapter also assesses the
fundamentals of such drug delivery systems form the standpoint of
fabrication as well as crucial physiochemical, biopharmaceutical, and
pharmacokinetic properties that need to be maintained constant during
the movement of a new drug product from the research phase to the
production phase.

II. PHARMACEUTICAL INDUSTRY TRADEWINDS: COMPELLING CHALLENGES

Through the rapid advances of recent years, the field of drug delivery has become a multidisciplinary science that is influenced by
numerous factors. These factors range from social behavior patterns
to stiff and fierce competition within various segments of the industry. Table 1 lists some of the dominant factors that are compelling the drug industry to assume a compromising position in the
entrepreneural marketplace. These factors collectively have been
the driving force for the current standing of the drug industry in
pharmaceutical innovation, which is more technically oriented as
compared to the basic hard-core science orientation of the recent
past.

A. Developmental Cost of a New Drug

Recently, a study conducted by the Department of Economics, Texas
A&M University, funded by the Pharmaceutical Manufacturers Association, concluded that the cost to develop a new drug has reached a

Table 1 Factors Responsible for the Current
Trends in Pharmaceutical Industry

Patent expiration

Cost of developing "new" drug entities

Consumerism

Geriatric patient population

Competition from generic drug companies

Prepaid health plans

Technical feasibility of controlled-drug levels

Impact of biotechnology

---

record high of $125 million [2]. This increase is nearly two and
one-half times the cost in 1976, when it averaged approximately $54
million. This increase can be traced to several changes in pharmaceutical research, the most significant one being the increasing research focus on degenerative and chronic diseases. More extensive
development and testing is required for drugs designed to combat
such ailments.

B. "Effective" Patent Life

The profitability of pharmaceutical research and development appears
to have decreased in recent years, and R&D is now on the brink of
becoming unprofitable [3]. While the average new chemical entity
(NCE) has failed to recovery its cost within 10 years of market introduction, less than 4% of 220 NCEs approved and marketed in the
United States achieved annual sales in excess of $50 million. Only
one-fourth of approved NCEs break even their R&D expenditures.
Most drugs will never recover their development costs.
   A study conducted by seven United Kingdom-owned research-
based pharmaceutical companies evaluated the trend of new drug development and innovation, focusing on NCEs evaluated in humans
between 1964 and 1980. The success rate as measured by the ratio
of new drugs tested in humans to those actually marketed was 6:1.
The total development time increased from 4.5 years for drugs
marketed during 1964 and 1968 to more than 11 years from 1976 to
1980 [4]. During this time, there was a corresponding decrease in
the effective patent life, from nearly 13 years to 6.5 years [4].
Usually, approximately 9 years are required to reach a breakeven
point to recover the expenses incurred during the development of a
drug.

Table 2 Patent Expiration Dates of 15 Top-Selling Prescription Drugs in the United States

Drug	Company	Patent expiration year
Zantac	Glaxo, UK	1995
Tagamet	Smith Kline Beckman	1994
Naprosyn	Syntex	1993
Cardizem	Marion Laboratories	1992
Dyazide	Smith Kline Beckman	Expired
Tenormin	Imperial Chemical	1989
Xanax	Upjohn	1993
Capoten	Squibb	1995
Ceclor	Eli Lilly	1992
Procardia	Pfizer	1991
Feldene	Pfizer	1994
Vasotec	Merck	2000
Clinoril	Merck	1989–1990
Lopressor	Ciba-Giegy	1993
Premarin	American Home Products	Expired

Source: *U.S. News & World Report*, June 6, 1988, basic data from Oppenheimer Company.

C. Competition from Generic Drug Companies

The passage of federal legislation to mandate the use of generic drugs whenever they are available, which is expected in the near future, would mean a marked impact of generic penetration on research-based pharmaceutical companies. Currently, the generics hold 35% of the prescription market (compared to 7% in 1980) and are expected to command almost 50% in the 1990s. More than 85% of the 15 top-selling prescription drugs in the United States will go off-patent by 1995 (see Table 2), which will give a significant boost to generic companies.

Additionally, it is observed that almost 90% of the growth in the U.S. drug industry is due to price increases that benefit the industry only in the short term [5]. Over the long haul, price increases could trigger the increased use of generics and fuel government intervention either directly via legislation or indirectly via reimbursement policies.

D. Geriatric Patient Population

While the 18-year-old population in the United States is decreasing, the 65-and-over population is swelling. Today there are 29 million elderly Americans in this country, and persons in that age group use three times as many prescription drugs as those under 40 [1,6]. Because the American health care system is designed for "the young," this nation's health care system is thoroughly and completely unprepared to cope with our aging population.

Currently, experts are developing a relationship between pharmaceutical R&D and the future of geriatric medicine. Many experiments are now attempting to explain the fundamental mechanisms of aging. Basic research into the aging process will reveal new approaches to the diagnosis and treatment of diseases now associated with aging. New opportunities are expected to arise for the pharmaceutical industry to design drugs that operate earlier in the disease process, before the symptomatic stages that are often found in old age [7]. Research and development in the pharmaceutical industry in the coming decade is going to be significantly affected by the current demographic picture of this country.

E. Technical Wizardry

Over the past two decades, research and development efforts by both pharmaceutical industries and universities have generated something of a critical mass of technical capabilities for controlling the rate of drug administration to humans and animals over extended duration. Technical wizardry at the bioengineering and pharmaceutical levels has now made it possible to overcome physiological adversities (e.g., first-pass effect, short gastric residence time, etc.) as well as frequent and timely dosing of drugs by incorporating drug entities in delivery systems with demonstrable sustained-release characteristics. More and more pharmaceutical companies are investing in technology development that can complement such advances. The advent of rate-controlled, extended-duration delivery systems has begun to show significant changes in the outlook of therapeutics as well as the future of the pharmaceutical industry.

F. Impact of Biotechnology

Analysts have predicted that the market for genetically engineered
therapeutic substances will exceed $1.5 billion in the next 10 years,
and clinicians have predicted considerable gains in their ability to
use these substances to treat a wide range of diseases [8]. However, these products will probably need improved delivery systems
to fulfill their market and therapeutic promises. Designing improved
ways to administer therapeutic entities has become almost as popular
as finding improved ways to manufacture them. Pharmaceutical/bio-
technological companies involved with innovative delivery system research are listed in Table 3.

Forces that will drive the expanded drug delivery industry include the growing biotechnology industry and the need for differen-
tiation among multisource drugs [8]. Opportunities for new companies with advanced ideas in drug delivery will grow as the biotechnology therapeutics market grows.

G. Health Plans and Health Care Costs

National health expenditures are projected to reach $1.5 trillion by
the year 2000—15% of the gross national product (GNP). National
health insurance is unlikely, but a minimum health insurance for
employees is expected. The increasing share of GNP used by health
care may reflect a conscious choice by the nation for increased quantity and quality of health care [9].

While the preferred-provider organization (PPO) is emerging as
the dominant system in the delivery of health care services, pharmacy
PPOs contain costs by substitution and prescribing protocols [10].
Very soon, providers will be paid at prospective prices for generic
products, regardless of the product actually dispensed or prescribed.
The PPO member is responsible for any price difference when either
the member or the prescriber insists on a particular brand of a
multisource product. This will force the pharmaceutical industry to
compete with generic drug houses for competitive pricing or to develop products that are so unique and/or specialized that they cannot be substituted. This task is becoming progressively monumental
as well as extremely costly, thus forcing the pharmaceutical industry
to look at viable alternatives to traditional drug delivery.

H. Consumers and Consumerism

The current consumer population at large is markedly different from
what it was over a decade ago from the standpoint of drug utilization
practices. The esthetic level of the consumer for a drug and the
delivery system in which it is contained is at a much higher level.
Questions and inquiries are being directed more toward the safety

and duration of efficacy of the drug product than the drug moiety itself. The acceptance of advanced drug delivery systems for routine use can be radily achieved. This aspect is indirectly forcing the drug industry to divery resources into nontraditional means for administering drugs, thereby enhancing the drug's efficacy and stretching its use maximally while adhering to safety requirements.

I. The "Old Wine in New Bottle" Concept

The aforementioned factors are posing formidable challenges to the pharmaceutical industry. They are forcing industry to make significant and serious adjustments in order to survive in today's marketplace. The escalating costs to develop new drugs coupled with the increasing time involved in their development, which reduce the effective patent life, are making it difficult for the drug industry to prosper. Current trends in the socioeconomic winds have significantly limited freelancing in research and development in the drug industry. The push toward generic substitution to contain sky-rocketing health care costs, coupled with the increased knowledge base of consumers, is changing the outlook of the pharmaceutical industry's futurists. The net compromise that could serve most of the basic interests of the pharmaceutical industry—survival and progress— would be to take a look at existing drug entities from a different perspective. Drug entities that have withstood the test of time from the standpoint of safety and use are being evaluated in new and improved drug delivery systems that enhance the efficacy of the drug product. This approach not only saves time, money, and effort in developing such drug products but also increases the patent life of these advanced preparations. Additionally, these new products are not only unique in themselves, thus overcoming generic challenge, but also are more appealing to the consumer. In this sense, the common theme currently being adopted by many pharmaceutical companies is of placing "old wine in new bottles, with significant advances and improvements imparted to the final drug product.

III. SPECIALIZED DRUG DELIVERY SYSTEMS: WHAT MAKES THEM SPECIAL?

The changes in the drug discovery and development process over the last decade have been supplemented by corresponding changes in the area of physical pharmacy and pharmaceutical research and development. Advances in analytical capabilities, formulation stability, sustained/controlled-release drug delivery devices, and more in-depth understanding of pharmacokinetics and drug metabolism have resulted in the development of the field of drug delivery.

Table 3 Pharmaceutical/Biotechnological Companies Involved with Innovative Drug Delivery System Research

External, portable, and programmable intravenous infusion

Abbott	Daltex	Kendall McGraw
Advanced Bio-Systems	Delta Medical Industries	Medfusion
Bard Med-Systems	Deltec	Muirhead Medical
Baxter Travenol	DRS Infusion Systems	Nissho
Becton Dickinson	Ferring	Orange Medical
Biomedical Devices	Fujisawa	Pancretic
Controlled Release	Hirata Sangyo	Pharmacia Nu Tech
Technologies	Hyco Aulas	Razel Scientific Instruments
Cormed	Intermedics	Siemans
CPI	Intelligent Medicine	

Implantable and programmable devices

Infusaid/Shiley	Medtronic	Minimed Technologies/Siemans

Transdermal, topical, and topical enhancers

Alza	Medtronic	Nitto Denko
Hercon	Membrane Technology & Research	Pharmaceutical Research
Key		SRI
Le Tec	Moleculon	Theratech

Macrochem	Motion Control	
Medi-Control	Nelson	

Inhalation, jet injection intramuscular, and at-site

Advanced Medical Inc.	Liposome Technology Inc.	Sumitomo
BTG	Pharma-Logic	Survival Technology
Derata Corporation	Sepracor	Viotech
Liposome Company	Squibb U.K.	Yissum

Subcutaneous implants

Alza	Endocon	Molecular Biosystems/Lilly
Amicon	Harvard Medical School	Polysystems
Bend Research	M.I.T.	Univerity of Utah
Dyrato Scientific, Inc.		

Novel oral delivery

BTG	Liposome Technology Inc.	Squibb U.K.
Liposome Co.	Medi-Control Corp.	

Mucous membrane research

California Biotechnology	Medi-Control Corp.	Nastech

Source: From Ref. 8.

Table 4   Some Examples of Advanced Drug Delivery Systems

Route of administration	System	Market drug
Oral	Balanced capsule	Valium
	Hydrodynamic	
	MODS	
	MODAS	
	Oros	Phenylpropanolamine
	Pennkinetic	
	Polymer-coated pellets	Indomethacin
Transdermal	Device control	Scopolamine
	Enhanced flux	Estradiol
	Skin control	Nitroglycerin
Ocular	Lacrisert	
	Ocusert	Pilocarpine
Implants	Poly lactide/glycolide	
	Poly [ortho ester(s)]	
	Silicone	Levo-norgestrel
Rumenal	Rumisert	
Prodrugs	Ophthalmic	Dipivaloyl epinephrine
	Oral	Clinoral
		L-dopa
		Aldomet

These advances can be implemented as strategic tools to enhance, if not ideally optimize, the efficiency of therapeutic agents resulting in one of a number of consequences [11]:

1.   Enhanced bioavailability
2.   Enhanced therapeutic index
3.   Reduced side effects
4.   Improved patient acceptance or compliance

Today it is possible to fabricate drug delivery systems or devices that not only prolong the release of the active principle over an extended period but also program the drug-release rate with a higher degree of predictability. Examples of some drug approaches and drugs that have been successfully incorporated into such advanced delivery systems are presented in Table 4. In effect, these systems can be designated as rate-controlled drug administration devices.

Most of the basic techniques employed to fabricate such specialized drug delivery systems are now relatively well established. However, a number of essentially new controlled-release technologies are being developed for pharmaceutical applications. In one such system the drug is delivered to a remote site of action at the required rate—this is the targeted delivery system. Another class of such systems are the feedback-controlled systems, in which the rate of drug delivery change in response to need.

A principal difference between the mechanisms of rate-controlled drug delivery divides the available systems into the two following groups [12]:

1. Open-loop delivery systems
2. Closed-loop delivery systems

The therapeutic system, as such, (platform) contains a drug reservoir, an energy source, and a therapeutic program governing the amount of drug passing the rate-controlling mechanism. In an open-loop system, the drug is delivered to the biological system without any influence on or feedback from the therapeutic effect. In a closed-loop system, the pharmacokinetic process is fed back to the therapeutic program by employing a very sensitive sensor in the biological environment that is capable of sending signals to the delivery program [13]. A schematic illustration of both an open-loop system and a closed-loop system is provided in Fig. 1.

Interestingly enough, even though there is a wide range of technology available for pharmaceutical development, only a few products employing this technology have reached and survived in the marketplace. The problems associated with the use of these approaches and the need to define the information required to devise successful dosage forms is examined in Table 5. Clearly, there remain numerous scientific issues to be addressed. Numerous attempts are currently under investigation [14], but they are still at the laboratory stage. The resultant systems have yet to stand the test of time through which they can safely progress from the laboratory bench to the production level and ultimately to the marketplace.

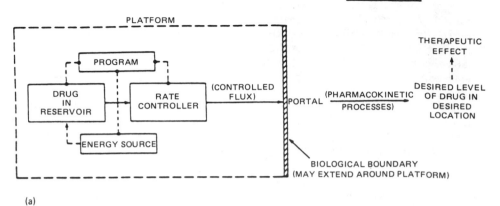

(a)

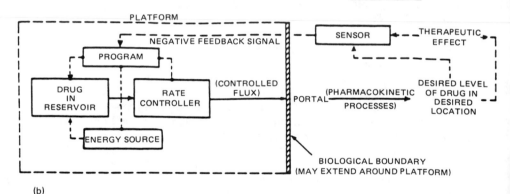

(b)

Fig. 1 Schematic illustration of (a) open-loop delivery system and (b) closed-loop delivery system. (From Ref. 12.)

IV. TECHNOLOGY TRANSFER: RESEARCH TO PRODUCTION

Transfer of technology from the research phase to the production phase of drug product development, for specialized drug delivery systems in particular, encompasses numerous considerations. Recently, more and more attention is being focused on streamlining the element of time involved to bring a product to market. This will result from containing the costs in this developmental process. Additionally, tangible rewards can be realized through appropriate planning for process commercialization. Often, development person-

Table 5 Problems and Needs for Current Drug Delivery Systems

System		
Oral	Absorption does not necessarily parallel release rate	Gastrointestinal transit control
Ocular	Patient acceptability—foreign body—stickiness of gels	Easily applied, long-lasting system
Implants	Erodibility	Chemical and biological information on implant erosion and rate and compatibility
	Reproducibility of erosion and release rates	
Transdermal	Transport rate	Understanding of transport processes
	Irritation	
	Wearability	Enhancer
	Depot effects	
	Tachyphylaxis	

Source: From Ref. 11.

nel—scientists, engineers, marketers—have stumbled on as well as struggled with perplexing problems during this transferral process.

At the outset, one must consider the development process as depicted in Fig. 2 [15], in order to rationalize planning of future efforts that are necessary. From Fig. 2, it is clear that the major point of decision in the so-called development pipeline appears at the juncture where the process is advanced from research-oriented status to commercialization. The critical path for success is dependent on successful completion of the transfer of technology at bearable as well as reasonable costs.

The primary issues that must be addressed include:

1. A feasible plan
2. Appropriate personnel
3. Stepwise procedural layout
4. Communication scheme connecting research, corporate-level administrators, and production site

It is imperative that effective communication exist between different parties involved to control the overall success of this transfer of

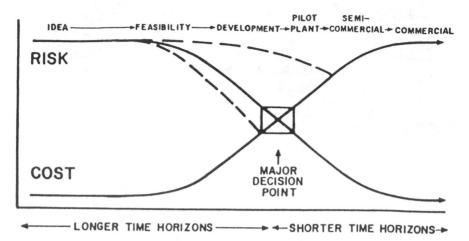

Fig. 2 An overview of the development process. (From Ref. 15.)

technology. Table 6 serves as a checklist for the various possible
activities involved in transferring technology from research to production, and Table 7 lists areas that should be addressed during
the planning of such a transfer [15].

From Tables 6 and 7 one can realize the expanse as well as the
intricate involvement needed for successful transfer of technology.
In addition to the aspects outlined, biopharmaceutical as well as
stability aspects need to addressed during scale-up of a product from
reserach stage to commercial production stage. Depending on the
resources available and the nature and type of special resources
necessary, the rate at which the product will move will be decided.
The interesting details of each activity and area listed in Tables 6
and 7, respectively, are discussed by Popp in Chapter 2.

Overall, the success of any such monumental undertaking is
highly dependent on the effectiveness of the communication preceding
its implementation. Consequently, the preparation and distribution
of a complete document summarizing raw material and equipment requirements, manufacturing and packaging processes, process validation parameters, quality control procedures, as well as a detailed
plan of action outlining expected results and time frames, must be
disseminated prior to scale-up [16]. In order to ascertain that the
right product is developed at the right price within the desired time
frame, input from marketing and manufacturing disciplines must be
integrated, as well. Various critical aspects pertaining to technology
transfer as they relate to specialized drug delivery systems are discussed in Chapters 2 and 3.

Table 6 Checklist of Activities in Transferring Technology from Research to Production

(i) Formulation selected	(ii) Site for trials finalized	(iii) Planning meeting	(iv) Date of plant trial	(v) Date of shipment	(vi) Post-production review	(vii) Assembling of final monographs	(viii) Final review monograph	(ix) First commercial batch production
		Manufacturing	Manufacturing	Confirmation of results		Manufacturing	R&D	
		Raw materials	Packaging	Stability		Packaging	Manufacturing	
		Packaging monographs	On-site review	Product evaluation:		Testing	Quality control	
		Packaging components	Shipment to R&D	Safety		Stability	Regulatory affairs	
		Testing monographs		Efficacy		Material safety data	Corporate	
		Process validation protocols				Shelf-life projection		
						Bibliography		

Table 7 Areas to Be Addressed During
Planning of a Technology Transfer

Formulation

Raw materials

Manufacturing

  Equipment

  Precautions

  Directions

Packaging

Process validation

Quality control/quality assurance

Rework procedures

Transportation

V. PHYSICOCHEMICAL PROPERTIES

For a drug to be a potential candidate for therapeutic use in specialized drug delivery systems (including devices), it is imperative to
carefully evaluate its physicochemical properties, especially when a
scale-up for a dosage is undertaken from laboratory development to a
pilot plant to large-scale production. This evaluation needs to be
based on the characteristics of the delivery device and the physiology
and/or anatomy of the administration site or the location in the body.
There is some overlap between the traditional physicochemical properties and the biopharmaceutical and pharmacokinetics aspects. Hence,
this section is a prerequisite for some of the aspects discussed in
the next section.
      Physicochemical properties discussed in this section refer to
solubility in various solvents, the rate of dissolution, the physical
state of the drug, the partitioning between media, solid-state
phenomena, etc. [17]. These properties, once determined for a drug
or vehicle substance, are expected to remain constant for the same
material. It is imperative that, if necessary, several batches of
raw materials are tested to set limits, and that the raw material is
well described and characterized. In order to maintain consistency,
it is understood that the raw material has strict specifications regarding the following aspects:

Organoleptic properties: color, taste, and smell
Purity: TLC, HPLC, IR
Density: true density, bulk density, tap density, packing
  density
Crystal form: polymorph, hydrate, or solvate
Particle size/distribution: statistical mean particle size, particle
  size distribution(homogeneity), shape (shape factor), surface
  area

A. Solubility

In general, for a drug to be absorbed it must be present in the form
of an aqueous solution at the site of absorption. This is true regardless of the mechanism of absorption, whether it be passive diffusion, convective transport, active transport, facilitated transport,
or ion-pair transport. The only exception is pinocytosis, the cor-
puscular or fat droplet absorption, which is very rare and applies
only to the fat-soluble vitamins A, D, E, and K, some fats, and
solid particles such as starch.

For all drug products, particularly for the new drug delivery
systems given perorally, it is necessary not to only to determine the
drug solubility in water but also at various pH values. During the
preformulation phase, pH-solubility profiles are established for at
least the following pH values: 1.5−3, characterizing the stomach
pH; 4.5, characterizing the acid mantle of the skin; 5.5, characterizing acidic urine; 6.5, characterizing the pH in the duodenum, bile,
jejunum, and saliva; 7.4, characterizing the pH in the plasma ileum
and cerebrospinal fluid; and 7.8, the pH of the rectum.

The pH-dependent solubility and the solubility of the drug in
various solvents other than water are sometimes important if the
drug is to be incorporated into special drug delivery systems. In
this case the release of drug will be due to partitioning between the
nonaqueous and the aqueous medium.

The dissolution rate, dQ/dt, is usually determined by exposing
one surface of a compressed disk to water at 37° under stirring at
50 rpm. The dissolution process can be described by Eq. (1):

$$\frac{dQ}{dt} = K \cdot SA \cdot (C_s - C_t) \tag{1}$$

where K is a constant depending on the material, temperature, and
stirring rate; A is the surface area; C_s is the solubility of the
drug; and C_p is the concentration of the drug at time t. If C_s is
much greater than C_p, Eq. (1) can be simplified to Eq. (2): That
is, if $C_s \gg C_t$, then

$$\frac{dQ}{dt} = K \cdot SA \cdot C_s \qquad\qquad\qquad (2)$$

If one plots Q/SA versus the time t [see Eq. (3)],

$$\frac{Q}{SA} = K \cdot C_s \cdot t \qquad\qquad\qquad (3)$$

then the slope represents the intrinsic dissolution rate KC_s, usually expressed in milligrams per minute per square centimeter. If the intrinsic dissolution rate is greater than 1 mg/cm^2, there is usually no problem with absorption because the drug is soluble enough to be absorbed by passive diffusion. However, if the intrinsic dissolution rate is less than 0.1 mg/cm^2, it is very likely that absorption problems or bioavailability problems will arise due to low solubility or slow dissolution rate.

The solubility aspect is of particular importance, because dissolution and drug release are likely to be different between drug delivery systems prepared in the lab and those manufactured on a large scale. Hence, often much development work needs to be done in scale-up.

B. Molecular Weight

Most drugs, probably more than 95%, are transported across membranes by passive diffusion. In this case the drug has to be present in the form of a true aqueous solution at the outside of the membrane, then dissolve in the lipid material of the membrane during transport across the barrier (hence the compound must also have some lipid solubility), and then be pushed out from the membrane and enter the aqueous compartment on the other side of the membrane.

The transport stream Q depends on the diffusion constant of the drug in the lipid material D, the surface area of the membrane A, the parittion coefficient of the drug between the aqueous material and the membrane material K, the membrane thickness h, and the concentrations outside the inside the membrane, C_o and C_i, as shown in Eq. (4):

$$Q = D \cdot \frac{A}{h} \cdot K \cdot (C_o - C_i) \qquad\qquad\qquad (4)$$

The diffusion constant D decreases with increasing molecular weight, hence, transport stream is directly proportional to molecular weight. The majority of drugs have molecular weights between about 200 and 500. Yet there are some important drugs with much larger molecular weights, such as digoxin, which has a molecular weight of 781, and amphotericine B, which has a molecular weight of 924. It seems that absorption is limited for drugs having molecular weight of 1000 and more. Other means, such as use of sorption promotors or ionto-phoresis, are necessary to facilitate transport of such large mole-cules [18].

In the case of convective transport of drug across membranes, which occurs through water-filled pores, it is believed that spherical compounds up to molecular weight 150, and chainlike compounds up to molecular weight 400, are considered to be permeable by this transport mechanism.

Molecular weight is also important for distribution of drug within the body. One has to remember that once a drug is in systemic circulation, it is distributed within the body by seeping out from the blood capillaries via pores. The pores in the capillary bed are not of the same size throughout the body. The pores in brain tissue are smaller than those in muscle tissue, and they are smaller than the capillaries in well-perfused tissue; these in turn are smaller than the capillaries in the glomeruli of the kidney, which again are smaller than those in liver parenchymal cells. The largest pores are found in the hepatic capillaries. One also has to be aware that in certain disease states, particularly in inflammation, the pore size may change. Epithelical membranes have a pore diameter between 7 and 10 Å.

C. pK_a

Many of our drugs are weak electrolytes, which means that they are ionized at a certain pH value. In general, it is assumed that the nonionized moiety is more lipid-soluble, and will therefore dissolve to a higher extent or more rapidly in the lipid material of the mem-brane, hence contributing to the transport process across membranes. The ionized moiety usually is not lipid-soluble. The percent of ion-ization depends on the pK_a value, and can be described by the so-called Henderson-Hasselbalch equation as shown in Eqs. (5) and (6):

$$\% \text{ ionized (acidic compound)} = \frac{100}{1 + \text{antilog}(pK_a - pH)} \tag{5}$$

$$\% \text{ ionized (basic compound)} = \frac{100}{1 + \text{antilog}(pH - pK_a)} \tag{6}$$

A significant change in the degree of ionization, which may be of clinical consequence, can be expected with any change of pH for acidic drugs having a pK_a between 3 and 7.5, and for basic drugs having a pK_a between 7 and 11.

Regarding intestinal absorption, it is believed that drugs are well absorbed by passive diffusion from the small intestine if at least 0.1% to 1% of the drug is in nonionized form, and from the rectum if at least 1% to 5% is in nonionized form. As mentioned before, passive diffusion is the most prominent mechanism of absorption. In the case of gastrointestinal absorption, one should use the pK_a of the drug for a preliminary estimate to determine the minimum amount of drug that will be in nonionized form throughout the pH range occurring in the intestinal tract.

D. Isoelectric Point

Amphoteric compounds, particularly peptides, are stimulating increasing interest for peroral administration. Peptides and proteins have an isoelectric point that is defined as the pH or hydrogen ion concentration at which the zwitterion concentration is a maximum and at which net movement of the molecule is negligible. At the isoelectric point a compound's solubility is at its minimum. Hence, for absorption purposes the pH at the absorption side should be at least one or two pH units away from the isoelectric point.

E. Apparent Partition Coefficient

The apparent partition coefficient, also called the lipid/water partition coefficient, is the ratio of the drug concentration in two practically immiscible phases. For biopharmaceutical purposes one usually uses a buffer of pH 7.4 (blood pH) as the aqueous phase, and n-octanol as the lipid phase. Prior to the experiment each phase is saturated with the other phase. The drug is dissolved in one phase and then the other phase is added and agitated for a minimum of 3 hr, usually at 37°C, and the concentration of the drug in the aqueous phase prior to the experiment and after separation, at the end of the experiment, are determined as $C_{A(before)}$ and $C_{A(after)}$, as shown in Eq. (7):

$$APC = \frac{(C_{A(before)} - C_{A(after)}) \cdot V_a}{C_{A(after)} \cdot V_1} \tag{7}$$

where V_a and V_1 are the volumes of the aqueous and the lipid phase, respectively. Drugs being absorbed by passive diffusion must have a minimum APC. With increasing APC the drug will increasely enter lipid material; i.e., it will enter brain tissue (important for CNS drugs) and fat tissue, and will be retained longer in obese and geriatric patients.

APC must also be considered for drug release from drug delivery systems. For instance, the partitioning of a drug of high APC from a fat-based suppository, a fat matrix tablet, or from a lipophilic ointment base will be slow and may be incomplete. On the other side, this very principle is often utilized for sustained drug-delivery systems.

F. Binding

Binding of drugs to biological material may occur in blood and in tissue. In blood, binding occurs primarily to plasma proteins (molecular weight 67,500), to α1-acid glycoprotein (molecular weight 41,000−45,000), and to erythrocytes. In tissue, binding may occur to all types of tissue protein, nucleic acid, cartilage, and bone material (particularly those compounds that form complexes with Ca and Mg). Considering human adults of 70 kg body weight, there are about 100 g of plasma protein, about 12 g of α1-acid glycoprotein, and in tissue about 10 kg of protein.

The extent of protein binding is not constant but is concentration- and temperature-dependent, and displacement from binding can occur by endogenous substances as well as by drugs. The extent of protein binding may also change due to disease, particularly liver and kidney disease. The amount of protein may also change due to diseases. It may be increased, such as in benign tumors and neurological diseases, or decreased, as in cancer and burn patients. The binding to α1-acid glycoprotein is particularly for basic compounds. During pathological conditions, such as fever, surgery, and inflammation, the α1-acid glycoprotein content in plasma may increase 10-fold.

Erythrocytes may take up drugs to an appreciable extent, as has been found for meperidine, where 70% of the drug in blood is bound to red blood cells. It should be noticed that for very potent drugs the binding to erythrocytes might be of future importance to a drug delivery system.

VI. BIOPHARMACEUTICAL AND PHARMACOKINETIC PROPERTIES

The physicochemical parameters as discussed in the previous section may give some reasonable information on the potential for absorption of a drug from a given site of administration. This information may even be sufficient for some routes of administration in delivery systems, such as for administering the drug by the intervenous, intramuscular, or subcutaneous route. For most other routes, particularly for the peroral route of administration but also for others such as buccal, nasal, and rectal administration, additional biopharmaceutical and pharmacokinetic information is required to decide on the feasibility of the use of the drug for a particular drug delivery system or device.

In this section we will deal with general biopharmaceutical considerations, mainly the general absorbability of the drug from a given
site of administration, the routes of administration, and some special
biopharmaceutical manipulations to increase or decrease the rate of
absorption. Also in this section we will discuss the pertinent pharmacokinetic parameters for the design of a drug delivery system/
device, mainly the elimination rate constant and the corresponding
elimination half-life, the area under the curve, clearance, and the
apparent volume of distribution [17,19]. The biopharmaceutical
and pharmacokinetic properties characterized for a dosage form or
drug delivery system are the same regardless of whether it is a
developmental preparation or a large-scale-manufactured product.

A. General Absorbability

A prerequisite for absorption of drug is its presence in the form of
a true solution at the site of absorption (with the rare exception of
pinocytosis). But being present in the form of a true solution does
not necessarily mean that the drug is absorbed across a membrane
into systemic circulation. This will depend on, among other things,
the size of the molecule, the lipid solubility, the partition coefficient,
and the pK_a. All this information applies to about 95% of all drugs
for their absorption by passive diffusion. However, about 5% of
drugs are absorbed by other absorption mechanisms, either in part
or exclusively, such as active transport, facilitated transport, convective transport, ion-pair transport, or pinocytosis. Practically
all mechanisms are present only in the small intestine. Hence, if a
drug is absorbed predominantly by active transport, then a peroral
controlled-release system or device is not feasible, because such a
system or device should release the drug over a long period of time,
say about 12 hr. The slow release, however, may not be relevant
because the drug is absorbed from only a very small segment of the
intestine. Hence, it is important to test each drug for its general
absorbability. This means that the drug is absorbable from all GI
segments, the stomach, duodenum, jejunum, ileum, cecum, colon,
and rectum. Beside having different absorption mechanisms, some
drugs are only specifically absorbed from a segment; for example,
griseofulvin is absorbed only from the duodenum. Also, for other
routes of administration a general absorbability is necessary, since
from those routes absorption occurs practically only by passive diffusion and convective transport.

Several models for studying general absorbability have been described in the literature.

B. Routes of Administration

The most important route of administration at present for controlled-release drug delivery systems and devices is the peroral route. However, other routes also seem to be very promising, and their utilization is under investigation by numerous research groups.

Peroral Route

The time span for effective drug release from a peroral (PO) controlled-release drug delivery system is limited by the gastrointestinal transit time, which is about 16 hr in humans. Hence, controlled-release drug delivery systems are feasible for 12- and 24-hr administration. One has to realize that there are not only wide interindividual but also intraindividual variations in the transit time, which also is influenced by physical activity, food and liquid intake, type of food, psychological stress, etc.

Attempts have been made to keep delivery systems, in the GI tract for an extended period of time, such as tablets that adhere or stick to the stomach wall, or tablets and capsules that float in the GI fluid, or using sizes and shapes of those forms that retain them in the gaster for a long period of time. However, in the latter case careful studies must reveal that no lodging of such systems occurs at the pylorus, which might be dangerous, particularly in case the drug exhibits irritant properties. To circumvent this it was suggested to use controlled-release pellets of different coating thickness and size, and type of coating, to achieve a more predictive GI transit time and to reduce the danger of dose dumping.

Another problem often encountered in PO dosage forms is the fact that many drugs exhibit first-pass effect, which is the presystemic loss of drug due to metabolism or the presystemic loss of drug to instability at a given pH, the hydrolytic degration in the contents of the GI tract, or the microbial inactivation by the gastrointestinal flora.

It is generally believed that a zero-order delivery-rate constant is ideal for all drug delivery systems. However, many very effective first-order or square-root-of-time-release-type dosage forms are on the market. Regarding zero-order kinetics, one has to realize that in vitro achieved zero-order release may not necessarily result in vivo zero-order absorption. This will happen only if the entire GI tract behaves as a one-compartment model. This would mean that the various segments throughout the GI tract are homogeneous with respect to absorption and that the drug release rate is the rate-limiting step in the absorption process.

Intramuscular or Subcutaneous Route

The intramuscular (IM) and subcutaneous (SC) routes of administration are widely used for aqueous and oleaginous solutions, suspensions, emulsions, and implants. The advantage of these routes of administration is that the duration of effect may be not only for hours or days, but for weeks, months, or even a year or longer. The limitation for a drug to be used by these routes of administration is the amount of drug that can feasibly be incorporated into the delivery system, and nonirritability to the tissue. At the present time the tendency is to increasingly use biodegradable material for such systems. The factors that influence the drug release are pK_a, molecular weight, diffusion coefficient, and blood flow rate at the absorption site. The rate-limiting step for such systems is the contact surface area between delivery system and surrounding tissue.

Transdermal Route

Transdermal drug delivery systems have gained wide acceptance. They are used particularly for drugs of high potency so that only milligrams have to be administered to result in effective therapeutic concentration, to be nonirritable, and upon peroral administration usually exhibit a high first-pass effect. The rate-limiting step in transdermal absorption is usually the *Stratum corneum*, but in some cases it can be the entire skin. Skin permeability is a passive process of dissolution and molecular diffusion. The rate and extent of transdermal absorption depends on many factors, such as the drug concentration, the type of system, the surface area of contact, occlusion, the anatomic region of application, skin condition, age, metabolism in the skin, skin blood perfusion rate, etc.

Intravenous Route

The intravenous (IV) route of administration can simply be used for controlled administration by infusion of the drug at a zero-order delivery rate. The intravenous route of administration is also used for specialized drug delivery systems to administer liposomes, nanoparticles, and other systems for tissue targeting.

Other Routes

In recent years some nonconventional routes of administration have received wide attention, such as buccal, ocular, nasal, rectal, and vaginal administration of drugs. In principle, their release mechanisms are similar to those of other routes, being based on drug dissolution, diffusion, and erosion. However, some specific physicological and anatomical aspects have to be considered, such as the pH, fluid volume, enzymes present, adhesive properties, and the blood flow rate at the administration site.

C. Desired or Required Therapeutic Concentrations or Concentration Ranges

Which type of special drug delivery system or device is most suitable for a given drug and a given indication is dictated by the desired or required therapeutic target concentration either in blood or in a specific target tissue. In some cases the desired target is to maintain a steady-state blood level throughout the entire dosing interval, C_{av}^{ss}, similarly to a drug level achieved after constant-rate intravenous infusion, or it could be a peak concentration, C_{max}^{ss}, or a drug concentration, C_{min}^{ss}, which needs not to be exceeded or undercut within any given dosage interval, meaning that the drug-level concentration fluctuates between $C_{ss(max)}$ and $C_{ss(min)}$. Another possibility is that within each dosing interval, a peak concentration, C_{max}^{ss}, is obtained, whereafter the drug concentraiton is not important—or vice versa, a minimum therapeutic concentration, MEC, is maintained throughout the dosing interval, which means that the drug level should be above the C_{min}^{ss} throughout the dosing interval. For some drugs a therapeutic window, TW, may apply, whereby the therapeutic concentration should fluctuate within the concentration limits of that window. For other drugs it might not be necessary to reach or maintain a given concentration at a strict periodicity; rather, a desired concentration is reached only upon request, such as if the blood glucose level falls, insulin shall be delivered. The latter case is for those special drug delivery systems based on drug targeting and trigger mechanisms.

An amount, A, is the product of volume, V, and concentration, C, as shown in Eq. (8):

$$A = V \times C \tag{8}$$

Translated into pharmacokinetic terminology, Eq. (9) is applicable:

$$D \cdot F = V_z \cdot C(0) \tag{9}$$

whereby D is the dose size, F is the fraction of drug absorbed, V_z is the apparent volume of distribution, and C(0) is the fictitious initial drug concentration in blood plasma or serum. One needs to know the desired or target concentration, C, and the volume of distirubtion of the drug, V_z, in order to calculate the dose size to be administered, corrected for bioavailablity. The information on the target concentration needs to be established by the clinical pharmacologist, along with information as to whether a certain concentration or concentration range (therapeutic range) in blood is desired, or in a given tissue. The situation is complicated by the fact that even if the drug is released at zero-order kinetics, is completely absorbed, and follows in general a pattern like a constant-rate IV

infusion, there is no guarantee that the concentration at steady state
will exhibit a straight line parallel to the abscissa as a function of
time. Rather, this line may look like a sine wave. The reason is
that many of our body functions are under circadian rhythm, with
fluctuations in blood flow rate, plasma volume, pH, etc. In other
words, even if a certain concentration is desired, in reality it may
fluctuate within a range of biological variation.

D.   Pharmacokinetics Aspects

Even though some drugs follow so-called two- or higher-compartment
models, for relating the principles we will, for practical reasons,
consider the one-compartment open model only.

   In a one-compartment open model, the drug, either injected or
absorbed after an extravascular route of administration, distributes
more or less instantly to all the space of the volume of distribution
of the drug. A two-compartment model or higher-compartment model
is characterized by the fact that the drug, reaching systemic circulation after intravenous or extravasuclar administration, stays for
a measurable period of time in the systemic circulation and all those
tissues that are in immediate equilibrium with it, and then slowly
seeps out from systemic circulation and enters the space of the
apparent volume of distribution.

   A drug given by rapid intravenous injection will reach a peak
concentration within one circulation time (1.5 to 3 min) and then
decay, usually in first-order fashion. A drug extravascularly (PO,
IM, SC, etc.) has no measurable drug concentration in blood at the
time of administration; the drug concentration will rise to a peak
concentration and then decay, usually in a first-order fashion. If
consecutive doses are given, at time intervals shorter than it takes
to eliminate about 90% of the drug from the body by either metabolism
or renal elimination, then an accumulation will occur to steady state.
This is shown in Fig. 3.

   Most dosage forms, and particularly most drug delivery systems
and devices, are designed to reach a certain steady-state concentration or concentration range. In order to predict such a steady-state
concentration one needs to determine some basic pharmacokinetic
parameters, which are usually calculated from single-dose concentration-time profiles. Only in the cases of enzyme induction, enzyme
inhibition, dose dependency, and Michaelis-Menten kientics is it
necessary to derive these parameters from steady-state concentration-time profiles.

   A simplified approach is discussed in the following subsections
for determination of the most important pharmacokinetic parameters:
elimination half-life, $t_{1/2}$; terminal elimination rate constant, λ_z;
total area under the curve, AUC; extent of bioavailability, F; total
clearance, CL; and apparent volume of distribution, V_z.

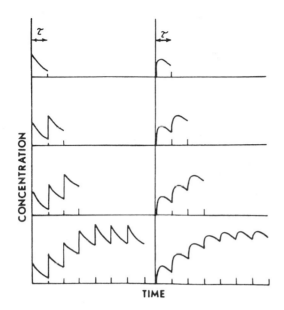

Fig. 3 Schematic diagram showing drug accumulation upon multiple
IV (left column) and extravascular administration (right column).
Identical doses are given at identical dosing intervals. The dosing
interval is shorter than it takes to eliminate the drug, hence accumulation occurs until a steady state (bottom panel) is reached. (From
W. A. Ritschel, *Graphic Approach to Clinical Pharmacokinetics*, 2nd
ed., J. R. Prous, Barcelona, Spain, 1984, p. 14, with permission of
the publisher.)

Terminal Half-Life and Terminal Disposition Rate Constant

The terminal slope after intravascular or extravascular administration
of a log concentration versus time plot shows a straight line, called
terminal phase. In most cases not all concentration-time points of
the terminal phase will be directly on a straight line but will be
scattered around it. Hence, one may use either eye fitting of these
points to a straight line or regression analysis to characterize the
best fit of line. If one selects any point on the terminal slope,
marked C_1 (see Fig. 4), and then marks the point on the same terminal slope when the concentration is one-half of C_1, the time span
between C_1 and $C_{1/2}$ is equal to the elimination half-life, $t_{1/2}$, as
shown in Fig. 4. If the time when concentration C_1 was chosen is
t_1, and that for $C_{1/2}$ is t_2, the $t_{1/2}$ is given by Eq. (10):

$$t_{1/2} = t_2 - t_1 \qquad (10)$$

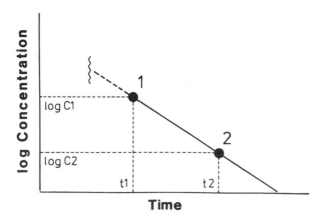

Fig. 4 Determination of elimination half-life. A concentration-time point (C1; t1) is selected on the terminal (straight) slope of a blood level-time semilogarithmic plot. The C2 is marked on that slope, where C2 = $C_{1/2}$. The difference between t2 and t1 is the elimination half-life.

The terminal disposition rate constant λ_z is calculated by dividing the ln 2(0.693) by $t_{1/2}$, as given in Eq. (11):

$$\lambda_z = \frac{0.693}{t_{1/2}} \tag{11}$$

Total Area Under the Curve

The total area under the cure, AUC, is calculated by the so-called linear trapezoidal rule. The principle of the linear trapezoidal rule is to convert the area between two concentration-time points to a trapezoid, as shown in Fig. 5. Usually, the concentration time curve is not followed up by blood sampling to zero concentration. The trapezoidal rule gives the area from time zero, drug administration, until the last blood sample is taken. In order to calculate the total area under the curve, one needs to estimate the remaining area after the last drug sample. This is obtained simply by dividing the last blood sample concentration by λ_z. The AUC is shown in Eq. (12):

$$\text{AUC} = \left[\sum \left(\frac{C_n + C_{n+1}}{2} \right) \cdot (t_{n+1} - t_n) \right] + \frac{C_{last}}{\lambda_z} \tag{12}$$

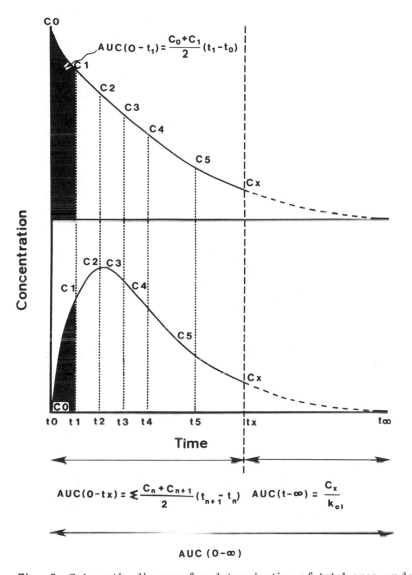

$$AUC(0-t_1) = \frac{C_0 + C_1}{2}(t_1 - t_0)$$

$$AUC(0-tx) = \sum \frac{C_n + C_{n+1}}{2}(t_{n+1} - t_n) \qquad AUC(t-\infty) = \frac{C_x}{k_{el}}$$

AUC (0-∞)

Fig. 5 Schematic diagram for determination of total area under the blood level-time curve. AUC = area under the curve; C_{index} = drug concentration; t_{index} = corresponding time for C_{index}; C_x = concentration of last blood sample taken; t_∞ = infinite time; λ_z = terminal disposition rate constant; $AUC(0 - t_x)$ = area under the curve from time zero to time t_x; $AUC(t_x - \infty)$ = area under the curve from time t_x to infinity; $AUC(0 - \infty)$ = area under the curve from time zero to infinity. [From W. A. Ritschel, Pharmacokinetics: Definitions, symbols and basic equations. *Rev. Farmacol. Clin. Exp. 1*: 23−28 (1984), with permission of the publisher.]

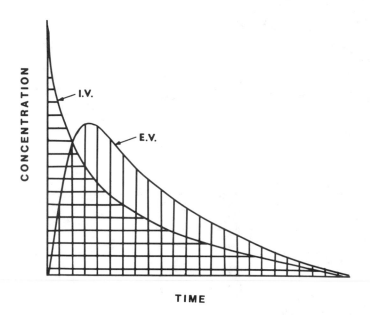

TIME

Fig. 6   Schematic diagram for determination of absolute bioavailability.   IV = intravenous administration; EV = extravascular administration.   [From W. A. Ritschel, General kinetics and bioavailability,
Rev. Farmacol. Clin. Exp., 1:29–32 (1984), with permission of the
publisher.]

Absolute Bioavailability

The absolute bioavailability, F, is calculated as the ratio of the total
area under the curve after extravascular (EV) administration to that
after intravascular (IV) administration, corrected for dose sizes, as
shown in Fig. 6 and Eq. (13):

$$F = \frac{AUC_{EV} \cdot D_{IV}}{AUC_{IV} \cdot D_{EV}} \tag{13}$$

Total Clearance

The total clearance is that volume of distribution which is cleared of
drug per unit of time.   It is calculated as the ratio of the dose
absorbed and the total area under the curve as shown in Eq. (14):

$$CL = \frac{D}{AUC} \tag{14}$$

In the case of extravascular administration, D has to be multiplied by the bioavailability, F.

Apparent Volume of Distribution

The apparent volume of distribution is not real volume but an artifact. It is that volume of blood theoretically needed if all of the drug were to stay in blood at the same concentration as found in the experiment. It is a proportionality constant relating the amount of drug in the body to the measured concentration in biological fluid. V_z is calculated from the dose given, the area under the curve, and the terminal disposition rate constant, as shown in Eq. (15):

$$V_z = \frac{D}{AUC \cdot \lambda_z} \tag{15}$$

In case a drug is given extravascularly, D has to be multiplied by F.

Dosing Equations

In Fig. 7 the relationship among IV constant-rate infusion, IV push, and extravascular administration is shown. Let us assume a drug is given to the same subject once as an IV constant-rate infusion (top panel in Fig. 7), once as an IV push injection (second panel in Fig. 7), and once extravascularly (PO, IM, SC, rectal, etc.) whereby the drug is completely bioavailable (third panel of Fig. 7). For IV and EV, identical dose sizes are used in identical dosing intervals. For IV constant-rate infusion, the total dose infused is equal to the sum of all doses given by IV push or extravascularly, and the duration of infusion TI is equal to the sum of all IV push or EV dosing intervals. No saturation kinetics, enzyme induction, or enzyme inhibition are present.

The IV constant-rate infusion will result in accumulation to a steady-state concentration C^{ss}. Since the input is at constant rate, no fluctuations occur (top panel of Fig. 7).

Upon IV push multiple dosing, the steady-state concentrations will fluctuate between C^{ss}_{max} and C^{ss}_{min}. The theoretical mean steady-state concentration C^{ss}_{av} will be the same as if the drug were given by IV constant-rate infusion (second panel of Fig. 7).

Upon EV multiple dosing, the steady-state concentrations will fluctuate between C^{ss}_{max} and C^{ss}_{min}. Note, however, that the fluctuation is less after EV than after IV administration. The mean steady-state concentration C^{ss}_{av} will be the same as if the drug were given by IV constant-rate infusion (third panel of Fig. 7).

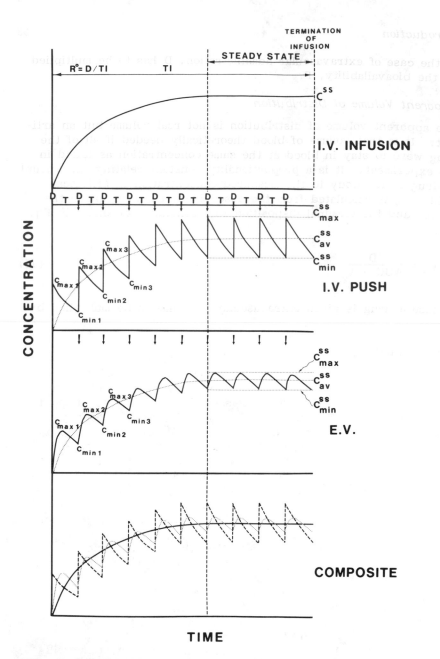

FIG. 7 Relationship between IV constant-rate infusion, IV push, and extravascular (EV) administration. R^0 = infusion rate; D = dose size; TI = duration of infusion; C^{ss} = steady-state concentration; C^{ss}_{max} = peak steady-state concentration, C^{ss}_{av} = mean steady-state concentration; C^{ss}_{min} = trough steady-state concentration. [From W. A. Ritschel, *Handbook of Basic Pharmacokinetics*, 3rd ed., Drug Intelligence Publications, Hamilton, Ill., 1986, p. 330, with permission of the publisher.]

A composition of the three routes of administration is given in the bottom of panel of Fig. 7.

The dosing equations for the three conditions are given in Eq. (16) through (17), where R^0 is the zero-order infusion rate constant and τ is the dosing interval. The other symbols are as defined in the previous sections.

IV constant rate infusion:
$$R^0 = C^{ss} \cdot V_z \cdot \lambda_z \tag{16}$$

IV push:
$$D = C^{ss}_{av} \cdot V_z \cdot \lambda_z \cdot \tau \tag{17}$$

EV administration:
$$D = \frac{C^{ss}_{av} \cdot V_z \cdot V_z \cdot \tau}{F} \tag{18}$$

VII. REFERENCES

1. K. R. Sheets and R. F. Black, *U.S. News & World Report*, June 6, 1988, p. 39.
2. "Trends and Forecasts," *NPC*, Reston, Va., Winter 1988, p. 6.
3. L. W. Charkin and D. A. Byron, *Pharm. Exec.*, July 1987, pp. 30−34.
4. S. R. Walker, M. K. Ravenscroft, and W. Wardell, 2nd World Conf. Clin. Pharmacol. Ther., Washington, D.C., 1983, Abst. No. 180.
5. *Chain Drug Review*, Oct. 26, 1987, p. 8.
6. K. Dychtwald, Amer. Soc. Hosp. Pharm. Ann. Mtg., Washington, D.C., June 1987.
7. "Pharmaceutical R&D and the Future of Geriatric Medicine," Foresight Seminars for Congressional Staff, Sept. 15, 1987.
8. R. C. Wade, *Pharm. Exec.*, Sept. 1987, pp. 62−68.
9. "National Health Expenditures, 1986−2000," *Health Care Financing Review*, Summer 1987.
10. F. R. Curtiss, *Amer. J. Hosp. Pharm.*, 44:1797 (1987).
11. C. R. Gardner in *Drug Delivery Systems: Fundamentals and Techniques* (P. Johnson and J. G. Lloyd-Jones, eds.), VCH Publishers, New York, 1988, p. 12.
12. F. E. Yates, H. Rensen, R. Buckles, J. Urquhart, and A. Zaffaroni, Designs for improved therapy among controlled delivery of drugs in *Advances in Biomedical Engineering* (J. H. Brown and J. Dickson, III, eds.), Academic Press, New York, 1975, p. 1.
13. U. V. Banakar, *Int. J. Pharm. Tech. Prod. Manuf.* (1989), in press.

14. Y. W.   Chein, *Drug Dev. Ind. Pharm.*, *9*:1291 (1983).
15. B. M. Rushton, *Res. Man.*, *29*:22 (1986).
16. K. F. Popp, *Drug Dev. Ind. Pharm.*, *13*:2339 (1987).
17. W. Ritschel, Pharmacokinetic and biopharmaceutical aspects
     in drug delivery, in *Drug Delivery Devices* (P. Tyle, ed.),
     Marcel Dekker, New York, 1988, p. 17–79.
18. P. Tyle, Iontophoretic devices, in *Drug Delivery Devices*
     (P. Tyle, ed.), Marcel Dekker, New York, 1988, pp. 421–454.
19. W. Ritschel, *Handbook of Basic Pharmacokinetics*, 3rd Ed.,
     Drug Intelligence Publications, Hamilton, Ill., 1986, pp. 43–
     281, 302–339.

Chapter 2

ORGANIZING THE TRANSFER OF PHARMACEUTICALS FROM RESEARCH TO PRODUCTION

Karl F. Popp*

Sterling Research Group, Rensselaer, New York

I. INTRODUCTION

An overview of issues to be considered when organizing the transfer of technology from the research arena to the production environment will be presented. The discussion will focus on the coordination and implementation of a transfer program for a product, with emphasis being given to those factors peculiar to the pharmaceutical industry. The success of any program is highly dependent on the effectiveness of the communication preceding its implementation. Therefore, the preparation and distribution of a complete document summarizing raw material and equipment requirements, manufacturing and packaging processes, process validation parameters, quality control procedures, as well as a detailed plan of action outlining expected results and time frames, must be disseminated prior to the scale-up experience. Input from the marketing and manufacturing centers must also be integrated into the plan to ensure that the right product is developed at the right price within the desired time frame. An outline encompassing these critical aspects of a transfer program will be presented.

Whether it is a tablet, a transdermal patch, or an injection, the transformation of a pharmaceutical prototype into a successful product requires the cooperation of many individuals. To complete the task efficiently, the transfer of the product from the research and development (R&D) area to production must be organized. Planning for process commercialization is one area where tangible rewards can be realized. The successful transfer of a project from the research arena to a production site does not happen on its own. Organizing

*Current affiliation: A. C. Stiefel Research Institute, Inc., Oak Hill, New York.

the transfer of a technology or new product from research to production may be one of the most perplexing problems that development
scientists, engineers, or marketers may encounter during their
careers. This presentation will provide some insight into what issues should be considered during the transfer program and offer a
sequence of events toward completing the task.

One major decision focuses on that point where the idea or process
is advanced from a research-oriented program to that targeted toward
commercialization. Generally, the cost of product development rises
dramatically during the pilot scale-up and initial production batch
efforts. In other words, the critical path for success is dependent
on the completion of the technology transfer to the production site
at a livable cost.

Three major issues must be addressed to implement an effective
transfer. Namely, a plan must be devised to organize the people
and process steps involved. Once prepared, the plan must be communicated to the parties involved at the R&D site, at the corporate
level and at the production site. The success of any program is
highly dependent on the effectiveness of the communication preceding
its implementation. Therefore, identifying the parties involved in
the development process is an important issue to be considered.

II. PERSONNEL

Let us first discuss the people involved in the transfer program.
Informing the proper personnel of their involvement, desired contributions, and responsibilities up front helps to identify potential
problem areas that may hinder the accomplishment of the task at
hand.

From the research and development group, a project leader is the
focus of the communication pattern. It is the responsibility of this
individual to coordinate the assembly of the necessary information
to support the product's advancement for process development. Information from the product development area would be gathered from
the formulator, analytical, and microbiology testing groups, as well
as the packaging development unit. A safety evaluation from the
toxicology group should be completed prior to a scale-up effort.
Reviews should be also solicited from the patent department and drug
regulatory affairs units to ensure that proper legal protection has
been secured and that an agreement as to how much of what information is needed either to submit for a drug approval or to introduce
a cosmetic to the marketplace. The goal here is to collect the proper
amount and kind of data necessary to support the prerequisite fill-
ings, either internal or external to the company.

At the corporate level, it is common to involve personnel from the
production planning unit, engineering group, new product coordina-

tion section, as well as marketing, as each of these divisions has a vested interest in the success of the venture. The effort to keep people informed becomes a critical accomplishment toward the final acceptance of the product by the corporation. Therefore, any time taken to explain the steps involved in the transfer program is time well spent.

At the manufacturing site, there are a number of individuals whose cooperation must be gained to ensure the timely and efficient completion of the transfer effort. The plant manager, technical director, production planning group, manufacturing area supervisor, quality control and quality assurance units, plant engineering, packaging, and transportation supervisors must be informed of their responsibilities. Personnel training must also be considered if the technology is new to this site. Last, but not least, do not overlook the contributions that line mechanics and chemical operators can make to the program. Remember, they perform the necessary functions day in and day out. Their insight and practical experience are an invaluable resource that should not be overlooked.

The success of the transfer is dependent on the ability of the project leader to motivate people to work together toward a mutually beneficial goal—that is, introducing a new product that may create jobs and profits for the company. It is of the utmost importance to remember that when you are presenting the worth of the project all around your company, what you are striving to do is to express yourself rather than to impress others.

III. MOTIVATING PARTICIPANTS

Return on involvement is one concept being promoted where changes in responsibilities and tasks are being implemented. Changes here include the manufacture of new products or using new procedures to produce existing products. By involving personnel in the planning of changes, in discussing the resources necessary to complete the tasks, and in creating an environment in which innovation can strive, the project manager should realize the completion of the program quickly and efficiently with reliable quality at livable costs. At the same time, people who have worked on the program to bring it to completion should share a feeling of teamwork, a taste of accomplishment, and, most of all, a sense of self-respect. Return on involvement encompasses the philosophy that employees are a key element in the successful introduction of any technology or entity. Project managers must keep this in mind, since they must frequently depend on the cooperation of individuals outside their control to accomplish their goals.

IV. PRETRANSFER CONSIDERATIONS

Prior to the advancement of any product for plant scale-up trials,
several requirements must be satisfied. First, the marketing division
should examine the proposed product prototypes and agree that the
product meets their needs. Second, the intended commercial package
configuration (color, size, shape, composition, etc.) should be selected. While it is not uncommon to package portions of the first scale-
up batch in a variety of packages, it is incumbent upon the project
leader to eliminate any unnecessary packages to minimize the dilution
of effort. Third, any constraints, such as cost or time, must be
identified so that they may be given due consideration.

Does the product meet the needs of the consumer? That is the
question that the development staff believes they have answered with
a prototype. The marketing and sales units must, however, concur.
The decision is generally theirs, as they are responsible for making
the product available to the consumer and, more important, they are
responsible for seeing that the product meets consumer demands,
either real or perceived. Focus groups or market research studies
should have been completed prior to the scale-up effort.

The cost of a development program rises dramatically as the number of package configurations to be advanced to commercialization increases. Selecting the proper sizes, shapes, closures, colors, and
finishes is compromised by package compositions, availability, and
last, but not least, the intended use and cost of the unit. For example, a smaller unit lasting about 1 month, such as a calendar pack,
makes marketing sense for oral contraceptives for several reasons.
Dispensing and units sales are generally cyclic and fairly predictable,
allowing for better profit projections. The calendar pack and monthly cost to the consumer not only position the product toward enhanced consumer acceptance, but also toward better patient compliance, especially with expensive medications. Suffice it to say, it
behooves the marketing unit to work with financial analysts to determine the optimal product configuration and cost profile that maxi-
mizes profits and resources.

Constraints always exist, but occasionally they are not communicated accurately or promptly. Competition in the marketplace frequently causes introduction deadlines and end-product cost constraints
that must be considered during the initial phases of a development
program. On the other hand, lead times for materials and personnel
resources must be appreciated when commitments are made to time
lines. Nobody wants to hear that the task cannot be done now.
The reality is that without some planning up front, the task may not
be possible at all. Factors that influence decisions may originate
from external as well as internal environments. Care must be exercised to address those issues that affect the timely completion of the
project.

Physicochemical properties of raw materials and the finished dosage form should be characterized prior to any scale-up effort. Having methodology available and validated to compare batches is essential to any scale-up effort. For example, drug release profiles and viscosities have the potential of being altered by manufactuing procedures as well as by equipment. Care must be exercised so that the desired profiles are maintained. The effect of batch size and process should be monitored closely.

Formulation and/or fabrication of the newer advanced drug delivery systems, such as microencapsulated molecules, transdermal patches, or liposomes, is frequently accomplished in the laboratory environment. However, large-scale production of these dosage forms may be problematic, as the conditions of manufacture may not be attainable or desirable in the plant setting. Consultation with process development personnel during the finalization of the prototype development phase is one means of minimizing scale-up difficulties.

One area occasionally overlooked by development staffs is the necessity of securing confidentiality agreements from vendors supplying technologies or services to a firm. All contractors should be required to execute a confidentiality agreement specifically encompassing the technology and product being shared. These documents should be prepared, reviewed, and executed by the appropriate legal and executive officers of both organizations. Especially when the science or product is not well defined and patent protection has not been secured, such as with the development of novel, new specialized drug delivery systems, this task must be completed expeditiously, and no work should be initiated until the signed instrument is in your hands.

V. THE TRANSFER PROGRAM

Any development program should be reduced to a written form. Figure 1 summarizes such a development program. An outline or checklist for the program must be compiled to ensure that appropriate consideration has been given to relevant issues. This also helps to ensure that all parties are approaching the task from the same perspective and priority. A manufacturing site must be designated and the appropriate personnel notified as to their involvement. Assembly of the collected necessary information must be disseminated to the involved parties. At a minimum, copies of the proposed formula and manufacturing directions should be distributed so as to allow sufficient time for review and comments to be generated. A planning review session should be convened with representatives from the research, corporate, and manufacturing sites in attendance. Selection of the time and location of this meeting should be such as to encourage maximum participation.

Activity	Completion Dates	
	Target	Actual
1. Formulation selected		
2. Site for trials established		
3. Planning meeting scheduled		
a. Manufacturing Monographs		
b. Raw Materials		
c. Packaging Monographs		
d. Packaging Components		
e. Testing Monographs		
f. Process Validation Protocols		
4. Date of plant trial established		
a. Manufacturing		
b. Packaging		
c. On-site Review of Experience		
d. Shipment to R&D Center		
5. Date of shipment delivery		
a. Confirmation of Results		
b. Stability Initiation		
c. Product Evaluation - Safety		
- Efficacy		
6. Post production review meeting		
7. Assembly of final monographs		
a. Manufacturing		
b. Packaging		
c. Testing		
d. Stability		
e. Material Safety Data Sheet		
f. Shelf-Life Projection		
g. Bibliography		
8. Review of final monograph		
a. R&D		
b. Manufacturing		
c. Quality Control (Testing)		
d. Regulatory Affairs		
e. Corporate		
9. Issue product monograph		
10. First Commercial Batch		

Fig. 1 Project transfer checklist.

The meeting should be chaired by the project leader. It is his or her responsibility to determine the relevant issues to be discussed, that an agenda for the meeting is distributed, and that minutes of the meeting are taken for later issuance. It is important that any concerns that arise during this meeting are noted and addressed, as the purpose of this gathering is to draw from the experience of the participants in identifying potential problem areas in the program. The tone of this session should be one of a team and not one of autocratic rule. Motivation, communication, and cooperation must be stressed in the voice and actions of the project leader. This is the first step to accomplishing the prime program objective: the timely and informed transfer of a new product from the research arena to the production site.

The following areas should be discussed at the planning meeting:

1. Formula
2. Raw materials
3. Manufacturing equipment
4. Manufacturing precautions
5. Manufacturing directions
6. Packaging
7. Process validation
8. Quality control and quality assurance
9. Re work procedures
10. Transportation

Each area should be reviewed to ensure that critical issues have been addressed. If the area is not relevant, state that this area is not applicable to the program. Do not omit an issue, as what may be perceived in one's own mind as unimportant may be a monumental task in another's domain. With the newer drug delivery systems, this effort is critical to a program's success.

A discussion of these elements may include some of the following thoughts.

A. Formula

As the base on which all effort is centered, understanding the formula, its derivation, and its constraints is the first prerequisite to any development program. The feasibility of the formula may be established by reviewing the ingredients of the composition and then explaining their function in the formula. It may be appropriate to review the claims and physical characteristics of the product while passing around a sample so that the participants appreciate what the product is to look like and why this product is being developed.

Comments about prestability and finished-product stability profiles should be presented as an overview of the new product's chemical

stablility. This will reinforce the formula's anticipated shelf life and
ability to withstand the "process shocks" normally encountered during production scale-up.

The toxicity of the finished product should be discussed. This
information ensures that a decision regarding handling of the formula
is made based on generated data and/or experience. A draft or
tentative material safety data sheet may be one avenue to disseminate
this information.

Review of any constraints, such as specific ingredients or sources,
and cost of goods or manufacturing equipment, should be made clear.
This aspect helps to explain why given actions or directions were
taken. Constraints must be considered when formula optimization is
undertaken. Optimizing formulas, however, may be best addressed
in the production environment, as batch size and manufacturing
equipment have been shown to render viable laboratory and small-
scale formulas virtually inoperative in the plant world. The experience gained during the manufacture of laboratory and scale-up
batches is invaluable and should be shared with the participants,
especially the production staff.

B. Raw Materials

Sources of raw materials, especially those critical to a new product's
functionality, should be identified. Availability and costs should be
ascertained to aid in the planning process. Testing monographs,
including methods to ascertain a lot's chemical and, if necessary,
microbiological integrity, should be provided to the selected manufacturing site in advance so that the methods may be applied to the
incoming supplies. Handling of materials, including storage, disposal, and employee precautions, should be documented, especially
for new or potentially hazardous materials. Again, material safety
data sheets (MSDS) for all materials used should be available and
disseminated to the plant prior to their exposure.

C. Manufacturing Equipment

With newer drug delivery systems developed in the laboratory, the
correlation of the necessary production equipment may be very difficult indeed. For example, the shear needed to create the desired
particle size of an emulsion using laboratory equipment may pose
serious problems in the selection of the plant equipment necessary
to reproduce the product's attributes. Recording a lab mixer's
rpm is not sufficient for this task.

The availability, size, and surfaces or composition of the required equipment needs to be specifically identified so that the

scale-up effort may be representative of a production run. A preliminary compatibility screen of contact surfaces should be completed
where appropriate prior to the selection of scale-up equipment. The
location of the equipment to other needs such as services or the
filling area may be a factor in the selection of equipment. A cleaning validation study should be conducted on this batch to ensure
that no residue of active ingredient or detergent remains and that
the equipment is suitable for production use once again.

Alternative equipment may be considered and used. However, experience will dictate its suitability.

D. Manufacturing Precautions

While pretty much self-explanatory, any concerns regarding the
manipulating of equipment or product by employees should be voiced
at this time. This is especially important if the areas of concern are
environmental (such as particulate contamination or sterility) or
atmospheric (product's oxygen sensitivity).

E. Manufacturing Directions

Directions should be clear and concise. Flexible generic descriptions
should be utilized where possible. For example, "Pass the emulsion
through a suitable colloid mill such as an Eppenbach mill at a setting
of 0.005 in." is preferred to a description referencing a specific
piece of equipment. While process validation testing may be necessary for any particular piece of equipment, generic descriptions
simplify the regulatory filings by allowing flexibility in allowable
equipment.

Directions should be realistic. Remember that any instructions
must be scale-oriented. Specific parameters may be necessary for
manufacturing areas. For example, cooling or heating times are
typically equipment-dependent. Cooling 1 kg in the laboratory in
15 min may mean 4 hr for a 40,000-kg batch in the plant.

Based on the experience gained during the pilot scale-up effort,
a process flowchart should be constructed. A process flowchart
helps to identify steps and issues in need of process validation review. Also, the timing of activities toward the scheduling of personnel needs, such as for in-process testing, generally are more
apparent when viewed in context with the total process.

Process optimization parameters identified during the pilot scale-
up effort should be monitored during the production scale-up batch.
This way appropriate recommendations based on experience may be
integrated into future batches. Many optimization experiments may
be efficiently incorporated into the process validation program.

F. Packaging

The description, specifications, and test methods for any package to be processed should be available to the plant prior to the production scale-up. Unit functionality and fit should be included as a practical use test in any specification. The plant equipment to be utilized in packaging this batch needs to be evaluated for its feasibility, speed, and, if it is critical, contact surface compatibility. Preliminary evaluations on surface compatibility, discussed previously, should suffice as an early indication of packaging equipment suitability. Finally, the cleaning of the packaging equipment should be checked prior to the equipment being used for other products.

The availability of or lead time to secure the necessary packaging components frequently places stress on the project time line. Package costs and possible alternative packaging could be evaluated with bulk produced from this batch. Therefore, a course of action to minimize project failure due to an unsatisfactory package may be appropriate. The resultant dilution of resources and increased project expense must be weighed in accepting this course of action.

Directions for filling the batch, including fill tolerances and precautions such as aseptic handling or nitrogen gassing, should be reviewed to state the requirements for success up front. As a part of this production scale-up effort, it may be desirable to evaluate the product's bulk stability in the storage tank in order to establish limits on the length of time a batch may be held prior to filling. Storage container compatibility may be a crucial issue here and deserves appropriate attention.

Finally, the personnel involved in packaging the product should be instructed about any safety or handling issues that might affect them or compromise the product's integrity. Whether it is for the development of newer packages, such as for intranasal drug administration or transdermal patches, or for more traditional delivery systems, such as aerosol cans, the need to educate the employees involved in the manufacturing process is essential to the transfer program's success. Identifying and controlling process variables is necessary while experience is gained and the process is optimized and validated.

G. Process Validation

Each class of products needs specific issues to be addressed. In general, process steps that may be variable, such as mixng times and temperatures, need to be validated. Many articles have been written regarding the validation of processes affecting pharmaceutical products. Protocols to evaluate those parameters that may affect a product's integrity should be agreed upon by both the R&D and production staff. During the preparation and packaging of the pilot production batch, generation of data toward improving the efficiency of these processes, as well as minimizing batch-to-batch variations, is very important, as this information will serve as documentation to support the new product's commercial feasibility.

There is no magic number of batches required to prove a process validated. The technical complexities of and product sensitivites to variable parameters will dictate how extensive a validation program will be needed. Suffice it to say that the process must be controllable, reproducible, and yield product that meets the desired specifications.

H. Quality Control and Quality Assurance

One of the purposes of the pilot production batch is to introduce the manufacturing site's functional areas—manufacturing, packaging, and testing—to the new product in its entirety. That is, the release of raw materials and packaging components, as well as in-process, bulk, and finish product testing, should be completed at the site as if this were a commercial batch. In many organizations, the pilot production batch does, in fact, become the first batch offered for sale.

Formula issues to be discussed are those concerning the in-process testing, bulk release prior to filling, and finished product specifications. These limits are proposed based on the experience gained with the smaller laboratory and scale-up batches. Essentially, any comments or concerns regarding the test methods and specifications should be aired at this time. Reagents and equipment to complete the required testing must be available at the plant. A contact at the R&D analytical laboratory should be established so that explanations to questions or aberrant values may be expeditiously secured.

Communication of requirements of time and personnel needs to the quality control department is a critical issue that must not be overlooked. It is their prompt attention to your analysis needs that helps keep the pilot production batch process moving forward.

Sampling must be scheduled for release and for stability testing using a statistically valid sampling program where appropriate. This is especially important for samples to be used for stability studies. This way the chosen samples are documented as representative of the entire batch.

Batch documentation is also an important factor to be considered. Preparation of master batch records in accordance with standard plant operating procedures should be followed by an approval of the document by the sponsoring division, usually the formulator or process development staff of the R&D unit. Upon completion, review of the batch records by the quality assurance group ensures compliance to Good Manufacturing Practices (GMPs) and that all necessary modifications to the manufacturing records are properly explained and documented.

I. Scheduling Date for Manufacturing Trial

At the conclusion of the planning meeting, any actions that must be undertaken prior to the scale-up should be documented and a responsible party identified. When the data for the trial is being discussed, time constraints must be considered along with the availability of raw materials, packaging components, plant time, and required personnel. Coordination of the people and supplies is the responsibility of the project leader. An ability to lead and to negotiate another individual's priorities helps to bring the trials to completion on schedule.

Lastly, arrangements for transporting raw materials, if necessary, and filled product must be set up to ensure that the scale-up effort is completed on schedule and that stability studies are initiated expeditiously.

Participants should leave the meeting with a feeling that someone is in charge of the project, that the program has been well thought out and documented, and that their commitments and the commitments made by others will be honored. The issuance of meeting minutes promptly after the meeting will reinforce the importance of each individual's responsibilities and serve as notice to the participants and their superiors that their cooperation has been solicited, is needed, and is expected.

J. Completing the Manufacturing Trial

In review, the activities to be completed at the manufacturing site are

1. Release of raw materials and packaging components
2. Manufacture and packaging of the trial batch
3. Generation of data from in-process, bulk, and finished product samples
4. Process validation, batch record, and on-site experience reviews
5. Shipment of finished product to the research facility for testing

An exit interview with involved plant personnel offers a mechanism for their comments to be aired. Their efforts should be acknowledged and their input seriously considered and incorporated into the manufacturing document where appropriate. Any differences that cannot be resolved at this time should be noted and studied further. The art of listening and diplomacy must be employed, as this forum must be one of cooperation and not one of confrontation.

At this meeting a discussion about possible re-work procedures may be appropriate. The ability to recover materials, especially ex-

pensive drug actives, is desirable. Early identification of steps
where re-work may be possible allows for procedures to be tested
and verified and in place should they be needed. For pharmaceuticals, re-work procedures may be utilized only if they are appropriately documented and approved by the responsible corporate and
government bodies. Re-work procedures are not a means for handling sloppy manufacturing but a means for identifying where a salvage
effort may be implemented successfully. Logistics and economics,
as always, will dictate whether a re-work will be implemented.

K. Postproduction Activities and Evaluation

Once the plant experinece has been concluded, confirmatory analyses
on duplicate samples for in-process, bulk release, and finished
product, previously tested at the plant site, should be completed at
the R&D center. In this way, the proposed methods are challenged
to yield similar results in the hands of different analysts in different
locations. Discrepancies in values generated at this point must be
investigated and resolved.

Samples should be placed into the stability testing system as
per the organization's policies. Samples may be also submitted, if
necessary, for efficacy and/or toxicity testing.

Finally a report must be prepared and issued expenditiously summarizing the experience, reviewing each area's involvement, and
proposing, if necessary, changes in the process or control methods.
Timely and factual communication of project progress to the other
corporate areas not directly involved in the scale-up, such as the
marketing, finance, and purchasing units, aids in the commitment
of resources. By fostering informed decision making through directed written communication, the time required to plan or complete
those activities to bring the product to market is minimized and the
resource usage optimized.

A formal postproduction trial review meeting should be scheduled
and held, with representatives from the R&D, corporate, and manufacturing centers invited. Plans to commercialize the product, or to
submit documentation for government approval, if this is the next
step in the development scheme, are outlined contingent upon the
successful completion of a defined stability program. Agreement as
to the suitability of all the factors involved in the preparation of
the product should be the result of this meeting, with a substantiat-
ing document in the form of meeting minutes or a signed "statment
of concurrence" being generated and distributed.

A product monograph of all pertinent sections to support the
product's introduction is assembled, reviewed, and disseminated to
the appropriate parties as per the organization's policies.

The transfer of the project is considered complete when the first commercial batch of product is produced solely under the control of the manufacturing site without problems.

VI. SUMMARY

This presentation has reviewed issues to be considered when organizing the transfer of technology from the research arena to the production environment. Critical areas affecting the manufacture, packaging, and quality of pharmaceutical products have been discussed in relationship to their impact on the transfer process. The necessity of the communication of a plan with input from the research, corporate, and manufacturing centers was emphasized. The success of the program is highly dependent on the communication and cooperation shared throughout the transfer process.

VII. REFERENCE

1. K. F. Popp, *Drug Dev. Ind. Pharm.*, *13*(13):2339—2362 (1987).

Chapter 3

FDA REGULATIONS FOR THE PRODUCTION OF SPECIALIZED DRUG DELIVERY SYSTEMS

John F. Stigi and Andrew Lowery

Center for Devices and Radiological Health, Food and Drug Administration, Washington, D. C.

I. QUALITY ASSURANCE SYSTEMS

A. Quality Assurance

This chapter will discuss FDA requirements for drug delivery systems starting with their relationship to the firm's total quality assurance (QA) system.

Manufacturers of drug delivery systems may be required to meet the Good Manufacturing Practices (GMP) for Medical Devices (21 CFR 820) or the Good Manufacturing Practices for Drugs (21 CFR 211), depending on whether the system more closely meets the definition of a medical device or a drug.

This chapter will focus on the application of the GMPs for medical devices. However, after reviewing the comparison of the device and drug GMP requirements in Table 1 in this section, you will note that there is commonality between the two programs.

Quality assurance must be an integrated effort—a total systems approach to satisfy the particular safety and performance needs of a specific manufacturer, product, and user-market. It must not simply consist of inspection and testing, spot solutions, or "fire fighting," no matter what the product is or how small the manufacturer. In all cases, quality must be considered at the earliest stages in every significant area that has an effect on the quality, safety, and effectiveness of the drug delivery device. These areas include product development, design evaluation, component and/or vendor selection, documentation, development of labeling, design transfer, process development and validation, pilot production, routine manufacturing, test and inspection, history record evaluation, distribution, service, and complaints. Complaints and, of course, favorable comments constitute customer feedback.

Most important of all factors, management and employees must have the correct attitude if their quality assurance (QA) program is to be effective. Quality consciousness must be developed in every employee. Each person must be made aware of the importance of his or her individual contributions in the overall effort to achieve an acceptable level of quality.

After a QA program is in place and checked, it must not be allowed to stagnate—it must continue to be dynamics. A QA program remains dynamic through continuous feedback; "big-picture" monitoring by system audits; "micro-picture" monitoring by flowcharting and operational analyses; and by corrective action. Sufficient personnel with appropriate eduction, background, and experience must be in all departments to make certain that QA activities are properly and adequately performed.

The result is an organization that is operating in a known state-of-control for the device, manufacturing processes, and records. A properly functioning quality assurance system results in increased safety and effectiveness of the device, reduced liability exposure, reduced regulatory exposure, increased customer satisfaction, less scrap, lower costs, less confusion, higher employee morale, and, of course, higher profits.

An ideal QA system is composed of an organization that executes a QA program according to documented policy and specifications in order to achieve stated objectives.

The written policies and objectives are set by management and are influenced by outside factors such as customer requirements, standards, and regulations. The objectives are to produce safe and effective (quality) devices at a profit. Ideally, the organization is everyone in the company, as everyone supports the program; in addition, however, organizations are established to achieve specific objectives. Tasks to be performed to meet the objectives are described in procedures and other documents.

Documentation is composed of: product-specific technical documentation, such as engineering drawings, labels, etc.; and general documentation, such as standard operating procedures (SOPs). All activities and product quality are monitored; and any deviations from policy and specifications are fed back into the system, where the deviations are corrected. If the required activities including the feedback are performed, the system is self-correcting and, thus, it is operating in a state-of-control. The Food and Drug Administration (FDA) requires manufacturers of medical devices to operate in a state-of-control.

In order to fully comply with the requirements and intent of the Good Manufacturing Practices (GMP) regulation and the Food, Drug and Cosmetic (FD&C) Act, manufacturers will need a QA program that approaches this ideal system. The system nearest to the ideal is a total QA system, which, of course, incorporates the requirements of the GMP regulation.

B. Good Manufacturing Practices

The majority of the Food and Drug Administration's rules deal specifically with a type or class of product. However, a growing number of significant FDA regulations relate to what may be called good practices, including testing and manufacturing of FDA-regulated products. To date, these rules include current good manufacturing practice regulations for foods, drugs, medical devices, and blood-derived products, as well as good laboratory practices, better known as GLPs. Unlike other FDA rules, these are systems-oriented requirements for quality assurance and compliance, which serve the FDA's enforcement purposes and give operational "guidance" to FDA-regulated firms.

Viewed in the context of eight decades of FDA regulation, good manufacturing and good laboratory practices are recent developments. The FDA originally concentrated on product detection, surveillance, and enforcement; then it chose to work through good manufacturing practice regulations on the *establishment of systems*; and later, as this systems concept developed and the regulations were adopted, the FDA became concerned about the validation of systems. The shift of FDA focus from catching bad products to monitoring "out-of-control" systems is a major historical shift deserving special attention. It was a realignment from random apprehension by the FDA of noncomplying manufacturers to coordinated, published systems planned to avoid hazards. With this shift has grown the presumption, with varying degress of statutory support, that system weaknesses are grounds for enforcement challenges against a firm without specific proof that one or more bad products has emerged from that system.

An adequate and properly implemented quality assurance program such as a GMP program, because of its broader scope, has a much higher probability than a quality control program of preventing the manufacture and shipment of defective products. Quality controls, however, such as inspection and testing, are important parts of a quality assurance program because they provide information that should be fed back into the quality problems. Identifying and solving quality problems is a core requirement of the GMP regulation. This action is in contrast to merely applying superficial corrections by pass/fail quality control inspection, including re-work of finished product or in-process assemblies.

The GMP regulation requires every finished device manufacturer to prepare and implement a quality assurance program that is appropriate to the device manufactured and that meets the requirements of the GMP regulation (section 820.5). Manufacturers who implement all applicable requirements of the GMP regulation will have in place a significant quality assurance program. Such a program does not completely meet a company's needs, however, because the GMP regulation has limited coverage of the initial product design stage and does not consider the needs of the user—hence the need for a total QA system.

Adequate Organization and QA Management

A specific organizational structure for executing a QA program is not prescribed by the device GMP regulation, but the regulation states that, where possible, one or more designated individuals not having direct responsibility for the performance of a manufacturing operation shall be responsible for the quality assurance program. The FDA is more concerned with the adequacy and appropriateness of quality assurance activities than it is with organizational structure. Larger firms will tend to have independent QA management.

The device GMP regulation requires quality awareness training for manufacturing and quality assurance personnel [820.25(a)]. Personnel involved in any quality assurance activities must be properly trained, both by education and experience. No matter how effective quality assurance and production systems are as concepts, people still play the major role in producing a quality product. Lack of training—as reflected in instances of negligence, poor operating techniques, or inability of employees to discharge their functions properly—can lead to defective products and, sometimes, to regulatory or liability problems. Management should be diligent in looking for factors that indicate a need for employee training.

A quality assurance system should include an ongoing formal program for training and motivating all personnel. All personnel should be made aware that product quality is not solely the responsibility of management. Quality is the responsibility of every employee— any employee can potentially generate a quality problem through negligence. It is extremely important to understand the following points with respect to typical quality-related functions.

Research and development has primary responsibility for designing quality into the device.

Technical services or an equivalent functional group has primary responsibility for documenting the design.

Manufacturing, process or "scale-up" engineering has primary responsibility for designing quality into the manufacturing processes.

Manufacturing personnel have primary responsibility for producing devices that have the maximum level of quality that can be achieved based on the product and process designs.

Quality assurance has primary responsibility for QA program management, status reports, audits, problem identification, data analysis, etc., as described in the GMP regulation, the Premarket Notification Regulation, and this book.

A medical device manufacturer must *never* try to operate on the basis that the quality assurance organization has primary and direct responsibility for the quality of the products. To do so means that quality problems will not be solved in a timely manner because attention is directed toward the wrong organization. In reality, it is part of the responsibility of the quality assurance organization to see that attention is directed toward the correct department if a quality problem arises.

Where necessary, employees should be certified to perform certain manufacturing or quality assurance procedures. Records of training and/or certification should be maintained. Personnel performing quality assurance functions must:

Have sufficeint, well-defined responsibilities and authority
Be afforded the organizational freedom to identify and evaluate
  quality problems
Be able to formulate, obtain, and recommend possible solutions
  for quality assurance problems
Verify implementation of solutions to quality problems

Formal and Documented QA Program

The device GMP regulation requires that each manufacturer prepare and implement quality assurance procedures adequate to assure that a formally established and documented quality assurance program is performed (section 820.20). "Formally established" means not only formal documentation, but an obvious commitment to quality from top management. There must be manifest indications that management recognizes the need for a quality assurance program in order to assure quality products. In many firms, this commitment is accomplished through such means as: a management policy; assignment of responsibilities and authorities; and general statements and actions that define and support the goals of the quality assurance program. This policy is supported by a number of more detailed quality assurance documents such as qualification methods, sampling procedures, inspection/test procedures, product audits, and records indicating that measurement and monitoring of quality have occurred. The number of documents needed depends on the size and complexity of the operation and the characteristics of the product. A firm must have the various records required by the GMP regulation. These records include:

Device master records
Device history records
Maintenance schedules and records
Complaint files and failed device/component files
Audit reports

Distribution records
Personnel training records

Most of these records are discussed in more detail in later sections. In each case, the records should be appropriate for the device and the operation involved. Any changes to master records
must be made by a formal procedure and be formally approved.

Among other records, the device master record contains manufacturing procedures and SOPs. Some firms tend to write an excessive number of general SOPs. This chapter contains information that
should help some firms write and maintain adequate procedures without excessive paperwork. Firms should not generate and use procedures that are not needed. Also, standard operating procedures
tend not to match actual operations because the operations gradually
change as the company grows or as products are added without the
procedures keeping pace. Such procedures may require operations
that have no benefit or require excessive collection of data or collection of data that are never used. Thus, firms need to occasionally
flowchart and analyze their operations to determine, among other
things, if the existing procedures are inadequate, correct, or excessive. Flowcharting and analyzing operations is an excellent method
for improving operations and the associated quality assurance activities.

Approval of Materials, Components, and Finished Devices

The quality assurance organization is also responsible for assuring
that all components, packaging, labeling, manufacturing materials,
and finished devices have been approved for use; and that contracted
items and services are suitable. Likewise, the QA organization must
assure that rejected items are identified and properly disposed. Additionally, the QA organization should assure that production records
are reviewed before the product is distributed. These are records
required by the GMP regulation for the device history record.
Records should be reviewed to verify that the operations represented have been properly conducted and that the records are complete.

Adequate Quality Assurance Checks

The quality assurance organization must determine that all tests and
inspections are performed correctly [820.20(a)(4)]. Some of the
methods used to accomplish this are training of test personnel, QA
system audits, review of quality assurance records, and product
audits. However, simply instituting a quality assurance control program and checking that it is conducted correctly is not enough to
satisfy the device GMP regulation. The GMP regulation also requires
that quality assurance controls be qualified to make certain they are
appropriate and adequate for their purpose. The qualification should

be done during final product development, pilot production, and, of course, whenever products and/or processes are modified. In cases where quality cannot be adequately measured by in-process or finished-product testing and inspection, the qualification must include validation of processes that have a significant bearing on product quality.

Identify and Solve QA Problems

As set forth by the device GMP regulation, one of the most important responsibilities of the QA organization is to identify quality assurance problems, to recommend and provide solutions, and to verify implementation of the solutions [820.20(a)(3)]. Other personnel are also identifying and solving quality problems, and the QA organization must support such activities.

Typically, the QA department identifies problems with device quality through review of inspection and test data, trend analysis of history and repair records, failure analysis, analysis of complaints, and review of other objective data. In this regard, reduction in productivity is often an indicator of quality problems. Low morale and confusion are indicators of inadequate device master records and poor management. Also, measurement of scrap and re-work is an effective method of detecting quality problems and reducing costs. These are examples of sources that provide feedback to the quality assurance organization. Feedback is necessary to verify the adequacy of the manufacturing process and the controls used. It also helps trigger corrective action to solve root causes of quality problems rather than just performing re-work.

Periodic QA System Audits

The GMP regulation requires (820.20) that each manufacturer must prepare and implement quality assurance procedures adequate to assure that a formally established and documented quality assurance program is performed. Many activities are required to fulfill this requirement; and management is aware of the overt aspects of the program as they perform their routine duties. However, to make sure that all aspects, overt or subtle, of the required program exist and are operating correctly, the GMP regulation requires [820.20(b)] planned and periodic audits of the QA program.

C. Total Quality Assurance Systems

Total quality assurance systems extend from customer requirements through development and production and on to customer use and feedback. Thus, total QA systems encompass the medical device law and regulations, particularly the drug and device GMP regulations. The Food, Drug and Cosmetic Act, and its implementing regulations

such as those for Labeling, Premarket Notification, Investigational
Device Exemptions (IDE), Premarket Approval (PMA), and Good
Manufacturing Practices impact at various times during the product
lifecycle on the design and quality of drug delivery devices. For a
few devices, the IDE, PMA, GMP, and labeling regulations with their
preproduction and production requirements essentially constitute a
total quality assurance program. For other devices, preproduction
or design quality receives limited attention until after a problem
occurs. For example, section 501(c) of the act states that a product
is adulterated if it does not have a quality equal to the quality stated
or implied by the product labeling. Analysis of device recall problem
data by the FDA has shown that such problems are divided about
equally between design and production. Thus, compliance with the
device GMP regulation is not sufficient to produce safe and effective
drug delivery devices—design must also be covered. The quality
requirements implied by 501(c) and the history of regulatory actions
taken thereunder are sufficient reasons for manufacturers of drug
delivery devices to implement a total quality assurance system.

    Two other reasons for having a total quality assurance system are
21 CFR Part 803, Medical Device Reporting (MDR); and product liability. MDR requires manufacturers of medical devices to report to the
FDA serious complaints that they receive from any source. Complaints
and product liability actions generally result from poor design, labeling, and manufacturing. Serious complaints, reporting and liability
exposure are reduced by the use of a total quality assurance system.

    Intrinsic, or desired quality is established by the design spec-
ifications for the product, its components, and the manufacturing
processes. Complying with the GMP regulation assures that the
manufacturing processes can consistently achieve desired levels of
quality and that the finished drug delivery device meets its design
or master record specifications. This result is a significant quality
step. However, if the device as designed is of poor quality, the
GMP controls will only assure that a poor-quality device is produced.
To overcome this limitation, many firms use an overall quality assurance program that embraces: evaluation of customer needs;
product design, development and evaluation; labeling development
and control; all manufacturing and control activities; and customer
feedback. The GMP regulation covers all of these areas except
customer needs and initial product design. The GMP regulation has
a significant impact on the control of product design after production
starts because of GMP requirements on changes to master records,
data feedback, complaint processing, and corrective actions.

Design Quality

Because the intrinsic quality level is established during the design or
preproduction phase, the quality assurance program *must* include this

phase if the program is to assure overall quality, meet customer requirements, meet company quality claims, and comply with the intent of the FD&C Act. The term "product assurance" is often used to identify the quality assurance activities related to product design. A product assurance system or design QA system combined with a GMP system constitutes a total QA system. (Design QA or preproduction quality is covered in Section III. The remaining sections cover good manufacturing practices in detail.) Quality assurance personnel should participate in the review, evaluation, and documentation of the data established during this preproduction phase from which all other activities derive; i.e., processing, purchasing, and testing. Development and evaluation data are also useful in cases of regulatory or product liability actions to show that the design and manufacturing processes were well conceived and properly qualified, reviewed, and documented.

Component Selection

Component and raw material specifications developed during the design phase must be well conceived and adequate for their intended purpose. In some cases where large quantities of components of raw materials are involved, the specifications must include valid and well-understood methods of sampling and acceptance. These specification and sampling/acceptance plans must also be accessible and acceptable to vendors.

Labeling Content

The regulations in 21 CFR Part 801, Labeling; Part 809, In Vitro Diagnostic Products for Human Use; and Part 812, Investigational Device Exemptions; are intended to control the content of labeling. Likewise, 21 CFR Part 807, Premarket Notification, and Part 814, Premarket Approval, help control the content of labeling through premarket submissions. The intent of these regulations and the FD&C Act is for manufacturers to have a labeling control program such that their labeling always complies with the regulations and meets the needs of the users. Under a total QA system, clear, concise, and correct printed and software labeling is developed during the design phase by a formal process. Such labeling is designed to meet customer and regulatory requirements. Thereafter, the procurement, use of the correct label, and correct attachment of labels is assured under a firm's GMP program.

Process Quality

Manufacturing methods and processes to be used must be developed, equipment selected, and processes and method qualified. In some cases, such as sterilization processes and packaging/sealing, the qualification must include a full validation of the processes. Production specifications and methods employed in manufacturing must result in standard in-process and finished products without excessive sorting or reprocessing. Inspection and test methods must be developed that will adequately monitor product characteristics to make certain they are within the acceptable specifications. These methods should be developed, verified, and documented during the product and process development phase. They must be implemented at the *beginning* of routine production.

Any adverse effects the manufacturing processes, manufacturing materials, or equipment may have on device safety and performance must be identified. Where necessary, procedures have to be developed, implemented, and monitored to control these characteristics. Quality assurance personnel should participate in the timely (i.e., early) development of special controls, test or inspection methods, or training programs needed to ensure product quality. Acceptance methods must be developed for accurate measurement of outgoing product quality.

D. QA Program Maintenance and Improvements

After the GMP program or total quality, assurance program is operational, quality assurance and other personnel must continue to look for problem areas or factors that can have an impact on product quality. Many factors can have an impact on the quality program, such as:

> Changes in, or absence of, personnel
> Uncomfortable working conditions (e.g., breakdown in air conditioning)
> Increases in workload or production rates
> Introduction of new production or inspection equipment
> Changes in company incentive techniques (e.g., placing hourly employees on piecework can cause deterioration of product quality)
> Changes in sources for purchased components and materials, as well as changes in components, devices, or process techniques

As noted, QA system audits and flowcharting of operations are excellent methods for determining the status of QA programs. Correcting problems or responding to conditions identified by audits, operational analyses, and customer feedback data can result in quality assurance program improvements.

Table 1 is intended as a quick comparison between the Current Good Manufacturing Practices for Human and Veterinary Drugs and those for Medical Devices. The longer GMP regulation addresses many points that are specific to all drug manufacturing operations;

Table 1 Comparison of Drug and Device Good Manufacturing Practice Regulations[a]

DRUGS 21 CFR 211.1 - 211.198	DEVICES 21 CFR 820.1 - 820.198
GENERAL PROVISION	GENERAL PROVISIONS
211.1 This section addresses CGMP's for the preparation of drug products for humans and animals. Over the counter drugs are specifically excluded. (820.1)	820.1 This section addresses CGMP's for the manufacturing, holding, packaging, storage, and installation of finished devices for human use only. (211.1)
	820.5 Quality Assurance Program The section states that every finished device manufacturer must implement a quality control system that is appropriate to the specific device manufactured. (211.22)
ORGANIZATION AND PERSONNEL	ORGANIZATION AND PERSONNEL
211.22(a) There shall be a Quality Control Unit having the responsibility and authority to approve or reject components, containers, in-process material, packaging, labeling, drug products, etc. (820.20)	820.20 There shall be a Quality Assurance Unit to assure: review of production records, approval or rejection of all components, in-process materials, packaging, labeling, finished devices, etc. (211.22(a))
211.25(a) Persons engaged in the manufacturing, packing, processing, or holding of a drug product shall have education, training, and experience to enable that person to perform the assigned function. (820.25(a)	820.25 There shall be an sufficient personnel to assure that the tasks are performed correctly. (211.25(c))
211.25(c) There shall be an adequate number of personnel to perform the assigned tasks. (820.25)	820.25(a) Persons engaged in the manufacturing, packing, processing, or holding of a drug product shall have education, training, and experience to enable that person to perform the assigned function. (211.25(a))
211.28(a) Personnel shall be properly attired as necessary to prevent products from contamination. (820.25(b))	820.25(b)Personnel shall be in good health and properly attired. (211.28(a)(b))
211.28(b) Personnel shall be in good health. (820.25(b))	

Table 1   (Continued).

211.34 Consultants advising the firm shall have sufficient education, training, and experience to advise on the subject for which they are retained. (NCS)

BUILDINGS AND FACILITIES

211.42(a) Buildings used in the manufacture, process, packing, or holding of a drug shall be of a suitable size, construction, and location to facilitate cleaning maintenance and proper operations. (820.40)

211.42(b) Buildings shall have adequate space for the orderly placement of equipment and materials to prevent mixups. (820.40)

211.42(c) Operations shall be performed within specifically defined areas. (820.120(b))

211.44 Adequate lighting shall be provided. (820.46)

211.46 Adequate ventilation, air filtration, air heating and cooling shall be provided. (820.46)

211.50 Sewage and refuse shall be disposed in a safe and sanitary manner. (820.46)

211.52 There shall be adequate washing facilities, easily accessible to work areas. (820.56)

211.56 Buildings shall be maintained in a clean and orderly manner.
There shall be written procedures for the cleaning of equipment and facilities and the use of rodenticides and insecticides to preclude contamination. (820.56)

BUILDINGS

820.40 Buildings used for manufacturing, assembling, packaging, holding, testing, or labeling operations shall be of suitable design and contain sufficient space to facilitate cleaning, maintenance, and other operations. There shall be adequate space designed to prevent mixups for the handling of incoming components, in-process and finished devices, labeling, reprocessing, equipment, etc. (211.42 (a),(b))

820.46 Environmental conditions which can adversely affect the product are to be controlled including: lighting, ventilation, temperature, humidity, air pressure, filtration, airborne contamination, and other contamination. Any controlled environmental condition shall be periodically inspected, and the inspections shall be documented.
(211.44, 211.46, 211.50)

820.56 There shall be written cleaning procedures and schedules necessary to meet manufacturing process specifications. This includes personnel sanitation, contamination control, personnel practices, and sewage and refuse disposal. (211.52, 211.56)

Table 1 (Continued).

211.58 Buildings shall be maintained in a good state of repair. (NCS)

EQUIPMENT

211.63 Equipment shall be appropriately designed, of adequate size, and suitably located for use, cleaning, and maintenance. (820.60)

211.65 Equipment surfaces shall not be reactive, additive, or absorptive so as to alter product strength. No operational fluids such as coolant of lubricants must come into contact with product. (820.60(d))

211.67(a) Equipment and utensils must be cleaned to prevent contamination of malfunctions. (820.60(a))

211.67(b) Written procedures are to be established for the cleaning and maintenance of equipment. (820.60(a))

211.67(c) Records of cleaning and maintenance of equipment are to be kept. (820.60(a), 820.60(b))

211.68(a) There shall be written procedures, and records maintained, for the calibration and inspection of automatic, mechanical, and electronic equipment. (820.61)

211.68(b) Backup files and hardcopy are to be maintained for computer operated equipment. (820.61)

211.72 Fiber releasing filters are not to be used in liquid filtration unless a non fiber releasing filter of 0.22 microns is located downstream of such a filter. (820.60(d))

EQUIPMENT

820.60 Equipment used in manufacturing shall be appropriately designed, constructed, placed, and installed for maintenance, adjustment, and cleaning. (211.63)

820.60(a) Where necessary a written schedule for the cleaning, adjustment, and maintenance of equipment is to be visibly posted near each piece of equipment. Maintenance activities are to be documented. (211.67(a),(b), (c))

820.60(b) Periodic documented inspections are to be made to assure adherence to maintenance schedules. (211.67(c))

820.60(c) Any inherent limitations or allowable tolerances on equipment shall be posted or readily available to persons performing adjustments. (211.160(b))

820.60(d) Manufacturing materials such as lubricants or mold-release agents shall be removed or reduced to a specified amount that does not affect the device's fitness for use.
Removal of manufacturing materials shall be documented. (211.65)

820.61 All production and quality control mechanical, electronic, or automated equipment shall be routinely inspected, calibrated, and checked according to written procedures.

Table 1 (Continued).

CONTROL OF COMPONENTS AND DRUG
PRODUCT CONTAINERS AND CLOSURES

211.80 There shall be written
procedures to control the
receipt, identification,
storage, sampling, handling,
sampling, and testing for
components and product
closures. (820.80(a))
Components are to be stored in
a manner to prevent
contamination, be properly
stored, and identified with a
lot number. (820.81(b))

211.82 Upon receipt prior to
testing, all components are to
be visually inspected and
stored under quarantine.
(820.80, 820.80(a))

211.84 A lot of components is
not to be used until they are
first tested.
Representative samples are to
be collected for examination.
Samples are to be collected ion
accordance with written
procedures that provide for:
sterile or aseptic sampling
where necessary; identification
of the sampling containers,
identification of the
containers sampled; and
subdivision of samples where
necessary.
Samples of components and
closures shall be examined for
identity and strength and
include, where appropriate, a
microscopic examination.
(820.81(a))

Records shall be maintained of
these activities. (211.68(a))
All computer software programs
shall be validated. (211.68(b))

820.61(a)   Calibration
procedures shall include
specific directions and limits;
820.61(b)   Where possible
equipment calibration is to be
traceable to NBS; and
820.61(c) Calibration records
are to be maintained.
(211.160(b))

COMPONENTS

820.80 Components used in
manufacturing are to be
received, handled, and stored
in a manner designed to prevent
damage, contamination, mixups
or other adverse effects.
(211.82, 211.89)

820.80(a) Written procedures
for the acceptance of
components. Records shall be
maintained of component
acceptance or rejection. Upon
receipt all components are to
be visually examined.
Where necessary, components are
to be sampled, inspected, and
tested for conformance to
specifications.   (211.80,
211.82))

820.80(b) If components are
subject to deterioration with
time, stock shall be rotated.
Component control numbers shall
be easily visible.
Records are to be maintained of
all obsolete, deteriorated, or
rejected material. (211.86)

Table 1 (Continued).

211.86 Stock of components, closures, and drug product containers is to be rotated so that oldest stock is used first. (820.80(b))

211.87 Product is to be retested after long periods of storage. (NCS)

211.89 Rejected components, containers, and closures are to be quarantined. (820.80)

211.94 Drug product closures shall not be additive or subtractive from the product and provide adequate protection.
Where indicated closures shall be sterile sterile and non pyrogenic. (820.130)

820.81 CRITICAL DEVICES–In addition to the above:

820.81(a) All critical components are to be tested using a statistical rationale for conformance to specifications.
Each lot of critical components shall be assigned a lot number upon receipt. (211.84)

820.81(b)Where possible there shall be a written agreement with suppliers to notify the manufacturer of any proposed changes in components. (211.80)

PRODUCTION AND PROCESS CONTROLS

211.100(a) There shall be written procedures for process and production control to assure that the drug products have the identity, strength, quality, and purity that they purport of are represented to possess. (820.100)

211.100(b) Any deviation from written procedures shall be reported. (820.100(b))

211.101 Written production and Control procedures are to provide for:
Formulation compounding to achieve at least 100% of the labeled active ingredients.
Components removed from their original containers are to be identified with their name, control number, weight, and batch identification.

PRODUCTION AND PROCESS CONTROLS

820.100 Written manufacturing specifications and processing procedures shall be established, implemented, and controlled to assure that the device conforms to its original design or any approved changes in that design. (211.100(a))

820.100(a) Procedures for specification control measurement shall be assure that the design basis for the device, components, and packaging is correctly translated into approved specifications.
Specification changes shall be subject to controls as stringent as those applied to the original design specifications of the device. (211.110)

Table 1   (Continued).

Weighing, measuring, or subdividing operations are to be monitored to assure to assure that the component was tested, properly weighed, and properly identified.
Each component shall be weighed by one person and verified by another. (820.101)

211.103 Actual yields and the percentage of theoretical yield shall be calculated at each phase of the manufacturing, processing, packaging, or holding operation. (NCS)

211.105 All compounding and storage containers, processing lines, and major equipment shall be identified at all times to indicate their contents and where necessary the phase of processing. Major equipment used in manufacturing shall be identified in the production records. (820.101)

211.110 Written procedures shall be established and followed that describe the in-process controls, and tests, or examinations to be conducted on appropriate samples of in-process materials of each batch. (820.100(a), 820.100(b))

211.111 When appropriate, there shall be time limits for the completion of each phase of production. (820.100(b))

211.113(a) There shall be appropriate written procedures to prevent objectionable microorganisms in products not designed to be sterile. (820.100(b))

211.113(b) There shall be appropriate written procedures

820.100(b) Where deviations from device specifications could occur as a result of the manufacturing process, there shall be written procedures describing any controls necessary to assure conformance to specifications.
Processing control operations shall be conducted in a manner designed to assure that the device conforms to applicable specifications.
There shall be a formal approval procedure for any change in the manufacturing process. (211.100(b), 211.110, 211.111, 211.113(a))

CRITICAL DEVICES – In addition to 820.100, 820.101 applies:

820.101 Any critical operation shall be performed by a suitable designated person on suitable equipment and be verified. (211.101, 211.105)

820.115 Reprocessing procedures shall be established to assure that the reprocessed device or component meets the original, or subsequently modified and approved specifications.
Any device rejected during finished device inspection and later reprocessed shall be subject to another final device inspection for any characteristic that might be affected by reprocessing. (211.115)

CRITICAL DEVICES – In addition to 820.115, 820.116 applies:

820.116(a) Written procedures for the reprocessing of any critical component or critical device shall include the equipment used in reprocessing

Table 1 (Continued).

to prevent microbiological contamination of drug products purported to be sterile. There procedures are to include validation of any sterilization process. (820.120(b))

211.115 Written procedures are to be established for reprocessing batches not conforming to specifications. The procedures are to include a listing of all steps necessary to bring the batch into conformance. Reprocessing must include the review and approval of the quality control unit. (820.115, 820.116(a), 820.116(b))

and any special quality assurance methods or tests.
The procedures shall be designed to prevent adulteration due to the reprocessing.
Devices or components to be reprocessed shall be clearly identified and separated from those not being reprocessed. (211.115)

820.116(b) Any critical device or component subject to reprocessing shall conform to the original or subsequently approved changes in design.
Any prior quality assurance check shall be repeated if the reprocessing procedure could adversely affect any performance characteristic previously inspected. (211.115)

PACKAGING AND LABELING CONTROL

211.122 There shall be written procedures for the receipt, identification, storage, handling, sample examination and/or testing of labeling and packaging materials.
Any labeling not meeting written specifications shall be rejected.
Records shall be maintained for each shipment of packaging and labeling material indicating receipt, examination or testing and whether accepted or rejected.
Different labels shall be stored separately.
Obsolete and outdated labels and packaging shall be destroyed.
Gang printing for different drug products or different dosage forms is to be avoided.
Machinery used for printing drug or drug packaging labeling shall be monitored. (820.120)

PACKAGING AND LABELING CONTROLS

820.120 Labeling controls shall be adequate to maintain label integrity and prevent mixups. (211.122)

820.120(a) Labels shall be applied so as to remain legible during the customary conditions of processing, storage, handling, distribution, and use. (211.130)

820.120(b) Each packaging or labeling operation shall be physically or spatially in a manner designed to prevent mixups. (211.42(c), 211.130(a))

820.120(c) Prior to any packaging or labeling operation there shall be an inspection of the area where the operation is to occur by a designated individual to assure that no devices or labels from prior operations remain in the area. (211.125)

Table 1 (Continued).

211.125(a)-(f)
Labeling materials issued for a batch shall be carefully examined for identity and conformity to the labeling specified in the master of batch production records.
There shall be procedures for reconciliation of the quantities of labeling issued, used, and returned and any discrepancies outside normal operational limits shall be investigated.   (820.120(c), 820.120(d). 820.120(e))

211.130(a)-(d)
Written procedures to assure that correct labels, labeling, and packaging materials are used for drugs shall be followed which shall include: prevention of mixups, identification of a drug product with a lot number traceable to the batch records, examination of labels and packaging for suitability prior to use, and the inspection of packaging and labeling facilities prior to use to assure that all non suitable packaging and labeling have been removed.
Results of these inspections shall be documented. (820.120(b),   820.121(a), 820.121(b), 820.121(c)

211.132 This sections contains specific requirements regarding tamper resistant packaging for over-the- counter human drug products including packaging requirements, requests for exemption, and effective dates for implementation. (NCS)

211.134 Packaged and labeled products shall be examined during the finishing operations to assure that containers and packages have the correct label.

820.120(d) Labels and labeling shall be stored in a manner designed to prevent mixups. (211.125)

820.120(e) Labeling materials issued for devices shall be examined for identity, and where necessary, the lot number, storage conditions, and handling instructions. (211.125)

CRITICAL DEVICES - In addition to the requirements of 820.120 the following applies:

820.121(a) Labels must contain a control number. (211.130)

820.121(b) The signature of the proofreader and the date recorded, (211.130)

820.121(c) Access to labels shall be restricted to authorized personnel. (211.130)

820.130 The device package and any shipping container for a device shall be designed and constructed to protect the device from alteration or damage during the customary conditions of processing, storage, handling, and distribution. (211.94)

Table 1 (Continued).

At the completion of operations a representative sample of units shall be visually examined for correct labeling, the results of which are to be recorded in the batch production or control records. (820.120(e)

211.137 Products shall bear an expiration date appropriate to: the results of stability testing required by 211.166 and storage conditions on the label. (NCS)

HOLDING AND DISTRIBUTION

211.142(a)-(b)
Written procedures describing warehousing of drug products shall be established to include:
Quarantine of drug products before release by the quality control unit.
Storage of drug products under appropriate conditions of temperature, humidity, and light so that the identity, purity, strength, and quality are not affected. (820.150)

211.150 Written procedures describing the distribution of drug products shall be established to include:
A procedure whereby the oldest stock is distributed first.
A system whereby the distribution of each lot of drug product can be readily determined to facilitate a recall if necessary. (820.151, 820.152)

HOLDING, DISTRIBUTION, AND INSTALLATION

820.150 There shall be written procedures for warehouse control to assure that only those devices approved for release are distributed.
Where a device's fitness for use or quality deteriorates over time, there shall be a system to assure that the oldest approved devices are distributed first. (211.142(a)-(b)

CRITICAL DEVICES -In addition to the requirements of 820.150, the following is required:

820.151 Distribution records for medical devices shall include or make reference to the name and address of the consignee, the quantity and date shipped, and the control number used. (211.150, 211.196)

820.152 Where a device is installed by the manufacturer or his representative, they shall inspect the device after installation to make certain that it performs as intended. If installed by other than the manufacturer or his representative, the

Table 1 (Continued).

LABORATORY CONTROLS

211.160(a) The establishment of
any specifications, standards,
sampling plans, test
procedures, or other laboratory
control mechanisms or changes
in them shall be drafted by the
appropriate organizational
unit, and reviewed and approved
by the quality control unit.
(820.160)

211.160(b) Laboratory controls
shall include the establishment
of scientifically sound and
appropriate
specifications, standards,
sampling plans, and test
procedures designed to insure
that components, drug product,
closures, in-process material,
etc. conform to appropriate
standards of identity,
strength, purity, and quality.
This provides for:
written specifications for
acceptance of lots of
components, closures, and
labeling, and in-process
materials.
Collection and testing of
representative samples.
Calibration of instruments,
apparatus, gauges, and
recording devices at suitable
intervals.
(820.160(c),(820.160)

211.165 For each drug product
there shall be appropriate
tests prior to release for
distribution.
Lots failing to meet test
specifications shall be
rejected; reprocessing may be
performed. (820.161)

manufacturer shall provide
adequate instructions and
procedures for adequate
installation. (211.150)

DEVICE EVALUATION

820.160 There shall be written
procedures for finished device
inspection to assure that
finished device specifications
are met.
Prior to the release for
distribution, each production
run, lot or batch checked, and
where necessary tested, for
conformance with device
specifications.
Sampling plans shall be based
an an acceptable statistical
rationale.
Finished devices shall be
quarantined prior to release.
(211.160(a), 211.160(b),
211.167)

CRITICAL DEVICES — In addition
to 820.160, 120.161 applies:

820.161 A critical device or
component which does not meet
its performance specifications
shall be investigated, and a
written record of the
conclusions and followup shall
be made. (211.165)

820.162 After a device has been
released for distribution, any
failure of the device or its
components to meet performance
specifications shall be
investigated and a written
record of the investigation
including conclusions and
followup shall be maintained.
(211.198)

Table 1 (Continued).

211.166 There shall be a written stability testing program designed to assess the stability characteristics of drug products.
An adequate number of batches shall be tested to determine an appropriate expiration date. (NCS)

211.167 Each batch of drug product purporting to be sterile and/or pyrogen free shall be appropriately tested to determine conformance with such requirements. (820.160)

211.170 An appropriately identified reserve sample that is representative of each lot in each shipment of each active ingredient shall be retained. (NCS)

211.173 Animals used in testing components, in-process, or drug products for compliance with appropriate specifications shall be maintained and controlled in a manner suitable for their intended use. (NCS)

211.176 If a reasonable possibility exists that a non-penicillin drug product has been exposed to penicillin, it shall be tested for penicillin. (NCS)

RECORDS AND REPORTS

211.180 Any production, control, or distribution record that is required to be maintained in compliance with the drug GMP's and is specifically associated with a batch of a drug product shall be maintained for a period of a least one year after the expiration date of the batch.
Records for components, drug product containers, closures,

RECORDS

820.180 Device master records, device history records, and complaint files are to be maintained at the manufacturing establishment or other location that is reasonably accessible to designated FDA employees.
The manufacturer may mark records "confidential" to aid FDA in determining confidentiality.
All records are to be

Table 1 (Continued).

and labeling must be maintained for at least one year after the expiration date. (820.180)

211.182 Written records for the cleaning and use of all major pieces of equipment shall be maintained in individual equipment logs. (820.61)

211.184 Written records of component, drug product container, closure, and labeling records shall include the following: the identity and quantity of each shipment, name of the supplier, suppliers lot number, date of receipt, and a receiving code; results of any tests performed; inventory control records; documentation of the examination and review of labels and labeling; and, the disposition of rejected product. (820.80(a))

211.186 Master production and control records shall be maintained to assure uniformity for batch to batch. Information required includes: name strength, and dosage of the product; name and weight of each active ingredient; a complete list of components and their weight or measure; theoretical weights during processing; theoretical yield of product; description of label, packaging, and product closures; and complete manufacturing, sampling, and control instructions. (820.181)

211.188 Batch production and control records shall be maintained for each batch of drug product produced and shall include the following: an appropriate reproduction of the master production and control record; documentation of each significant step of

maintained for period equal to the expected life of the device or a minimum of two years which ever is greater. (211.180)

820.181 The device master record shall be maintained for each type of device and signed and dated by an authorized individual. It shall contain or refer to the location of the following: device specifications including appropriate drawings, composition, formulation, and component specifications; production process specifications; quality assurance procedures, checks, and equipment; and packaging and labeling specifications. (211.186)

820.182 CRITICAL DEVICES – In addition to the above:

820.182(a) The device master record must include full information concerning critical components and critical component suppliers, complete labeling procedures for the individual device and copies of all approved labels. (211.184)

820.184 The device history record shall be maintained to demonstrate that the device has been manufactured in accordance with the device master record. (211.188)
It shall include the dates of manufacture, quantity manufactured, quantity released for distribution, and any control number used.

820.185 CRITICAL DEVICES – In addition to the above:

820.185(a) The device history records for critical devices

Table 1 (Continued).

manufacture; dates; identification of processing equipment used; identification of components and their weight or measure used; in-process control results; results of the packaging and labeling area inspection; statements of theoretical and actual yield; labeling control records; description of the containers and closures; identification of the individuals performing the operations; and the results of any investigations or examinations made on the batch. (820.184, 820.185(c))

211.192 All drug product production and control records shall be reviewed by the quality control units to determine compliance with all established and approved written procedures. (820.20(a))

211.194 Laboratory control records shall be maintained to compliance with established specifications and standards and include the following: a description of the tested sample; statements of the test methods used; statements of weights used in testing; a record of all data secured; record of all calculations; statement of test results; initials of persons performing the tests; and a signature verifying that a second individual has reviewed the results. (820.180, 820.184)

211.196 Distribution records shall contain the name and strength of product, dosage form, name and address of the consignee, quantity shipped and the lot or control numbers used. (820.151)

shall include: a control number on each device traceable to the complete information on the production unit; the control number of each critical component within the device; the acceptance record of the critical component;
(b) the record or reference to each critical operation identifying the date performed, individual performing the operation and, when appropriate, the major equipment used in manufacture; and
(c) the inspection checks, results, date, and signature of the inspecting individual. (211.188)

820.195 When automated data processing is used for manufacturing or quality assurance purposes, adequate checks shall be designed and implemented to prevent inaccurate data output, input, and programming errors. (211.68(b))

820.198 Written and oral complaints relative to the identity, quality, durability,, reliability, safety, effectiveness, or performance of a device shall be reviewed, evaluated, and maintained by a formally designated unit which will determine whether or not an investigation is necessary. Any complaint involving the possibility of failure of a device to meet any of its performance standards shall be reviewed, evaluated, and investigated.
Where a formally designated unit is located at a site different from the manufacturing site, a duplicate copy must be transmitted to the manufacturing site. (211.198)

Table 1 (Continued).

211.198 Written procedures shall be established for the handling of all written or oral complaints regarding a drug product.
A file shall be maintained for these complaints at the place where a drug product was manufactured, processed, or packed and shall include:the name and strength of the drug product, lot number, name of the complainant, nature of the complaint, and the reply to the complainant.
If an investigation is conducted the results will be documented in the file. If no investigation is conducted the record will include the reason why it was determined that an investigation was not necessary. (820.198)

RETURNED AND SALVAGED DRUG PRODUCTS

211.204 This section governs the quarantine and suitability for reprocessing of returned drug goods. (NCS)

211.208 This section governs the salvage of merchandise that has suffered damage as a result of adverse storage conditions in excess of the labeled limits.   (NCS)

---

aNote: Section cites in the CFR, and subparts which follow the section number separated by a decimal are arranged in ascending numerical order; however, the composite number is not to be viewed as a whole number with a decimal fraction. An ascending sequence would be: 820.3 - 820.5 - 820.20 - 820.25 - 820.100 - 820.152 etc. The easiest way to locate a specific cite within a specific part, e.g., 820, is to ignore the decimal and view only the digits following it. The above would become 3 - 5 - 20 - 25 - 100 - 152 etc.

in contrast, the device GMP needs more flexibility to adapt to the
myriad of different products and manufacturing schemes encountered
in device manufacturing operations. In addition the medical device
GMPs have a two-tier structure that imposes additional requirements
on a select group of critical devices; whereas the Drug GMPs specifically exclude over-the-counter (OTC) drugs from regulation. The
medical device GMPs must also be able to adapt themselves to the
manufacture of In Vitro Diagnostic Products, which closely resembles
drug manufacturing operations.

In those instances where no corresponding sections exist under
the same subsection, any applicable areas of other subsections will
be indicated. In addition, the corresponding CFR section of the
drug or device GMP is listed at the end of each specific GMP point.
Where there is *no corresponding section*, (NCS) will be indicated.

II. PREPRODUCTION QUALITY

A. Regulatory Requirements

Developing a new drug delivery device and introducing it into production are very complex tasks. For many new devices and associated manufacturing processes that use software, these tasks are further complicated because of the importance of every minute characteristic of the software, and the possibility of subtle software errors.
Without thorough planning, program control, and design reviews,
these tasks are virtually impossible to accomplish without errors or
leaving important aspects undone. The planning exercise and execu-
tion of the plans are complex because of the many areas and activities
that must be covered. Some key activities are the following:

    Determining and meeting the customer's requirements
    Meeting regulations and standards
    Developing specifications for the drug delivery device
    Developing the device
    Evaluating prototype devices
    Developing, selecting, and evaluating components and vendors
    Developing specifications for manufacturing processes
    Developing and validating manufacturing processes
    Developing and approving labels and user instructions
    Documenting the details of the device design and processes
    If applicable, developing a service program

Most of these topics are discussed in this section. Section IV
covers equipment, including automated production and quality assurance equipment, and thus discusses preproduction activities such as
validation. Other topics, such as component selection, and labeling
content and approval, are covered in Section VI and IX, respectively.

There are various programs for assuring that appropriate preproduction activities are correctly performed in the listed areas so that
the result is the orderly development and transfer into production of
a new or modified device. These programs include using a product
assurance program and complying with the GMP regulation, using a
total quality assurance program, etc. This section emphasizes preproduction quality or product and process assurance—the first half
of a total quality assurance system.

An adequate quality assurance system requires coordination of all
quality-related activities from initial concept of each specific drug
delivery device through production and postmarketing activities;
hence, such a system is called a total quality assurance system. A
product assurance system plus a GMP system constitutes a total QA
system. The primary goal of a total QA system is to produce quality
products by assuring both intrinsic quality and achieved quality.

Intrinsic quality is the inherent quality designed into a drug
delivery device and the associated manufacturing processes. Intrinsic quality is accomplished by having the design or formulation,
process or process modification, and related documentation for a new
or modified device or process comply with appropriate requirements
of the company, customers, standards, and regulations. As a result,
the device design has the desired level of quality designed into it
and the associated processes have the desired capability designed
into them.

The intrinsic safety and effectiveness of a drug delivery device
is established during the design phase and is a direct function of:

Awareness of the design goal by management, research and development, production, and quality assurance
Review and analysis of the proposed design
Correct selection and application of parts and materials
Performance of normal and worst-case testing to evaluate and
assure that the device and manufacturing processes will perform as intended under all reasonable circumstances

Worst-case testing for a drug delivery device design must be
reasonably and *prudently* interpreted based on the anticipated use,
use with other devices, environmental conditions, and review of the
literature for past problems with similar devices. For a manufacturing process, worst-case conditions are derived from operational limits
established by the firm, environmental conditions, process equipment
capabilities, maintenance requirements, employee changes, and the
like.

Achieved quality is assured through procedures for orderly
transfer of the design information into the production department
followed by controlled manufacturing of the new or modified device.
Some key activities are listed below and discussed later:

Adequate device master record and change control
Process validation
Review of total development and manufacturing programs
Pilot production
Detailed review of the pilot devices

Application of the GMP Regulation

The device GMP regulation applies to the design and control of facilities, production and measurement equipment, design transfer, and to production processes, including controls for packaging and labeling design. A manufacturer who follows the GMP regulation is working toward maintaining the intrinsic safety and effectiveness established during the design phase by using a formal QA program to assure that all manufacturing activities that affect quality are controlled. The GMP regulation is intended to provide a high degree of confidence that a manufacturing process will consistently produce finished devices that conform to their specifications.

Manufacturers may transfer design specifications that result in unsafe or ineffective drug delivery devices if the manufacturers fail to make certain that the design basis for a device is correct; that is, if they adopt design specifications that have not been properly qualified and verified. GMP section 820.100(a)(1) controls transfer by requiring manufacturers to establish procedures to make certain that:

The approved design is *accurately* transferred into written
  specifications.
There are *sufficient* specifications, which accurately describe the
  drug delivery device, its components, and packaging.
These specifications are *adequate* to assure that the design configuration and performance requirements can be met if the drug
  delivery device is manufactured and assembled according to
  specifications.

Typically, assuring accuracy, sufficiency, and adequacy are accomplished through a formal evaluation and review process, as discussed in this section, to verify that the design or design change is adequately translated into specifications. If the design is *not* adequately translated into correct specifications as needed to procure components and manufacture finished devices, the resulting product may be unsafe and ineffective. The need for a written procedure for adequate transfer of specifications should be determined on the basis of the need for communication, complexity of the activity, etc. The GMP regulation does not mandate a written procedure for transferring a design, but, as noted above, it does require that the design be correctly transferred into production.

The GMP regulation addresses design retrospectively through the Complaint File requirements, Failure Investigations, and through the Quality Assurance Program requirements. These GMP sections require drug delivery device manufacturers to:

Review and investigate all complaints (820.198).
Investigate failure of released devices to meet performance specifications and take corrective action (820.162).
Identify, recommend, or provide solutions for quality assurance problems [820.20(a)(3)].

In the context of the total GMP regulation, particularly the scope in 820.1 and the QA program in 820.20, the follow-up (corrective) activities in 820.162 refer to solving the quality problem regardless of its origin or nature. That is, design and labeling content deficiencies are not excluded.

After production starts, GMP section 820.100(a)(2) requires manufacturers to subject all changes to the original device design to stringent controls. Change control for devices or processes is covered in Section V.

B. Product Assurance

Product assurance is a quality assurance program that assures quality is designed into a product. Under it, drug delivery manufacturers determine customer needs and expectations or specifications, if specifications exist. These are documented by the manufacturer in device specifications that, to the technical and economic extent feasible, reflect the customer needs and expectations. In addition, to device specifications, a product assurance program encompasses employee responsibility, safety standards, component selection, label content and physical characteristics, design evaluation, design analysis, design review, adequate documentation, and correct transfer into production. Meanwhile, under the GMP regulation, employees are being trained, and manufacturing processes are being developed and validated for the new product. During pilot production, the product assurance and GMP programs work together to make certain that design and production quality goals have been achieved.

One of the first steps in the transfer of a design into specifications and production is to inform the quality assurance manager or other designee about all new or significantly modified devices or processes. Also, management should designate appropriate persons to be responsible for directing, monitoring, and reporting all activities from device concept through associated postmarketing activities, with nothing left to chance (see 820.20, Organization). Preproduction quality planning for a specific device by the quality assurance manager and other managers must include consideration of all significant aspects of that device, the manufacture of it, and its ultimate use. These activities result in many documents, the first of which is usually a device specification.

Device, Software, and Process Specifications

An important goal in a preproduction program is to have all of the involved personnel working toward developing and manufacturing the same drug delivery device as outlined by the device, software, if any, and process specifications. Preliminary device specifications that identify the characteristics of the new or modified device should be drafted at the very *beginning* of the development program. A major value of specifications is to aid communications between various departments working on the project. The major value of specifications is lost if they are written after the product is developed; however, belated device specifications are still useful for developing accurate catalog sheets or other marketing aids.

At the start of the development project, performance standards and general safety standards to be met should be identified by management and included as part of the device specifications. The document, "Preproduction Quality Assurance Planning: Recommendations for Medical Device Manufacturers," available from the FDA , lists several standards and books on product development and product quality. If international sales are planned, then appropriate foreign standards and marketing requirements should be considered. For example, the International Electrotech Commission has a draft review standard. "Guide on Formal Design Review," which should be helpful to product assurance personnel. Information about national and international standards may be obtained from American National Standards Association (ANSI), 1430 Broadway, New York, New York 10018. ANSI is a private organization that monitors most of the standards activity in the United States and foreign activity in which U.S. citizens "offically" participate. Thus, ANSI can supply addresses and other information about all well-established standards-writing groups. Also, ANSI has many different types of standards for sale.

Designing and design evaluation are expensive and time-consuming. Therefore, to control these and increase the probability of achieving desired safety and performance characteristics, device, software, and process specifications should be thoroughly reviewed *before* development commerces. As the hardware and software designs evolve, they should be evaluated versus their specifications.

Design Evaluation Versus Specifications

The original design of devices and any subsequent changes should
be evaluated by appropriate and formal laboratory, animal, and
clinical testing. Appropriate laboratory and animal testing followed
by evaluation of the results must be carefully performed before clinical testing or commercial distribution of drug delivery devices. Such
testing includes normal operation, operational limits, environmental
limits, sensor failures, operator errors, etc. Where data inputs are
involved, these must encompass none, normal, low, high, and extremely high positive and negative data. The company must be assured that the design is safe and effective to the extent that can be
determined by various scientific tests and analysis before clinical
testing on humans or use by humans. For example, the electrical,
thermal, mechanical, chemical, radiation, etc., safety of devices
usually can be determined by laboratory tests.

Clinical testing is not needed for many substantially equivalent
devices (see 21 CFR Part 807 Subpart E—Premarket Notification Procedure). Where it is needed, such as for complex, substantially
equivalent devices or new devices, clinical testing on humans must
meet the applicable requirements in the Investigational Device Exemption (IDE) regulations (21 CFR 812 and 813).

The general IDE regulation (812) exempts a manufacturer during
the "premarketing phase" from the following provisions of the FD&C
Act:

Misbranding
Registration of the establishment
Premarket notification [510(k)]
FDA performance standards
Premarket approval
Good manufacturing practices
Color additives
Banned devices
Restricted devices

Don't be misled by this list of exemptions—being exempted from
these provisions does not mean that a company may develop a new
device under uncontrolled conditions and then test it on humans.
The situation is just the opposite—development and testing must be
highly controlled (i.e., formal). Devices being clinically tested are
not exempt from section 501(c) of the FD&C Act, which states that
a device is adulterated if it does not meet company quality claims.
In addition, the IDE regulation has labeling requirements in section
812.5 and quality assurance requirements in section 812.20(b)(3)
that must be met. Further, manufacturers should remember that
human subjects are also protected through the courts via product

liability laws and actions. In summation, protection of company interests, human test subjects, practitioners, and patients requires
that all medical devices be developed, evaluated, and manufactured
under a total QA system.

Laboratory testing of a drug delivery device to force a failure
takes considerable time, and the "culprit" may not fail during the
testing. Another evaluation technique is *failure mode and effects
analysis* (FMEA), in which failures are assumed to occur. FMEA is
useful for evaluating reliability, safety, and general quality where,
for example, the evaluator assumes that:

> Each component fails.
> Each subsystem or subassembly fails.
> The operator makes errors.
> The power source is interrupted and immediately restarted.

The probability of each failure actually occurring and, if it does,
the resulting effect, are analyzed. Then, where needed and feasible,
hazards and faulty performance are designed out of the drug delivery
device; or compensated or prevented/reduced by interlocks, warning
signs, explicit instructions, alarms, etc. Risks, of course, cannot
always be removed from medical devices, but they should be known
and controlled to the extent feasible with existing technology.

Failure mode and effects analysis is a very powerful and cost-
effective technique. Note that it takes very little time to assume
that a component or subsystem is going to fail versus the time required to test to failure. The idea is not to promote one method
above the other, because a reasonable amount of both actual testing
and failure mode and effects analysis should be done before a drug
delivery device is clinically tested and/or placed into production.

All evaluation results must be reviewed by product development
personnel who compare the test and FMEA results with specifications,
including safety and performance standards, to make certain that
the desired level of intrinsic quality has been designed into the drug
delivery device.

Software Validation

Software is evaluated and reviewed versus the software specifications
during the ongoing development of the device design. When a "final"
prototype(s) is available, the software and hardware are validated
to make certain that company specifications for the device and process are met. Some aspects of hardware evaluation were discussed
above. Aspects specific to software are covered below.

Before testing the software in actual use, the detailed code should
be visually reviewed versus the flowcharts and specification. All
cases, especially decision points and error or limit handling, should
be reviewed and the results documented.

In all cases, algorithms should be checked for accuracy. Recalls
have occurred because algorithms were incorrectly copied from a
source and, in other cases, because the source algorithm was incorrect. During the development phase, complex algorithms may have
to be checked by using a test subprogram written in a higher-order
language, if the operational program is written in a low-level language.

The validation program is planned and executed such that all
elements of the software and hardware are exercised and evaluated.
The testing of software usually involves the use on an emulator and
must include testing of the software in the finished drug delivery
device.

The testing includes normal operation of the complete device;
and this phase of validation program may be completed first to make
certain that the device meets the fundamental performance specifications. Concurrently or afterward, the combined system (hardware
and software) should be challenged with abnormal inputs and conditions. As appropriate, these include such items as:

> Operator errors
> Induced failure of sensors
> Induced failure of output equipment
> Exposure to static electricity
> Power loss and restart
> Simultaneous inputs or interrupts
> As appropriate, deliverate application of none, low, high, positive,
>   negative, and extremely high input values

The results of the software and combined system validation are
included in the design reviews discussed later.

Labeling Evaluation

During evaluation, the complete drug delivery device is exercised
such that all labeling, displays, and outputs are generated, reviewed, and the results documented. During the evaluation, all
displayed prompts and instructions are checked versus company and
FDA labeling requirements and versus the operator's manual.

Printed labeling and screen displays should be checked to see if
they are directed to the user and not to the system designers,
which is a common fault found in labeling. Displayed text should
be short and to the point. Because displays are brief, keywords
should be carefully selected to match system characteristics and yet
transfer the maximum information to the user. The text and references to controls or other parts of the system *must* match the labeling on the drug delivery device. Data, identifications, or other
key information displayed must be current, complete, unambiguous,
and accurate.

During the evaluation, all prompts and instructions should be followed *exactly* by the device operator and such action must result in correct operation of the device. Prompts and instructions must appropriately match the instructions in the operator's manual. The evaluation should include verification that the screen displays meet the requirements of and have been approved per the company policy/procedure for control of labeling.

Patient and procedure data on printouts must be correct; therefore, printouts must undergo an evaluation similar to that performed for the screen displays. In addition, the printouts should be evaluated with respect to their "cold" information-transfer characteristics. Will the printouts be quickly and clearly understood a few weeks later when the reader is not reading the screens, operating the device, or looking at the patient? All printouts should also meet the company policy/procedure requirements for labeling. Likewise, patient data or other key information transmitted to a remote location must be correct; therefore, it must be checked for accuracy, completeness, and identification.

The overall device specifications usually have requirements that cover operator error prevention and control. Along with operator training, such errors are controlled by:

Adequate instruction manuals
Display of adequate prompts and correct instructions
Status (history) reports
Exclusion of certain erroneous inputs or actions
Human factors
Ergonomics

Also, for some devices, it may be important to control the order in which data can be entered by the operator. In emergency situations or because of distractions, it may be important to present the operator with a brief history or status report of recent actions. During the evaluation, the listed items should be evaluated versus the specifications, and checked for completeness and appropriateness.

Design Reviews

During the development program and especially after the device is formally evaluated as noted above, and after associated manufacturing processes have been developed as discussed below and in Section VII, progressive design reviews should be performed in a group setting by all affected company managers or designees. Reviews should be performed for all new designs or formulations and for device or process revisions to make certain that the following two goals are fully met:

   The desired level of intrinsic quality is in or is being designed
      into the drug delivery device and/or processes before the
      start of production.
   The designs are appropriately reflected by the device master
      record documentation as verified by ample evidence that the
      device specifications (i.e., the company labeling claims) are
      met.

C.   Adequate Master Record

Most of the documents in the device master record should be drafted
before process validation or pilot production begins. Of course,
these documents may be changed later due to changes in requirements, corrections, and results from validation, pilot production, etc.
A complete and adequate device master record, including all labeling
and data forms, must be drafted and approved before full-scale production and before commerical distribution of the device. Details
of device master records and their control are described in Section
V.

   A device master record document plan, which is basically an index
or table of contents, should be drafted to support product specifications and improve communications among involved personnel. By
reviewing the document plan, one can see which drawings and procedures are completed, in-process, or need to be drafted.

D.   Adequate Manufacturing Process

Production processes should be planned, developed, validated, and
documented to assure that they will routinely achieve the intrinsic
level of quality designed into the new or modified device. Manufacturing, customer, and vendor problems associated with previous
device designs should be analyzed to eliminate or reduce similar
problems in new or modified devices.

   The evaluation of a new design and its associated manufacturing
processes usually includes pilot production of a few units or batches.
Pilot production is recommended, as it helps debug the device design
and overall production program. Thus, pilot production should be
planned so that manufacturing activities are monitored, problems are
discovered and resolved, and documentation is updated.

   The adequacy of facilities and equipment for manufacturing a new
or modified device must be determined as discussed in Sections III
and IV. Included in this determination should be the facilities used
in, and equipment used for, environmental control, inspection, testing, labeling control, device and component handling, etc.

   Where finished device testing cannot adequately measure desired
attributes of a device, assurance of quality must be derived by
other means—a method acceptable to the FDA is validation of each

process used in production and consideration of the interaction of these processes.

E. Process Validation

Process validation is a formal program to determine with a high degree of assurance and documentation that a specific process will consistently meet its predetermined specifications and thus produce devices that meet their predetermined specifications and quality attributes. Process validation is intended to be a terminal activity because it is performed on production equipment and processes that, along with a new or modified device design, are expected to meet their specifications based on previous phase-by-phase evaluations and reviews during their development.

Thus, the device and, as appropriate, the packaging must be defined in terms of the desired attributes, such as physical, chemical, and performance characteristics. The device and packaging attributes must then be translated into written device specifications, as discussed, and manufacturing specifications to assure that the finished device conforms to the approved design. Acceptable ranges or limits must be established for each attribute. The validity of the acceptance specifications should be verified through testing and challenge of the device, package, and manufacturing processes during their respective development programs and later during pilot production. These specifications are needed because validation is performed versus predetermined specifications. If specifications do not exist, they should be written before continuing with the validation.

The need for validation is indicated in situations where the desired characteristics of the finished device cannot be readily measured. Where in-process and finished device testing is not adequate or practical, a manufacturer can assure, through careful design of the device and packaging, and careful design and validation of both the process and process controls, that there is a very high probability that all manufactured units from successive lots will be acceptable.

Validating a process also reduces the dependence on intensive in-process and finished device testing and is particularly indicated when such testing is destructive or is done on a sampling basis for an important parameter such as the package integrity of a sterile device. Thus, for some devices and processes as listed below, validation may be the only practical means for assuring that these processes will consistently produce devices that meet their predetermined specifications.

The finished device tests have insufficient sensitivity to determine the desired safety and efficacy information.

Clinical or destructive testing would be required to show that
the manufacturing process is adequate to produce the desired
device.

The finished device testing does not reveal all safety- and effec-
tiveness-related variations that may occur in the device.

For practical reasons, the finished device or package needs to be
tested on a sampling basis. (Sampling is valid only when a
process is operating in a state-of-control, which in the case
listed here means that the process has been validated.)

The process uses software that contains so many interactive elements that the system behavior under all reasonable circumstances might not be known.

The process capability is unknown, or it is suspected that the
process is barely capable of meeting the device specifications.

For some devices, such as those that use certain biological raw
materials, finished device testing is *sufficient* to show effectiveness, but the variability of the biological raw materials renders
adequate testing impossible or the testing of incoming biological
materials is not technically feasible. (Thus, some batches of
finished devices will fail and must be discarded. In this
situation, it is important that appropriate processes be validated so that failures will be due to only the one known but
nonmeasureable cause—the raw material—and not due to unknown causes.)

General programs for validating these processes include planning,
written protocols, equipment qualification, process performance qualification, revalidation considerations, and documentation of the results of the validation program. In some cases, such as for sterilization processes, process-compatible devices and packaging must be
available for use during the validation program.

Validation Planning and Protocol

A manufacturer should evaluate and document all factors that affect
device quality when designing and performing a validation study.
These factors may vary considerably among different devices and
manufacturing technologies and could include, for example, component
specifications, air and water handling systems, environmental controls, process equipment functions, and process control operations.

Validation documentation should include evidence of the suitability
of materials, the performance and reliability of process equipment
and control systems, the suitability of buildings, and the competence
of personnel.

Prospective validation includes those considerations that should
be made before an entirely new device is manufactured or when there
is a significant change in the manufacturing process that may affect

the device's attributes, such as uniformity and identity. It is usually not sufficient to process a device using procedures that were either established for another device or that are preconceived, without actually qualifying the specific device. There is an inherent danger in relying on perceived similarities between devices, processes, and equipment without appropriate analysis and/or challenges. Some key elements to consider are the validation protocol, device specifications, equipment and processes qualification, challenges, performance qualification, documentation, and revalidation.

It is important that the manufacturer prepare a written validation protocol that specifies the procedures to follow, the tests to be conducted, and the data to be collected. The purpose for which data are collected must be clear, the data must reflect facts, and data must be carefully and accurately collected. A protocol should specify a sufficient number of replicate process runs to demonstrate reproducibility. The number of runs should be selected to yield a valid measure of variability among successive runs and include a full challenge of the process.

The challenge of the process should encompass those operational limits of actual production *allowed* in the firm's written standard operating procedures. These constitute conditions most likely to result in a few devices that do not conform to specifications.

Process variables should be monitored during the validation runs. Analysis of the data collected from monitoring will establish the variability of process parameters for individual runs and will help establish if the equipment and process controls are adequate to assure that device specifications are met.

Equipment and Process Qualification

The process(es) and equipment should be designed and/or selected so that in-process and finished device specifications are consistently achieved. This selection should be done with the participation of all appropriate groups concerned with assuring a quality device, e.g., engineering design, production operations, and quality assurance. The next step is to obtain, install, and qualify the equipment. Then the performance of the overall process including the qualified equipment is qualified.

Equipment: installation qualification. Installation qualification studies establish confidence that the process equipment and ancillary systems are capable of consistently operating within established limits and tolerances. After process equipment is designed or selected, it should be reviewed, calibrated, evaluated, and tested to verify that it is capable of operating satisfactorily within the operating limits required by the process specifications.

The installation qualification phase of process validation includes:

Examination of equipment design
Determination of calibration, maintenance, and adjustment require-
     ments
Identification of important elements that could affect the device

Information obtained from the installation qualification studies of
process equipment and ancillary systems should be documented and
used to:

Establish written equipment calibration and maintenance procedures
Establish manufacturing procedures for the monitoring, operation
          and control of the equipment including the minimum number of
          operators
Establish any needed environmental controls and procedures
Assure that the work area has sufficient space to perform the
          processing associated activities

Equipment fabricators perform qualification runs at their facilities
and analyze the results to determine that the process equipment is
ready for delivery. Device manufacturers should obtain copies of
the suppliers' qualification studies to use as a guide, to obtain basic
data, and to reduce their own qualification studies. However, it is
usually insufficient to rely solely on the representations and studies
of the equipment supplier, or on limited experience in producing
another device. The ultimate decision regarding equipment suitability
should be based on collection of data from appropriate evaluation,
challenge, and testing of the equipment as applied to the specific
device in question, before the equipment is used for routine production.

Tests and challenges of equipment operation should include the
operational range in the written standard operating procedures. It
is important that test conditions simulate actual production conditions
within and at the established operating limits of the equipment for
the device and process involved. In most cases it is important that
tests be performed at the upper and lower limits of the operational
range, because the intent is to include those allowed conditions that
pose the greatest chance of the process or device not meeting specifications. When establishing challenges, events such as loss of
electricity, air pressure, vacuum, steam, water, etc., and failure of
valves, sensors, etc., may need to be considered.

In evaluating an entire processing system for a device, it may be
necessary to study the interaction of several process elements to
determine the cumulative effect on the attributes of the finished
devices.

When necessary, the tests and challenges should be repeated a sufficient number of times to assure reliable and meaningful results. If the equipment is shown not to perform within its specifications, then the equipment and related systems must be evaluated to identify the cause. Corrections should be made and additional test runs performed to verify that the equipment performs within specifications.

All acceptance criteria *must* be met during the final acceptance tests or challenges. The observed variability of the equipment between and within runs can be used as a basis for the total number of trials selected for the subsequent performance qualification studies of the process.

After the equipment configuration and performance characteristics are established and qualified, they should be documented.

During the qualification phase, planning for eventual maintenance can reduce or prevent confusion during emergency repairs, which could lead to improper repairs, such as use of a wrong replacement part. Therefore, the installation qualification should include a review of pertinent maintenance procedures, repair parts lists, and calibration methods for each piece of equipment. If necessary to prevent inadvertent manufacture of nonconforming devices, postrepair cleaning and calibration requirements should be developed. The objective is to assure that all repairs can be performed in a way that will not affect the characteristics of material processed or devices manufactured after repairs.

Process: performance qualification. The purpose of performance qualification is to rigorously test the process to demonstrate effectiveness and repeatability in producing in-process or finished devices. Each step where variability can affect device specifications should be challenged. In entering the performance qualification phase or validation, it is understood that:

The device, packaging, and process specifications have been established, documented, and essentially proven acceptable through laboratory or other trial methods.
The process and ancillary equipment has been judged acceptable on the basis of suitable installation qualification studies.

Challenges must simulate those conditions that will be encountered during actual production. A range of conditions at and within established process specification limits for a given process should be used. The challenges must include the range of conditions allowed in written standard operating procedures and should be repeated enough times to assure that the results are meaningful and consistent.

At this step of validation, some function tests may be needed to establish that finished devices meet the device specifications. As stated earlier, routine function testing for desired attributes of some types of finished devices is generally not practical. Therefore, during validation some finished devices may need to be evaluated by special test methods and test equipment, which are not practical for use on a routine basis. For example, the tests may be destructive.

Validation Documentation

It is essential that the validation program results be documented and that the documentation be properly maintained. Each process must be defined and described in sufficient detail so that employees understand what is required for control, routine production, and maintenance (also see Section V, "Master Records"). Approval and release of the process for use in routine manufacturing should be based on a review of:

    All the validation documentation
    Data from the equipment qualification
    Process performance qualification data
    Finished device and/or package function testing

Devices from validation runs may be distributed if all devices and process specifications are met. After the process is validated, routine production may start. The process *must* be operated according to the device master record specifications. These, of course, contain the setpoints, parameters, and procedures determined and documented during the validation program.

For routine production, it is important to record process details such as time, temperature, and equipment used, and to record any changes that have occurred. Also, a maintenance log can be useful in failure investigations of a specific manufacturing lot if the need arises.

Revalidation

As long as the process *routinely* operates in a state-of-control, it does not have to be revalidated. Whether the process is routinely operating in a state-of-control is determined by comparing the day-to-day process control data and any feasible finished device and package evaluation data (i.e., device history record data) with the master record specifications. If control problems develop, or if the device, packaging, or processing is modified, information regarding the device, package, production control, and original validation program and results must be carefully analyzed. If indicated by the analysis, all or parts of the process must be revalidated. Processes may also be validated on a periodic basis but, as noted, if problems develop or changes are made, the need for immediate revalidation must be considered.

Revalidation is performed using applicable portions or all of the same program as described from the original validation.

F. Personnel Training

The firm must assure that there are properly trained personnel or programs to train personnel as needed to produce a new or modified drug delivery device. In one very valuable training technique, manufacturing personnel assist research and development personnel in assembling and evaluating engineering prototype drug delivery devices. This technique:

Achieves advance training for manufacturing personnel
Reduces production problems by improving the producibility of the device based on the expertise and input of the manufacturing personnel.
Improves communications and technology transfer among the various departments—important and valuable side benefits.

G. Device Evaluation and History Record

The research and development programs for the device and manufacturing processes, and pilot production, if needed, *must* result in the development of verified procedures for in-process and finished-device inspection and test. These inspection and/or test procedures *must* not be deliberately allowed to evolve during full-scale production—to do so is a violation of the GMP regulation, particularly Subpart F, Production and Process Controls, and Subpart I, Device Evaluation. *All* devices placed into commercial distribution *must* be manufactured under a quality assurance system that meets the requirements of the GMP regulation—not just the devices that are produced several months after the first lot or batch is produced. The GMP regulation, of course, allows devices, processes, and master records to be changed after initial production; however, a manufacturer is *not* allowed to deliberately produce and commercially distribute drug delivery devices without an adequate device master record.

During pilot production it is very important that device evaluation and other device history record information be collected and analyzed to make certain that the specifications of the device intended to be produced, the device master record, and the actual finished devices *agree* with one another. This conformance is a fundamental objective of the GMP regulation, and additional information on this topic is presented in Sections VII and VIII.

Finished Device Release

An adequate quality assurance program for new or modified devices
requires that final prototypes or pilot production models be formally
evaluated by the product development group to determine that the
devices conform to specifications. Then the evaluation data and associated records for the pilot devices should be reviewed by the
design review group. Any discrepancies in the finished devices
versus the specification and other elements of the master record *must*
be resolved before drug delivery devices are released for full-scale
production. If pilot models are to be commercially distributed, the
firm *must* make certain that pilot units meet master record requirements and are approved for release. Most firms, however, use the
pilot models in training programs for technical writers, production
and service personnel, etc. Pilot production models are also used
in early marketing displays.

III. BUILDINGS AND ENVIRONMENT

A. Buildings

Facilities of drug delivery device manufacturers and their contractors
in which components, in-process devices, accessories, and finished
devices are handled, processed, and stored must have sufficient
space and be designed to allow proper cleaning, maintenance, and
other necessary operations in order to meet the requirement of section 820.40 of the Good Manufacturing Practices regulation. Buildings
should be suitably designed so that there is adequate space for manufacturing, receiving, packaging, labeling, storage, etc., to minimize
contaminants, assure orderly handling procedures, and prevent mixups. As the company grows or the product line is changed, existing
facilities may become inadequate. Thus, as part of the quality assurance program audit, existing buildings must be reviewed to determine
if these are adversely impacting quality assurance requirements.

Contamination Control

Typical problems in manufacturing and storage facilities include environmental contamination and insufficient space for receiving and
holding incoming components and materials before test and inspection.
For each area in the building where components or devices are
processed, any elements such as particulates (cardboard dust, slitter
byproducts, etc.), microorganisms, humidity, temperature, static
electricity, etc., which a manufacturer has determined might cause
contamination must be controlled. Buildings should be approximately
constructed to prevent, reduce, and control these parameters and
support the firm's environmental control program as discussed later.

For example, the control of dust may require that driveways and parking lots be paved. Crowding causes mixups and can result in contamination or in the use of unapproved components, materials, or rejected in-process assemblies. Designated areas should be assigned for various production activities such as receiving, inspection/testing, manufacturing, labeling, packaging, recordkeeping, etc. Traffic by personnel who do not work in or manage the designated areas should be held to a minimum.

Orderly Operations

In addition to having sufficient space, the facility must be designed and arranged so that all operations can be performed in an orderly manner. This will facilitate the satisfactory performance of all operations and, in manufacturing areas, prevent confusion that can lead to unsatisfactory job performance and mixups.

To preclude mixups, distinct operations or processes should be separated either physically—for example, by walls or partitions—or spatially—by providing enough room between operations to indicate that separate activities are being performed. An appropriate degree of separation, or walls, curtains, etc., must exist so that no activity will spray, dust, or otherwise have an adverse effect on other adjacent activities. For example, there must be a handling and storage system to preclude the mixup of labeled "sterile" but not-yet-sterilized devices from the devices with the same labeling that have been sterilized. Likewise, samples of labeled "sterile" devices to be given away must be sterile because they may be used. Firms that have more than one labeling operation must maintain adequate separation of these to prevent any mixups occurring between various products and their specified labeling. Labeling mixups are a major cause of product recalls, and a number of these mixups can be traced to inadequate separation of operations during the labeling of devices.

B. Environmental Control

One of the variables that can significantly affect product quality and employee performance is the environment. A controlled environment is, to various degrees, an integral part of most production facilities. Some environmental factors to be considered are lighting, ventilation, temperature, humidity, pressure, particulates, and static electricity. Section 820.46, Environmental Control, of the GMP regulation is considered by FDA to be a "discretionary" requirement; that is, the degree of environmental control to be maintained must be consistent with the intended use of the device, and details of how to achieve this control is left to the manufacturer to decide. "Discretionary GMP requirements" are those that may or may not apply to the manufacturer of a specific device. In these cases the manufacturer must make use of a prudent decision as to whether such requirements are necessary to assure the quality of the finished drug delivery device made by a particular manufacturing operation. These requirements are modified in the GMP regulation by phrases such as "where . . . could have an adverse affect" or "where . . . necessary."

General Controls

General air conditioning is normally not regarded as an environmental control; however, changes in temperature and lighting can have an adverse effect on employee performance and, in turn, on assuring that the device is properly assembled, inspected, and tested. Air conditioning can control humidity which, in turn, can reduce static charges. Static charges on the hands of employees can damage some electronic components and, in such situations, need to be controlled. Production workers are a major source of particulate contamination, and standard operating procedures for personnel are often necessary in order that employees not adversely affect the environment.

Analyze Operation

If the environment in which components or devices are manufactured or held can have an adverse effect on the devices' fitness for use, that environment must be controlled. For each operation, the manufacturer should analyze the manufacturing operations in order for the finished device to meet the device specifications, be fit for the intended use, and to control costs. For example, in the manufacture of a sterile device such as an implant, or a device such as a diagnostic medium that requires aseptic filling, the environment must be controlled to reduce particulate matter and viable microorganisms. The packaging for these must be stored in a clean, dry, insect-free area. Components that support bacterial growth must be stored in a controlled environment which, in some cases, will include refrigeration. Because particles can bridge across submicron circuits and static electricity can rupture semiconductor junctions, microcircuits for use in devices should be manufactured in a clean-room environment where particulates and humidity are controlled.

When analyzing the production of a device to determine the degree of control needed, the manufacturer should identify exactly what needs to be controlled: the device itself; area for one task; or large production area. For example, if the device can be cleaned after production, there usually is no need for extensive environmental control during production. The cleaned devices are stored in clean containers or are immediately packaged. The environment usually must be controlled where the device is being packaged. If the work area needs to be controlled, how much must be controlled—

a workbench, a room or a factory? For example, a HEPA-filtered laminar-flow bench maintains a low-particulate environment that is large enough for many small tasks or operations. If a larger area is needed, then it may be possible to set a broad environmental specification for most of the room area and use a local laminar-flow unit and curtains to create a small very clean area. Considerations such as these can reduce environmental facility and equipment costs and reduce the activities required to maintain and monitor the controlled area and operations.

Specifications

When it is necessary to control the environment, specifications for parameters such as temperature, humidity, colony-forming units (CFUs), particulates per cubic foot, etc., must be established. No FDA guidelines for these parameters presently exist for environmentally controlled areas such as cleanrooms. Federal Standard 209b with its appendices and 209c are suggested as guidelines for developing cleanroom controls such as particle counts per cubic foot. Federal standard 209c defines various levels of environmental control such as Class 1000. A Class 1000 room contains no more than 1000 particles 0.5 µm in diameter or larger per cubic foot of air. Information may also be obtained from manufacturers of cleanroom equipment. Aseptic manufacturing and filling are usually done in a Class 100 or better cleanroom or bench. The Class 100 status is maintained during routine operations—during idle periods the particle count will generally be much lower than 100. Some manufacturers use a Class 10,000 clean room for the assembly and packaging of devices that will be terminally sterilized and where a low particulate count on the devices is desired. The specifications for such a room could be as follows:

Particulates: Maximum of 10,000 of 0.5 µm diameter or larger per cubic foot
Humidity: 45 ± 5%
Temperature: 72 ± 2.5° F
Air velocity: 90 ft/min ± 2%
Air pressure: 0.05 in. water between the cleanroom and other areas

For assembly of many types of convenience kits and assembly of medical devices that need to be free of visible particles, many manufacturers use an "industrially clean area or controlled environment area." Such rooms are air conditioned and use furnace filters; in some cases, prefilters (much better than furnace filters) are also used. The temperature is controlled by a normal room thermostat. Humidity variations are limited by the normal air conditioning (cool-ling below the dewpoint and reheat are not necessarily used). Air velocity is as established for the air conditioning; and the room is known to have positive pressure with respect to other areas by a flow or pressure indicator. A particle class is not specified; however, these manufacturers have established a controlled environment, and appropriate specifications for temperature, cleaning, and people control must be met. For example, filters must be replaced per schedule or as needed based on scheduled inspections. Any practices or factors from the following list that the manufacturer has deemed appropriate and elected to use must be specified and routinely performed or followed. Some additional factors that must be considered when planning and using a controlled environment include:

Proper attire and dressing anteroom
Controlled use of and entry into controlled areas
Prohibiting eating, drinking, smoking, or gum chewing
Preventing use of lead pencils
Regulating the storage of glassware and containers
Preventing or controlling the cutting, tearing, or storage of cardboard, debris, etc.
Cleaning the room and production equipment per written procedure
The original design and cleaning of work surfaces and chairs
Selecting correct furniture and eliminating use of extra furniture
Controlling room air quality, pressure, velocity, and exchange rate
Eliminating electrostatic charges by controlling work surface composition or grounding
Ensuring cleanliness of raw materials, components, and tools
Controlling the purity, sterility, and nonpyrogenicity of process water
Maintaining prefilters, HEPA filters, and electrostatic precipitators

Monitoring

An appropriate system for regular monitoring must be established and maintained for each of these factors to be controlled for a given operation. This will ensure that equipment is performing properly and that the quality of the environment is within specifications. When a particle count class is specified, monitoring of airborne particulates is usually done with an air sampler. Monitoring of work surfaces for microbes CFWs (colony-forming units) may be done with surface-contact plates or setting plates. However, settling plates should not be used for monitoring when horizontal laminar air flow is used. All sampling should be done per written procedure and the data recorded. Further, periodic inspections of environmental controls and documentation of the inspections are required by the

GMP regulation. The inspection checkoff form or other record should be kept simple. Appropriate action limits for particle counts and CFUs should be established. Action limits for surface CFUs should take into account that large counts from handprints occasionally will be encountered unless gloves are worn.

C. Cleaning and Sanitation

The GMP regulation requires, in 820.56, that every manufacturer have adequate cleaning procedures and schedules to meet manufacturing process specifications and prevent contamination. These process specifications are established by the manufacturer to ensure that finished devices will meet the company's quality claims. If necessary for the drug delivery device to meet company product specifications or labeling claims, cleaning procedures and schedules to meet the requirements of section 820.56 must be written. Each operation should be analyzed in order to write an appropriate procedure or determine that one is not needed. For example, written procedures are usually not required for cleaning floors and workbenches in areas where nonsterile and non-growth-promoting components or devices are processed and packaged.

The record of cleaning may be a checkmark, initial, or signature. Where a checkmark is used for repetitive work, companies commonly require that the person's name be on the record at least once. The schedule for cleaning may be posted or filed, as long as it is in a convenient location. As appropriate, manufacturers may use this procedure as is, modify it, or use it as a guide to develop a procedure to meet specific needs.

Personnel Sanitation Practices

Adequate bathroom, dressing, storage, and waste facilities must be provided, as appropriate, for personnel to maintain cleanliness. Such facilities must be maintained on a regularly scheduled basis. Where necessary, such as in a cleanroom, special clothing and an area in which to don and store the garments must be provided. Cleanroom clothing must *not* be worn into uncontrolled rooms or outside the facility.

Preventing Contamination by Hazardous Substances

If rodenticides, insecticides, or other hazardous substances are used, written procedures to limit their use or for their removal from work surfaces and devices must be established to prevent any adverse affect on the manufacturing porcess or the device.

Personnel Practices

If eating, drinking, or smoking could have an adverse effect on the
devices' fitness for use, manufacturing procedures must include instructions on how to avoid such adverse effects. For example, these
activities could be confined to specially designated areas. Directions
and containers or equipment must be provided for timely and safe
disposal of trash, by-products, effluents, and other refuse.

IV. EQUIPMENT AND CALIBRATION

A. Maintenance

The Good Manufacturing Practices regulation requires that all equipment used to manufacture a drug delivery be designed and installed
so that it can be adequately cleaned, serviced, and adjusted as
necessary to maintain the equipment's accuracy, performance, and
reliability (820.60). The degree of maintenance of all equipment and
frequency of calibration of measuring equipment will depend on the
type of equipment, frequency of use, and importance in the manufacturing process. The GMP regulation also implies that manufacturing materials such as mold-release compounds, cleaning agents, lubricating oils, and other substances used to facilitate manufacturing, be
procured and received as components. If any of these materials has
an adverse effect on the finished device, then it must be removed to
a safe level.

Device manufacturers must maintain, clean, and adjust equipment
used in the manufacture of medical devices where failure to do so
could have an adverse effect on the equipment's operation and hence
the device. For example, failure to maintain, clean, and adjust a
sealing and/or packaging machine used for primary packaging of
sterile devices will eventually result in defective packages and thus
nonsterile products.

A manufacturer must determine if the equipment requires maintenance and apply the appropriate parts of the GMP requirements
for equipment. The user usually can determine if specific equipment
requires maintenance by reviewing the equipment operations and
maintenance manuals usually supplied by the equipment manufacturer.
If failure to maintain equipment does not appear to adversely affect
the device, the FDA will not insist that the manufacturer meet the
maintenance requirement. Typically, a manufacturer will maintain
equipment simply because it prolongs equipment life and minimizes
the need for major service. If it is *necessary* to maintain, clean,
or adjust equipment, the manufacturer must:

Have a written schedule for performing these activities.
Post the schedule or make it readily available.

Document the activities.

Where adjustment is necessary to maintain proper operation, post
the inherent limitations and allowable tolerances of the equipment or make these readily available to personnel responsible
for making the adjustments.

Audit the activities and document the audit.

As appropriate, maintenance records should be maintained for
each piece of equipment. Maintenance records and schedules are
not needed for equipment such as lathes, presses, grinders, etc.,
that are used in a machine shop and maintained on a daily basis by
skilled employees. Automated machining equipment will require maintenance schedules.

There is no device GMP requirement for a written maintenance
procedure, although one is recommended to assure that all aspects
of maintenance are covered. An example of an operation and maintenance procedure, "P.C. Board Cleaning," is shown in Exhibit 1 in
this section.

The purchase of stable and accurate measuring equipment can
reduce the frequency of calibration and increase confidence in the
company's metrology program. Where economically feasible, equipment with more accuracy than needed for various measurements can
be used longer without recalibration than equipment that marginally
meets the desired accuracy requirements. Delicate instruments, however, that are "pushing the state-of-the-art" should not be used for
routine measurements unless no other approach is feasible.

B. Manufacturing Materials

The proper or optimum operation of manufacturing equipment often
requires the use of manufacturing materials. The GMP regulation
defines "manufacturing material" as any material, such as a cleaning
agent, mold-release compound, lubricating oil, or other substance,
used to facilitate a manufacturing process that is not intended by the
manufacturer to be included in the finished device [820.3(a)]. Manufacturing materials are specified, procured, inspected/tested, etc.,
the same as components.

The use of manufacturing materials that may adversely affect the
finished device should be carefully analyzed. Each process should
be designed to use a minimum amount of adverse materials so as to
reduce costs, reduce removal efforts, and increase the intrinsic
safety of the device. The fact that a manufacturing material has
been removed or limited below the adverse level may be determined
by either of the two general approaches below.

1. The adverse material may be measured directly and compared
    to the process specification.

2. If feasible, the component, in-process device, or finished
    device may be tested against its specification. If the item
    passes, it follows that the residue is not affecting the per-
    formance. The test specification *must* be appropriate for this
    method of evaluating residues and may need to include tests
    for toxicity, pyrogens, etc.

Section 820.60(d) requires a written procedure for the use and
removal of manufacturing materials that can have an adverse effect
on devices. Usually, the procedure used for routine cleaning of
the device and its assemblies can be used for this purpose. If so,
a special procedure is not necessary; however, when residues from
such agents as ethylene oxide must be removed, special instructions
usually are necessary.

When manufacturing materials such as oils, mold-release compounds,
gases, cleaning agents, etc., are used on or in equipment, manufacturers must:

Remove the material or limit it to a safe amount.
Provide written procedures for the use and removal of materials.
Document the removal.

The sample procedure, "P.C. Board Cleaning," in Exhibit 1,
covers the removal of flux (not mentioned in the procedure), finger
oils, etc., from printed circuit boards. In most cases, flux is an
adverse manufacturing material.

C. Automated Production and QA Systems

The hardware system, software program, and general quality assurance system controls discussed below are essential in the automated
manufacture of drug delivery devices. The systematic validation of
software and associated equipment will assure compliance with the
GMP regulation; and reduce confusion, increase employee morale,
reduce costs, and improve quality. Further, proper validation will
smooth the integration of automated production and quality assurance
equipment into manufacturing operations.

Medical devices and the manufacturing processes used to produce
them vary from the simple to the very complex; thus, the GMP
regulation needs to be and is a flexible quality assurance system.
This flexibility is valuable as more device manufacturers move to
automated production, test/inspection, and record-keeping systems.

One of the basic requirements of the GMP regulation is that
formal processing procedures be established, implemented, and controlled as necessary to assure that device design specifications are
met (820.100). Thus, among many other quality assurance elements,

processing methods and equipment [820.20(a), 820.60] must be selected, and specific operating parameters established and evaluated, in order to establish valid and reliable manufacturing processes. The activities conducted to verify process and equipment specifications are collectively referred to as process validation.

In addition to this general requirement for all significant processes, the GMP regulation has specific requirements in sections 820.61 and 820.195 for validating and controlling automated equipment used in the manufacture of medical devices.

Software Validation Guidelines

The GMP regulation requires (820.61) that software programs be validated by adequate and documented testing when computers are used as part of an automated production or quality assurance system. Software used in automated production and quality assurance systems consists of programs or codes that cause computerized equipment to perform desired tasks, plus operator manuals and instructions. The FDA has published general guidelines, "Principles of Process Validation," that can be used with the GMP regulation to establish a software validation program. There are also standards, books, and articles that can be used for guidance. Military Specification MIL-S-52779A and the Institute of Electrical and Electronic Engineers (IEEE) "Standard for Software Quality Assurance Plan" (IEEE Std 730) are examples.

Manufacturers, however, should not rely completely on such documents, but must examine their software needs and develop whatever controls are necessary to assure that software is adequate for its intended use [820.20(a)(4)].

Employee Responsibility and Training

The drug delivery device manufacturer should identify individuals or departments responsible for software quality and clearly specify their responsibilities. These individuals and/or department personnel should have sufficient training, authority, responsibility, and freedom of action to specify and evaluate the design and use of software and associated equipment.

A manufacturer probably will experience problems if employees operating the automated system or inputting data do not have adequate background and/or training. Employees must have adequate knowledge of the system through both on-the-job experience and formal training. Those responsible for data input should be able to recognize data errors (820.25). The GMP regulation requires that adequate checks be designed and implemented to help prevent inaccurate data input [820.20(a)(4), 820.195]. This requirement can be accomplished by the aforementioned training and by software controls. Where practical, software programs should have built-in error conrols such as prompts, alpha-only fields, numeric-only fields, length limits, range limits, and sign (+ or −) control to help eliminate mistakes during data entry. These error-control or human-factors requirements, as appropriate, should be part of the specifications for software being development or purchased.

Formal Development of Software

Manufacturers that develop their own software should follow a prescribed quality assurance plan and document each step of the development. The software should be appropriately structured and documented so that any future changes can be accomplished, even by a *different* programmer, with a minimum of difficulty and maximum reliability.

To validate software, it must be:

Structured, documented, and *evaluated* as it is developed
Checked to make sure that it meets specifications
Adequately tested with the assigned hardware systems
Operated under varied conditions by the intended operators
    or persons of like training to assure that it will perform consistently and correctly

Each module or routine of the program should be evaluated to make sure it performs the specified function. The main core of the program should be checked to make certain that all parameters are correctly initialized and that data is correctly transferred between the routines. The input-output routines should be checked for proper operation with the intended peripherals to the extent feasible at this stage of the development. The testing is performed with real or simulated input data. The input data should accurately represent the real data that will occur in the next phase of testing and should also represent data at the boundaries of acceptability. The test protocol, data, and results should be documented. The documentation should be made available to the party who will evaluate the software with the automated production or quality assurance equipment to be used in routine manufacturing.

The testing of the software with the actual drug delivery device production or testing equipment should exercise all program functions under all expected production conditions. The testing should include the input of normal and abnormal data to test program performance and error handling. The validation must assure to a high degree that the software and associated equipment meet the company specifications. Testing and results should be documented. Any serious deficiencies must be corrected.

Commercial Software and Equipment

When an outside contractor is engaged to develop software, the device manufacturer must make sure that the contractor clearly understands the software requirements and translates them into documented specifications with sufficient objectivity that compliance can be measured. The FDA recognizes that most of the validation may be done by the contractor; however, the device manufacturer is still responsible for the adequacy and the validation of the software. Therefore, the contract should require the contractor to develop the software according to a quality assurance plan that includes validation.

When possible, the purchaser also should conduct pre-award audits to verify adequacy of the contractor's quality assurance program. Two key elements that should be checked are the contractor's test plans and system for controlling changes to documentation. Subsequent audits should be conducted as needed to verify that the contractor is complying with the quality assurance plan. The manufacturer who has custom software prepared and validated by a contractor must ensure the software program is running properly and producing correct results before using the program to produce medical devices for distribution.

Drug delivery device manufacturers who purchase commercial equipment with incorporated software must still validate the software and associated equipment for the intended applications. If, however, the software has been validated by the developer and proven through use, the purchaser need not test it as comprehensively as new software. For example, automated production and test equipment that is controlled by software can usually be validated through use of a "dummy" device. This "dummy" device should exercise all functions and decisions in normal and worst-case situations that may reasonably be expected during production. In some cases, vendors provide test programs that may be used to assure that the equipment will appropriately and accurately perform all intended functions before it is used for routine production.

Validation of Equipment and Processes

Automated machine tools such as lathes, printed-circuit drills, and component inserters usually can be validated by conducting a first- and last-piece inspection of representative product lots. The record of this activity may be noted on the routine quality control or production records for the machine. Validation of complex microprocessor-controlled equipment, such as sterilizers, to verify satisfactory operation is generally a more extensive activity than the validation of machine tools. Typically, verification must be done by using calibrated measurement instruments to check the actual parameters achieved during trial runs, and comparing these measurements with

the setpoints and data outputs of the automated system. In all
cases, under the GMP regulation the user is responsible for:

Assuring the adequacy of automated equipment and software
Verifying that all intended functions will be correctly and reliably
    performed
Maintaining appropriate records

Validation records (820.61) for software and automated equipment
must be maintained by the user and, upon request, made available
to FDA investigators for review and copying during their audit
(820.180) of the manufacturer's GMP system. Likewise, specifications
for the hardware and software including directions for their use, if
any, must be included or referenced in the device master record
(820.181).

The device master record [820.3(i)] is a compilation of records
containing the design, formulation, specifications, complete manufacturing procedures, quality assurance requirements, and labeling
for a finished device.

All changes to specifications, software programs, and other
master record documents must be formally reviewed and approved
before implementation [820.100(a) and (b)]. Because changes in
one part of software can affect other parts of software, adequate
consideration must be given to side effects of these changes. Such
changes are much easier to make and evaluate when the original software is appropriately structured and thoroughly documented.

Automated Data Collection and Processing

In addition to aiding the production of devices, computers may be
used to collect and maintain quality control and production records.
These records are called the device history record in the GMP regulation. A device history [820.3(h)] is a compilation of records containing the production history of a finished device. When device
history records or master records are maintained by computer, appropriate controls must be used to assure that data is entered accurately, changes are instituted only by authorized personnel, and
records are secure. Hard copy or alternative systems such as
duplicates, tapes, or microfilm should also be used to avoid losing
records as a result of inadvertent erasure or other catastrophe. As
appropriate, access to records and data bases should be restricted
to designated individuals.

The GMP regulation requires (820.181) that device master records
be signed by designated individuals, and that changes to master
records be signed by individuals designated to authorize such

changes. In addition, signatures are required when certain data [820.185(a)(2), 820.185(c)] are recorded in critical device history records. The GMP regulation also requires (820.101) that only designated employees operate equipment used to perform critical operations on critical devices, and that the history record contain [820.185(b)] the names of these individuals.

The GMP regulation was promulgated when most records were hard copy, for which written signatures were appropriate; however, the increased use of computers and related input/output peripherals has affected FDA policy regarding GMP signature requirements. In response to the use of new electronic technology, the FDA has issued an advisory opinion stating that magnetically coded badges or other computer-compatible identifiers may be used in lieu of signatures as long as there are adequate controls to prevent inaccurate data input. If coded badges and the like are not controlled (i.e., not restricted to designated employees), they will not meet the applicable GMP requirements.

Manufacturers may wish to keep appropriate records such as master records and complaint files at central or corporate offices. If the overall data handling system is controlled as stated above, firms may maintain appropriate GMP records at central locations if they can transmit these records to the manufacturing establishment by FAX, electronic mail (computer plus modem), or other high-speed data transfer system.

Equipment Controls and Audits

Automated equipment and any peripheral equipment requiring maintenance and/or calibration must be included in a formal calibration and maintenance program (820.60, 820.61). Also, environmental factors such as temperature, humidity, cleanliness, static electricity, magnetic fields, and power supply fluctuations can adversely affect automated equipment and data storage mechanisms such as magnetic disks and tapes. Consequently, necessary precautions, environmental controls, and maintenance programs (820.46, 820.60, and 820.61) must be implemented to prevent adverse effects on the equipment and stored data.

During their quality assurance system audit [820.20(b)], manufacturers should audit the use and control of their automated production and quality assurance systems. The audit should include software and equipment maintenance procedures and records, and should evaluate the adequacy of security measures, change controls, and other controls necessary to maintain software quality and proper performance of associated equipment. The audit must be documented, important results reviewed with management, and corrective action taken as appropriate.

D. Equipment Calibration

The GMP regulation is intended to help assure that devices will be
safe, effective and in compliance with the FD&C Act. To support
this goal, each drug delivery device manufacturer must develop and
implement a quality assurance (QA) program that assures with a
high degree of confidence that all finished devices meet the company's
device master record specifications. These specifications should, in
turn, reflect the company quality claims [see section 501(c) of the
FD&C Act]. Such assurance is obtained by many activities including
the measurement of component and device parameters. These measurements must be made with appropriate and calibrated equipment.
   Each drug delivery device manufacturer must assure that production equipment and quality assurance measurement equipment
(mechanical, electronic, automated, etc.) are

   Suitable for the intended use in manufacture and testing of in-
      process and finished devices
   Operated by trained employees
   Capable of producing valid results
   Properly calibrated versus a suitable standard

   To succeed, the QA system must include a calibration program that
is at least as stringent as that required by the GMP regulation
(820.61). The intent of the GMP calibration requirements is to assure adequate and continuous performance of measurement equipment
with respect to accuracy, precision, etc. The calibration program
implemented by a company can be as simple or as sophisticated as
required for the measurements to be made. Some instruments need
only be checked to see that their performance is within specified
limits, while others may require extensive calibration to a specification.
   In establishing a quality assurance system, manufacturers should
determine which measurements are necessary to assure that finished
devices meet approved master record specifications, and that the instruments used to make these measurements are included in a calibration program. When measurement equipment that is part of the
calibration system is located in the same areas as instruments that
are not part of the system, the system equipment should be identified by label, tag, color code, etc., to assure that it is the only
equipment used in determining compliance of a component, in-process
devices, or finished device with specifications.
   Equipment used only for monitoring a parameter need not be
calibrated but should be identified (e.g., for monitoring). A monitoring function might be to indicate if a voltage or other parameter
exists, but the exact value is not important.

As appropriate, environmental controls must be established and monitored to assure that measuring instruments and standards are calibrated and used in an environment that will not adversely effect the accuracy required. Consideration should be given to the effects of temperature, humidity, vibration, and cleanliness when purchasing, using, calibrating, and storing instruments.

The device GMP regulation requires, in section 820.61(a), that equipment be calibrated according to written procedures that include specific directions and limits for accuracy and precision.

Records

Calibration of each piece of equipment must be documented to include the calibration date, the calibrator, and the date the next calibration is due. Many manufacturers use a system where each device has a decal or tag that contains the data of calibration, by whom calibrated, and the date the next calibration is due. Standard decals are available as catalog items, or a firm may use its own artwork to purchase decals with specialized wording.

Calibration information is entered onto cards or forms, one for each piece of equipment, or entered into a computerized data system. Most cards or data systems include the calibration date, by whom calibrated, the date recalibration is due, the reason for the calibration, comments, address of the manufacturer and calibration laboratory, equipment specifications, serial number, use, etc.

Schedules

Measuring instruments should be calibrated at periodic intervals established on the basis of stability, purpose, and degree of usage of the equipment. Intervals should be shortened as required to assure prescribed accuracy as evidenced by the results of preceding calibrations. Intervals should be lengthened only when the results of previous calibrations indicate that such action will not adversely affect the accuracy of the system, i.e., the quality of the finished product.

A firm should use a suitable method to remind employees that recalibration is due. For small firms, calibration decals on the measuring equipment may be sufficient, because recalibration can be tracked by scanning the decals for the recalibration date. For other firms, a computerized system, calibration cycle cards, tickler file, or the like may be used. Calibration cycle cards are maintained in a 12-month (12-section) tickler file. There is one card per item of measuring equipment. The cards in the section of the file for the current month are pulled and all of the equipment listed is calibrated. For example, in a 6-month calibration cycle, when an instrument is calibrated in May, the card is moved from the May section to the October section of the file. When the file is checked in October,

```
| CALIBRATION CYCLE CARD                                           |
|                                                                 |
|    MANUFACTURER: _____        |
|                                                                 |
|  INSTRUMENT: _____        |
|                                                                 |
|  _____          |
|                                                                 |
|  MODEL NO. _____  SERIAL NO. _____         |
|                                                                 |
|  CALIBRATION INTERVAL: _____         |
|                                                                 |
|  LOCATION OF EQUIPMENT: _____         |
|                                                                 |
|  _____          |
|                                                                 |
|  CALIBRATION CARD NO. _____        |
|                                                                 |
|  Form No. _____          |
```

Fig. 1 Calibration cycle card.

the cycle card will be there to remind the firm that calibration is due. The process is repeated until an event such as instrument wear-out occurs and the respective cycle card is removed from the file.

Cycle cards are used when a firm has many instruments to be calibrated. It would be rather difficult to keep track of the calibration of a large number of instruments by reviewing calibration record cards or scanning the decal on each instrument. It is easier to use a cycle card file. A cycle card file or equivalent also must be used if the calibration records are filed by type of instrument or manufacturer rather than due date. A typical cycle card is shown in Fig. 1. The "calibration card number" blank refers to the calibration record card for the same item of equipment.

Standards

Where practical, the GMP regulation requires that standards used to calibrate equipment be traceable to the National Bureau of Standards (NBS) of other recognized standards. Traceability also can be achieved through a contract calibration laboratory that in turn uses NBS services.

The meaning of traceability to NBS is not always self-evident. Two general methods commonly used to establish and maintain traceability to NBS are as follows:

NBS calibration of standards or instruments: When this method is used, private standards are physically sent to NBS for calibration and return.

Standard Reference Materials (SRMs): NBS provides reference materials to be used in a user's calibration program. These SRMs are widely used in the chemical, biological, medical, and environmental fields.

Information can be obtained from the *Catalog of NBS Standard Reference Materials*, NBS Publication 260, 1984-1985 Edition, available free from the National Bureau of Standards, Office of Standard Reference Materials, Chemistry Building, Room B311, Washington, D.C. 20234.

The GMP regulation states: "If national standards are not practical for the parameter being measured, an independent standard shall be used. If no applicable standard exists, an in-house standard shall be developed and used." In-house standards should be fully described in the device master record. Independent or in-house standards must be given appropriate care and maintenance and must be used according to a written procedure as is required for other calibration activities.

E. Audit of Calibration System

The calibration program must be included in the quality assurance system audits required by the GMP regualtion. These audits should determine the continuing adequacy of the calibration program and assess compliance with the program.

Many manufacturers utilize contract calibration laboratories to calibrate their measurement and test equipment. If this is the case, the FDA views the contract laboratory as an extension of the manufacturer's GMP program or quality assurance program. Normally, the FDA does not inspect contract laboratory facilities, but the agency would expect the manufacturer to audit the contract lab, if feasible, to verify that proper procedures are being used. If problems occurred due to inadequate calibration and the FDA needed to determine where the problems existed, the FDA could visit the contract laboratory. Either the contract laboratory or the manufacturer might be held responsible for inadequate procedures leading to a defective, unsafe device or false data. Generally, the manufacturer of the finished device is responsible for assuring that the device is manufactured under an acceptable GMP program.

When a drug delivery device manufacturer utilizes a contract calibration laboratory, the FDA expects the manufacturer to have evidence that the equipment was calibrated according to the GMP requirements. The manufacturer can do this by:

Requiring and receiving certification that the equipment was
   calibrated under controlled conditions using traceable standards
Maintaining an adequate calibration schedule
Maintaining records of calibration
Periodically auditing the contractor to assure that appropriate and
   adequate GMP procedures are being followed.

Certification notes and data should include accuracy of equipment
when received by the lab to facilitate remedial action by the finished
device manufacturer, if necessary. Certification should also include
accuracy after calibration, standards used, and environmental conditions under which the equipment was calibrated. The certification
should be signed and dated by a responsible employee of the contract
lab.
   The contractor should have in place the applicable controls called
for in the GMP regulation. For example, the contractor should
have:

Written calibration procedures
Records of calibration
Trained calibration personnel
Standards traceable to NBS, or other independent reproducible
   standards

If in-house standards are used by a contractor to calibrate device-related measuring equipment, these standards must be documented, used, and maintained the same as other standards.

F.   Integrating Measurements into the QA System

Proper and controlled equipment calibration can contribute to overall
quality by assuring that unacceptable items are not accepted and
that acceptable items are not rejected. If the appropriate product-
quality parameters are not checked, however, calibrated equipment
will have little impact on assuring quality.
   A good quality assurance program must include calibration activities. However, proper calibration will be of little use unless the
applications of the measurement equipment are properly developed
and qualified during the preproduction development of inspection
test methods and procedures. As stated, effectiveness depends on
the participation and influence of QA at the preproduction stage.
Calibration of equipment cannot correct poor design of products, nor
can it compensate for poor applications of equipment and techniques.
It is the continued use of a complete, integrated quality assurance
system that assures that safe and effective devices are produced.
   Examples of calibration cards, decals, and cycle cards have been
presented. An example of a cleaning procedure for a printed circuit
board washer is given in Exhibit 1. The procedure covers operation,

Exhibit 1 Printed Circuit Board Cleaning

TITLE: **P.C. Board Cleaning**   NO:___ REV:___ Sheet: 1 of 2

DRAFT: _____ APP: _____ DATE: ____

1.0 **PURPOSE:** The purpose of this procedure is to document production operations performed on the XXXXXX printed circuit board washer.

2.0 **SCOPE:** This procedure sequentially identifies all operations necessary to properly operate and maintain this equipment.

3.0 **OPERATING PROCEDURES:**

3.0.1 Switch the Exhaust Systems fan on.

3.0.2 Assure that the sump pump is on at the circuit breaker panel.

3.1 Turn the power switch to the "ON" position.

3.2 Push the main power "START" button (#21 on Control Panel Diagram).

3.3 Visually inspect all pump compartment and screen filters for debris - make sure they are clean before continuing.

3.4 Push the fill buttons on the rear control panel to fill the wash and rinse sections with water. Make sure all drain lines are closed. The incoming water will stop automatically when the tanks are filled to the correct levels.

3.4.1 Add 4 gallons XXXXXX detergent to the wash tank.

3.5 Depress the center knob on the temperature controllers (#30 on control panel diagram) and turn clockwise until the red pointer indicates 60 C (140° F) for the wash tank and 60 C (140° F) for the rinse tank.

3.6 Wait about 10 min. for water temperature to rise in the wash and rinse tanks. Wait until the red lights on the temperature controllers go off and the black needle aligns with the red pointer.

3.7 Push the START-STOP button (#25 on diagram) on for the conveyer.

3.7.1 Adjust the "SPEED CONTROL" (#27 on diagram) to the correct setting for the boards to be run. See the cleaning specifications for each family of boards for the setpoints.

3.8 Push the "START" button (#28 on diagram) on for the Dryer cycle. NOTE: conveyer belt **MUST** be moving when dryer section is on or the equipment will be damaged.

3.9 Turn Photocell Switch (on Rear Panel) to the "Automatic" position.

4.0 **SHUT DOWN PROCEDURES:**

4.1 Push the dryer cycle "STOP" button for the Wash and Rinse sections (#29 on control panel).

4.2 Turn Photocell Switch (on Rear Panel) to the "OFF" position.

4.3 Push the conveyer "START - STOP" button (#25 on diagram) to stop the conveyer.)

4.4 Pull the DRAIN buttons on the control panel for the wash and rinse sections. Using litmus paper, take a reading on the wash tank before draining it. IF the wash water has a reading of "10" or less drain it; otherwise, do not drain the wash tank. Always drain the rinse tank.

Exhibit 1 (Continued).

4.5 Pull the FILL buttons on the control panel for the wash and rinse sections to let water flush the equipment for 5 minutes. Using a soft cloth, wipe off any residue remaining on the equipment.

4.6 Pull the drain buttons on the control panel for the wash and rinse sections to let the water drain.

4.7 Remove the screen filter in the washer and remove any debris.

4.8 Wipe the exterior front section of the machine with a soft cloth.

4.9 Push the main power "STOP" button. (#33) to shut off the equipment.

5.0 **MAINTENANCE:**

5.1 Monthly

    5.1.1 Lubricate the conveyer drive chain with high temperature grease.

    5.1.2 Check the wear strips on the conveyer belt frame and replace if required. These are 2 white plastic strips located at the front of the equipment.

    5.1.3 Check conveyer belt tightness - using a wire cutter and needle nose pliers, remove links to tighten if required.

5.2 Quarterly

    5.2.1 Shut off power in main panel at rear of equipment.

    5.2.2 Lubricate pump motor ball bearing using standard bearing grease.

    5.2.3 Lubricate flange bearings on conveyer shafts with bearing grease.

    5.2.4 Check all wiring for loose connections and tighten if necessary.

    5.2.5 Check all heater contacts - replace worn contacts.

---

shut-down, cleaning, and routine maintenance. Drug delivery device manufacturers may use this procedure as presented if it matches their operations, or they may modify it to meet specific requirements.

V. MASTER RECORDS

A. Master Record Requirements and Guidelines

A device master record (DMR) is a term used in the device Good Manufacturing Practices regulation for all of the routine documentation required to manufacture devices that will consistently meet company requirements. Section 820.3(i) of the GMP regulation defines "device master record" as a compilation of records containing the design, formulation, specifications, complete manufacturing procedures, quality assurance requirements, and labeling of a finished device. The detailed requirements for master records are contained in sections 820.100, 820.181, 820.182, etc.; however, almost all sections of the

GMP regulation have requirements related to the DMR. The DMR must contain specifications for, or a full description of, the drug delivery device, and a full description of how to manufacture the drug delivery device including facilities, environment, and production equipment. In addition to the drug delivery device specifications, a DMR contains documents that cover typical manufacturing activities such as:

Procurement
Assembly
Labeling
Test and inspection
Packaging

Note that the listed activities and records or documents are required to produce any product—medical, industrial, or consumer. There is *nothing special* about device master records except the name! Also, note that in common usage, the term "device master record" is used for the total record or any of its individual records. Therefore, the term is singular for the total record, singular for a single document, and plural for a group of single documents. The term also may refer to an original record or copy of a record.

Master records must be technically correct, contain and/or reflect the approved device and process designs, be change-controlled, contain the release or other control date, contain an approval signature, and be directed toward the intended user. These requirements are in the device GMP regulation because the DMR is the "beginning and end" of a product—errors in the DMR will have a serious impact on the state-of-control of the manufacturing operation and may have a serious impact on the safety and performance of the device. The DMR must be accurate and complete, because the essence of the GMP regulation is a quality assurance program based on producing a finished device that meets the device master record requirements. In turn, the device master record must accurately reflect the drug delivery device intended to be produced by a firm.

Document for Intended Employees

The content, style, language, graphics, etc., of master records must be directed toward the needs of the intended employees and, if the record is for labeling, it must be directed toward users. A failure to consider the intended user leads to confusion and means that the company has not achieved the state-of-control intended by the GMP regulation. Therefore, applicable records must be directed toward the needs of procurement, processing, and test/inspection personnel, rather than the needs of drafting, technical services, or product development departments. Likewise, installation instructions

must be directed to installers. Labeling is often prepared by the
same employees who draft master records, and these employees should
also be aware that labeling must meet the needs of the user as directed in the labeling regulation, 21 CFR 801.6.

In any manufacturing activity such as assembly, labeling, processing, testing, etc., achieving and maintaining a state-of-control is
enhanced by appropriate personnel knowing:

> What task is to be done
> How to do the task
> Who is to do the task
> What task is being done
> What task was done and/or the results of the activity

In order for employees to perform a job correctly, they must know
exactly what is to be done and exactly how to do the work. Device
GMP sections 820.181 and 820.182 require that what is to be done be
documented in the device master record. The DMR also contains test
and inspection procedures and data forms that are used to help determine and record what was done.

Documents that instruct people how to fabricate, assemble, mix,
label, test, inspect, etc., or how to operate equipment should:

> Be directed toward the needs of the employees who will be using
>   them and not directed toward the draftsperson or researcher
> Match the tools and equipment to be used
> Be correct, complete, and current
> Depend on part numbers and basic drawings to transfer informa-
>   tion rather than almost photographic-quality drawings. If a
>   component is changed, the pictorial representations on the
>   drawings will no longer be correct and may be very confusing
>   to employees, particularly new employees.

The how-to-manufacture instructions must be adequate for use
by the intended employees and correct for the intended operation.
In the medium-to-large company, the instructions tend to be extensive technical (engineering) drawings and written procedures. In
any company, particularly small firms, the work instructions may
take several forms as discussed below.

> Engineering drawings may be used if employees are *trained* to
>   read and use them. Some of the how-to information comes
>   from employee training rather than from drawings.
> Assembly drawings may contain parts list and quality control
>   criteria. A separate quality control test and/or inspection
>   procedure is not always necessary. Some firms use large
>   sheets for assembly drawings and include the parts list on it.

The combination drawing results in instant availability of the
parts list and reduces the number of drawings to be controlled.
Exploded-view drawings are used when employees cannot read
   plan-view engineering drawings. Exploded-view drawings
   tend to be more "how to" than plan-view drawings. Exploded-
   view drawings are expensive to draft—in some cases it may
   cost less to teach employees how to read and use ordinary
   plan-view drawings.
Step-by-step written procedures may be used to detail how to
   perform specific tasks, with checkoff blanks to show that
   each specific task was performed. This type of procedure is
   commonly used for critical operations and where there is little
   or no visual indication of what has been done, such as for
   mixing chemicals.

Documentation may be supported by production aids such as
labeled photographs, videotapes, slide shows, assemblies, or sample
finished devices. All of these perform master-record functions and
must be current, correct, and approved for the intended operation.
   The most commonly used aids are models or samples. There are
two conditions that should be satisfied in order to use these aids.
First, a written specification for the sample must be contained in
the device master record. This specification, of course, may be the
same as the specification for the assembly or finished device to be
manufactured. This specification must be subject to a formal change-
control procedure. Even though a model is available, the specification is needed for present and future product development, and for
production control purposes. Second, the sample must:

Adequately reflect the device master record specification
Be identified as an approved acceptable sample, which means it
   should meet the company required workmanship standards
When appropriate, contain a drawing number, revision level, and
   control number (lot, serial, batch)

A card or tag may be used to identify and help control the use
of samples of assemblies or finished devices. Such tags are usually
covered by a clear plastic pouch and attached to the model or
sample.
   Samples and other aids such as photographs are subject to normal
wear and tear in a production environment. Therefore, such aids
should be adequately protected by a suitable means such as being
located in a protected area or covered by a protective pouch or
container. Production aids must be periodically audited to make sure
they continue to be suitable for the intended use (see sections
820.20, 820.100, and 820.181).

Adequate Information

Although a firm tries to document for the intended employees, there is a need to audit periodically to see how well the goal is being met. There are various means of determining if information in the device master record, production tools, and other production elements are adequate for a given operation and associated employees. These include analyzing the amount of:

> Assistance required by new employees
> Assistance required when a new device is manufactured
> Confusion and hesitation
> Exchanging of information among employees
> Drafting of "homemade" documentation by the line employee
> Re-work
> Products produced (productivity)
> Complaints from departments that subsequently process the device
> Device failures and customer complaints

If any of these factors persist and if they are out of line with industry norms or with the production of old designs, then the firm should take corrective action. The corrective action may include changes in supervision, documentation, adding new documentation, modifying the design, using different tools, modifying the environment, etc. Corrective action, other than necessary "fire fighting" to prevent shipment of defective devices, should not be taken, however, until the real problem is identified.

Preparation and Signatures

A separate device master record is required for each type or family of drug delivery devices. Also, a separate device master record is required for accessories to devices when these are distributed separately for health care purposes. Such accessories are considered to be finished devices. In practice, if the device and accessories are made by the same firm, the master record for the accessory may be incorporated into the master record for the primary device.

Section 820.181 of the GMP regulation requires that an individual(s) be designated to: prepare, date, and approve the DMR; and authorize changes. An individual(s) with the necessary technical training and experience must be designated to prepare and control master records. In addition to requiring approval signatures on device master records, the GMP regulation requires individual identification for a few other activities. For convenience, these activities along with the section numbers that require them are listed in Table 2.

The list is self-explanatory except for audit certification. When a firm certifies in writing to the FDA that GMP system audits have

Table 2 GMP Activities Requiring Individual Identification

820.20(b)	Audit certification
820.181	Device master record
820.181	Changes in master record
820.121	Proofreading critical device labeling
820.161	Release of finished critical devices
820.185(a)	Acceptance record for critical components
820.185(c)	Inspect/test records for critical devices

been performed, the certification letter is signed by a company official according to standard commercial practice.

If a record that requires a signature is maintained on a computer, it is best if the designated individual(s) maintains an up to date signed printout of the record. Where it is impracticable to maintain current printouts, computer-compatible identifiers may be used in lieu of signatures as long as there are adequate controls to prevent improper use, lack of employee identification, inaccurate data input, or other inappropriate activity. If identifiers such as coded badges and equipment keys are not controlled (i.e., not restricted to designated employees), then these identifiers will not meed applicable GMP requirements.

Location of Records

Device master records must be stored at the manufacturing establishment or at other locations (820.181) that are reasonably accessible to company employees responsible for the manufacturing activities and accessible to FDA investigators. Appropriate records may be maintained in computer data banks if the records are protected, change-controlled, and readily accessible for use by responsible employees at all relevant facilities. It is acceptable for a manufacturer to maintain records on microfilm and discard the original hard copies. Microfiche and/or microfilm reductions may be used in lieu of original record retention if the following conditions are met:

All reductions must be readily available for review and copying by FDA investigators and designated company personnel at any reasonable time.

All necessary equipment must be provided for viewing and copying the records.

Reproductions must be true and accurate copies of the original
record.

If the reproduction process results in a copy that does not reveal
changes or additions to the original record, the original must be
retained. In this situation, the reproduced copy and any image
shown on a viewing screen must note any alteration from the original
and indicate that the original record is available.

By maintaining master, complaint, and other records required by
the GMP regulation at the manufacturing establishment or other
reasonably accessible location, responsible officials of a company can
exercise control and accountability over the entire manufacturing
process and, thereby, maximize the probability that the finished
device conforms to its design specifications. This GMP requirement
helps assure that responsible officials at the manufacturing establishment have ready access to those documents essential for producing
devices and for conducting self-inspections, complaint investigations,
failure analyses, and audits. The device master record must be a
single source document or file, as stated in the preamble to the GMP
regulation. Portions of this file may be kept in various locations.
A device master record may exist as:

One or more files or volumes of the actual records containing
    the information required by the GMP regulation
A reference list of such documents and their location
Any combination of actual documents or reference lists

These documents must contain the latest revisions, be signed,
and be dated to show they have been checked for accuracy for
use.

The device GMP regulation allows use of reference lists as a means
to reduce the duplication of records, particularly duplication of general documents such as standard operating procedures. The use of
a reference list also allows filing of master record documents at several convenient locations. If the master record contains a list of
documents, the actual documents must be available for employee use
and FDA inspection at the manufacturing site or other reasonably
accessible locations. As noted above, this is a key and important
GMP requirement. Typical locations of various master records are
shown in Table 3.

Although the GMP regulation allows use of reference lists, FDA
investigators performing an inspection of a company must have access
to actual records for review and copying during reasonable business
hours. FDA investigators review these records to determine if a
firm is complying with the GMP regulation and with the Food, Drug
and Cosmetic Act. Records deemed confidential by a manufacturer
should be marked confidential to aid the FDA in determining whether

Table 3 Location of Device Master Records

| Type of DMR element | Typical locations of documents[a] | |
	Originals	Working copies
Reference list(s)	Engr. master file	
Component drawings	Engr. or Manuf. Engr. master file	Manuf. or Procurement
Component acceptance procedures	SOP master file	Receiving department
Device specifications	Engr. master file Engineering	Marketing or
Manufacturing procedures	Engr. or Manuf. Engr. master file	Manufacturing
Test specifications	Engr. master file	Engr. or Manuf. Engr.
Test procedures	Engr. or Manuf. Engr. master file	Manuf., QA, or QC
General inspection procedures	Manuf., QC, or SOP master file	Manufacturing or QC
Label drawings	Engr. master file	Engr., QA or Manuf.
Label artwork	Artwork master file	Engr., Procurement
Label control procedures	Manuf., QC, or SOP master file	Manufacturing
Cleaning procedures	SOP master file	
System audit procedures	SOP or QA master file	Quality Assurance

[a]SOP = standard operating procedure; QA = Quality Assurance; QC = Quality Control.

or not specific information may be disclosed under the Freedom of Information Act.

Record Retention

The GMP regulation, in section 820.180(b), requires that all records pertaining to a device shall be retained for a period of time equivalent to the design and expected life of the device, but in no case

less than two years from the data of release for commercial distribution by the manufacturer. For devices with very short lives, such
as radioimmunoassay (RIA) products, manufacturers may obtain a
variance from the FDA to reduce the two-year requirement to one
year. In some cases where maintaining records for the life of the
device may be overly burdensome or impractical, manufacturers may
decide the appropriate time to retain records beyond the two-year
minimum. Thus, manufacturers of long-life products should make
prudent decisions as to how long to keep records beyond two years.
For example, there is no value in keeping records for long-life devices such as stretchers, surgical tools, containers, etc., beyond
two years, as the probability is low that any postdistribution remedial
activity will occur. For devices that must be repaired or capital
equipment devices that probably will be updated, records must be
retained, as appropriate, to support these repairs or modifications.
Master record requirements apply to devices modified in the field by
the manufacturer's representatives after the devices are commercially
distributed. Modification of a device is manufacturing, and the GMP
regulation covers all manufacturing of devices where the result is
placed into commercial distribution. In any case, a manufacturer
must be prepared to provide a rationale for its decision to discontinue
recordkeeping. For example, the decision could be based on the
length of time beyond two years that records have been maintained
and on the fact that there has been no adverse feedback from customers during that period on the device's "fitness for use."

B. DMR Contents

As discussed above, the DMR shows and/or tells employees how to
perform specific and general functions related to the production of
a device. The GMP regulation does not dictate how this information
is to be arranged or filed except that it must be readily accessible.
In most firms, this information is contained in records that are
specific for the device being produced and in general records that
are applicable to all devices being produced. Because a drug delivery DMR may contain many documents, an index is usually needed.

DMR Index

A master record for a complex drug delivery device or a device manufactured by complex processes may contain many documents. For
convenience, many firms generate an index, which lists all of the
documents in a master record. An index, of course, is an overall
reference list. It may eliminate the need for other lists, incorporate
other lists, or refer to other lists. An index may be arranged according to the standard flow of manufacturing operations, by major
subassemblies in the device, or by specific operational area in a

factory. Using an index, employees can find related drawings and information even if they only know the correct name of the device. An index is a valuable communication tool, which increases the state-of-control of a firm and reduces costs by reducing the effort, time, and frustration required to locate a document or related documents. Thus, an index helps manufacturers meet the GMP accessibility requirement for records.

General Documents

General documents are used for many activities that are essential to operating a manufacturing establishment—these are *not* specific to any given product, even if the company produces only one product. Thus, the DMR includes general documents such as standard operating procedures (SOPs) and standard quality assurance procedures (QAPs). If the company adds another product line, the basic content of these documents would undergo none or only minor changes.

In a typical manufacturing operation, general SOP and QAP documents include the following:

Cleaning procedures	Product development protocol
Insecticide use-removal procedures	Component inspection procedures
	Workmanship standards
Air conditioning/heating procedures	Design review policy/procedure
	Label review policy/procedure
Tool kit policy	Sterile water system maintenance
Safety procedures	Calibration policy
Procurement procedures	Complaint procedure
Returned goods policies	Recall procedure
Drawing numbering system	Materials review policy/procedure
Change control procedure	
Service policy	

This list is not all-inclusive. Medium-to-large companies tend to have many of these general documents to guide management in maintaining consistent operations. A very small company would have only the most essential and appropriate of these documents, such as procedures for numbering drawings, change control, and use of hazardous materials.

The original master copy of each general procedure is filed in the department specified by management as having responsibility for maintaining each of them. The working copies of the above procedures are usually located in SOP manuals and QA manuals. The procedures are usually numbered and arranged in a logical order by topic. The device GMP regulation does not require firms to have SOP or QA manuals; however, the experience of many industries has demonstrated that such manuals are worthwhile if they are kept current, contain real working procedures, and do not contain useless puffery.

Specific Documents

Specific documents are drawings, prcedures, labels, data forms, etc., for a specific product or family of products. The originals of specific documents are usually located in files in engineering or technical service departments. In most firms, specific documents contain no general information; however, they often refer to general documents. The number of specific documents for a given product line may range from about 10 to several hundred. If large numbers of documents are needed, an index is usually needed to help locate them.

Device Specification

A device or product specification is a specific document in the device master record that briefly describes and gives all important details of the external characteristics of a drug delivery device. The specifications may also contain some internal characteristics of the drug delivery device that are important to the manufacturer and/or the users. For drug delivery devices, some of the external characteristics such as temperature tolerance are related to the environment in which the devices will function properly.

Generally a product specification will contain the drug delivery device's:

    Product trade and common name(s)
    Intended use(s)
    Performance characteristics and theory of operation
    Regulatory classification
    Physical characteristics
    Environmental limitations and product stability
    Important components and formula (if applicable)
    Manufacturing cautions
    User safety characteristics

Manufacturers should have specifications for all drug delivery devices being manufactured to help assure that manufacturing specifications are adequate to produce devices that conform to the approved design of the device. A preliminary drug delivery device specification should be written at the *beginning* of a project and updated as the device is developed or modified. Specifications are usually developed by the marketing and product development departments, with review and consultation by quality assurance, manufacturing, and other departments. The contents of the final specification must agree with the other elements of the device master record and with actual drug delivery devices when they are manufactured. Before the start of full-scale production and commercial distribution, the device specification must be dated, approved, and placed under change control.

In addition to defining and describing a drug delivery device, a specification is a communication tool that, if used in a timely manner, can help achieve some important results. First, it helps assure that everyone is talking about the same device and working toward the same objectives with respect to safety, effectiveness, human factors, configuration, etc. Also, it is used as a guideline for developing test and inspection procedures for the finished device.

Ultimately, the device specification or a condensed version of it should be used in catalogs, or other product documentation to aid communications between salespersons and customers.

The use of device specifications will result in:

Improved communications between employees on a departmental and interdepartmental basis
Less confusion and increased morale
An improved state-of-control
A higher probability of meeting cost, time, safety, effectiveness, and regulatory compliance objectives

Also, if the marketing department uses the specifications when preparing advertisements and catalog sheets, public relations with users will be enhanced because the marketing documents are based on proven scientific safety and performance claims for the actual drug delivery device. That is, the user has an opportunity to read the technical specifications of the item actually being offered for sale.

C. Written Procedures

Many sections of the GMP regulation require written procedures for guidance in performing various QA and manufacturing tasks. Some devices, because of the nature of the manufacturing operations and processes, tend to have a relatively large number of written procedures.

Written procedures are used for product development, manufacturing, and postmarketing activities to:

Improve communications and guidance
Assure consistent and complete performance of assigned tasks
Promote management of operations

In large manufacturing facilities involving many operations and people of various skill levels, written procedures are usually necessary. In a small firm, communication lines are usually short, few people are involved, and management is readily available to provide guidance, so the need for written procedures is usually considerably less than for a larger firm.

A firm, particularly a small firm, may conclude that device GMP requirements for written procedures are not applicable for a particular operation. Such a decision, however, must be supported by management observations that sufficient control is present to meet the intent of the written procedure, for example, on the basis of the limited number of rejects, lack of complaints, complaints, etc. If rework, confusion, or complaints are excessive such that unsafe or ineffective drug delivery devices are likely to be or are being distributed, then written procedures and/or other corrective actions are needed.

Often training and work experience alone or combined with drawings, photographs, and models are valid substitutes for written procedures. For example, machinists are typically skilled personnel who fabricate components and finished devices using dimensioned drawings for guidance rather than written procedures. The company and FDA investigator must evaluate each situation and determine the need for written procedures based on the training and knowledge of the operators and the control needed to meet device specifications. Typically, a written procedure is not necessary when:

The activity is very simple.
The activity is relatively simple and models are used as aids.
Straightforward quantitative rather than qualitative standards
    determine acceptability.
The operation is performed by personnel highly skilled relative
    to the task being performed.

Written procedures and associated history of status records, however, are often needed for filling, mixing, or other activities where there is no change, such as color, texture, or form, to indicate that the activity has been performed. Such procedures and records are needed for critical manufacturing operations.

When the device GMP regulation requires a procedure, but does not specify a "written" procedure as in section 820.115, manufacturers must evaluate their existing controls to determine if these are adequate without written procedures. Some firms, however, have found that they must use written procedures even if not required by the GMP regulation in a specific area in order to comply with the overall GMP regulation. For example, some firms have found that they cannot comply with 820.115, Reprocessing of Devices, unless they use a written procedure because reprocessing is not frequently done for some types of products. Thus employees tend to forget how to perform the reprocessing. Firms should determine that they meet all GMP requirements and, if necessary, ex-

ceed them in order to produce finished devices that meet DMR
specifications, because the FDA insists that firms meet their quality
claims [FD&C Act, section 501(c), and GMP 820.100 and 820.160].
To achieve this, state-of-control may require *fewer* or *more* written
procedures than specifically required by the GMP regulation.   FDA
does not insist that a firm meet GMP requirements or generate
records that do not contribute to assuring conformance to specifications simply because they are part of the GMP regulation.   Also,
section 519(a)(1) of the FD&C Act prohibits record-keeping requirements that are unduly burdensome to a device manufacturer.

Developing Procedures

Developing written procedures is relatively labor-intensive and time-
consuming, which may lead to use of "back-of-the-envelope" notes
instead of formal procedures.   Likewise, changing written procedures
is time-consuming, which may lead to delays or forgetting to make
the changes.   Drafting or changing written procedures is also prone
to errors.   Therefore, manufacturers are encouraged to consider the
use of microcomputers and low-cost printers as word processors to
aid in writing and changing procedures.   With the use of microcomputers these tasks become easier, thereby increasing the probability
that they will be performed correctly and when needed.   Microcomputers can also be used for generating and maintaining master record
indices, complaint files, and performing a host of other GMP-related
activities.

There is a method for developing procedures that will result in
short, clear procedures that help solve real problems.   The steps
are as follows:

1. Identify the problem to be solved.
2. Decide if new or modified procedures are needed to help solve
    or reduce the problems.
3. Make certain that the contents cover who, what, when, where,
    how, etc.

Events that point to a problem are excessive re-work, employee
confusion, and customer complaints.   These "pointers," however,
may not be the real problem—the real problem may be inadequate
design, components, equipment, maintenance, operational techniques,
documentation, environment, etc.   The real problem *must* be identified before it can be solved—a written procedure may or may not
be needed to help solve it.

The real problem can be identified by careful analysis of:

The "pointers" noted above
Device design

Process design
Process flow and employee work habits (operational analysis)
Test and inspection data
Any other activity related to the quality of the device

Operational analysis is aided by flowcharting, which is a step-by-step chart of the minute details of the operation. Thus, a flowchart is much more detailed than a QA audit report and is very helpful in determining what is actually happening in a particular manufacturing operation. This knowledge may lead to a solution of manufacturing and quality problems.

From a personnel management viewpoint, the problem, the reason for flowcharting the given activity, etc., should be discussed with affected personnel. Their input should be requested with respect to identifying and solving the real problem. By using the information presented by the flowchart and the experience gained while producing the chart, the auditor is better able to:

Analyze the particular operation with respect to process requirements
Determine what needs to be added, modified, or deleted to solve any problems or improve performance
If needed, write or modify a procedure to cover the new way of performing the activity

Content of Procedures

Written procedures are widely used, and industry experience has shown that these should contain the following items:

Company identification and a procedure title
An identification or control number with a revision level code
An approval signature, and date the procedure becomes effective
The number of pages (e.g., sheet 1 of 4) in the procedure, or another means to indicate that the employee has the complete document
A body that describes the activities to be performed

The effective date may be the same as the approval date. Also, the effective date may appear on a separate document, such as an engineering change order (ECO) form. The main body of the procedure should cover, as appropriate:

Subject, scope, and objectives
Who is assigned to perform the task
What activity or task is to be performed
When and *where* the task is to be performed

How to perform the task, including what tools, materials, etc., to use

Particularly for the new employee, it is important for the procedure to state the reason for performing a function and the reason it must be performed in a certain way. Background information such as this helps the employee to understand an assignment and remember how to perform it. For example, when working on CMOS integrated circuits that are easily damaged by electrostatic potentials, unskilled employees need to understand why they have to be grounded, work on grounded mats, and, especially, why they are not allowed to wear certain clothing while at work. Likewise, employees working in environmentally controlled, clean manufacturing areas need to be told about invisible microbes and particulates, and that humans are the major source of these unwelcome contaminates. If so informed, employees are more likely to follow the operational procedures for working in controlled areas.

The task description in each procedure should cover appropriate details such as:

The expected and actual results from performing the tasks, such as what data to collect and how to analyze, file, and report it

What to do with the component, in-process device, or finished drug delivery device if such is involved

Any related activities that need to be performed in order for the overall operation to remain in a state-of-control or for the drug delivery device to meet all of the device master record specifications

If the procedure being developed, for example, covers change control, the procedure must also cover related activities such as changes to labeling. Consider a change to a device where an analog meter is replaced with a digital meter—obviously the instruction manual (labeling) and service manual also need to be modified. Otherwise the finished device may not meet company labeling policies, may be *misbranded* because it does not meet the labeling requirements of the FD&C Act, and may be *adulterated* because the change does not meet the change-control requirements of the GMP regulation.

After the procedure is drafted, if appropriate, it should be reviewed with the affected personnel before it is approved and implemented. During the initial implementation, the use of the procedure should be monitored. Then, based on actual experience in using the procedure, if necessary, it should be modified to more exactly meet the need of the operation or process.

D. Change Control

Change control applies to: components, including software; labeling
and packaging; devices; processes; production equipment; manufacturing materials; and all associated documentation such as standard
operating procedures, quality assurance procedures and data forms,
and product-specific documentation. These documents constitute the
device master record (DMR). The DMR is defined in 21 CFR 820.3(i)
as "a compilation of records containing the design, formulation,
specifications, complete manufacturing procedures, quality assurance
requirements, and labeling of a finished device." In addition to the
master record, the FDA allows manufacturers to use production aids
such as labeled photographs and models or samples of assemblies and
finished devices. Because these are used to support or in lieu of
more extensive master records, these production aids must also be
under change control.

A given design and associated manufacturing process for a drug
delivery device must be documented in the device master record. It
follows that changes in components, design, labeling, etc., of a
device, or changes to processes, equipment, etc., used to produce
a device for commercial distribution, must result in a changed device
master record. Therefore, most of the discussion herein is centered
around the master record.

Change Control Procedure

The device master record should be managed and controlled according to documented procedures. For the medium to large company,
a change control procedure is one of a family of standard operating
procedures used to produce, number, size, change, and control documentation.

The written change control procedure should describe the company-
approved procedures to be followed *from the time the master record
is first released* for production of a device, or a change is requested
for an in-process device or the associated manufacturing processes,
through examination of the change in relation to other appropriate
documents, activities, and implementation.

The company procedure should have an appropriate degree of
flexibility integrated into it. That is, all changes do not require the
same degree of evaluation and approval. The GMP rule is a flexible
regulation that allows firms to develop and use procedures that meet
their specific needs.

All changes *must* be made according to the approved company
policy and procedure. A trap that is easy to wander into is the
situation where a company, knowingly or unknowingly, allows research and development personnel or other appropriate personnel to
make changes to a drug delivery device that is already in production
or make changes to an ongoing process without following the approved

procedure. Such changes generally do not receive the necessary evaluation and review and, therefore, they may and *have* resulted in hazardous or ineffective devices. Making such uncontrolled changes is a violation of several sections of the GMP regulation, particularly sections 820.20, 820.100, and 820.181. Such a company is not operating in a state-of-control. It bears repeating: All changes *must* be made according to approved company policy and procedure.

A change control procedure may be long because of the large number of activities that must be covered, as discussed in detail later. This fact may also be seen by reviewing the example policy and procedure exhibited at the end of this section. All firms should analyze their operations and determine whether or not a written procedure for change control is needed. For example, if a very small firm has only a few manufacturing procedures, the person(s) designated to change and approve master records may use the following procedure.

1. Draw a black line through but do not black out the old information.
2. Ink in the new information.
3. Date and sign at the change or place a mark at the change that refers the user to the date and signature.
4. See that the modified documents are placed into use and the old documents are removed from production.
5. See that in-process and old finished devices are reprocessed or discarded.

The above procedure obviously depends on the devoted attention and knowledge of the designee. It is easy to see that for a larger firm, or for complex operations, the designee would not or could not "pass the word" to everyone who has a need to know. Hence, the need for written procedures. Small firms, with short communication lines, usually need a less extensive procedure than a large firm; however, the use of a change control form, as described below, by a small firms is highly recommended. As the firm grows, all procedures, particularly the change control procedure, should be analyzed and modified to meet current needs. Such a review should be part of the quality assurance systems audit.

A typical change control procedure for a device, manufacturing processes, equipment, and associated DMR should cover: identification of what is being changed; effective data; responsibility; revision levels; evaluation of the change and affected documentation; communication; updating documentation, document distribution and disposition; in-process control; finished-device remedial action; regulatory submissions; coherence of the DMR with device and processes; and business factors. These elements of a typical change control system are explained below.

Identification

The written procedure must cover the identification of the changed drug deliviery device, assembly, component, labeling, software, process or procedure, and other related details. The change control form should have blanks for recording this data and other data discussed below.

Effective Date

The procedure must cover the effective date of the change, which is usually a completion date, or action to be performed when a specific event occurs, such as "implement the change when the new mixer is installed and operational." The blank on the change control form for recording the effective date should not be left empty.

Responsibility

The change control procedure should state which department or designee is responsible for each function to be performed. One of these is the issuance, use, and control of blank and completed change control forms.

Revision Level

The way the revision level is to be incremented and which code should be used needs to be covered by the change procedure for components, including software, assemblies, and devices, and for associated documentation such as labeling, process procedures, and assembly drawings.

Evaluation

Each changed device or process must be thoroughly tested and evaluated by the appropriate department. Then the test results and all information related to the change should be reviewed by the change control board or other designated review group. This procedure is the same as needed for introducing a new product or process into production. The change control procedure must state the details of the evaluation and review process. It must define the responsibilities of the various departments and members of the review board.

Communication

The change procedure must cover the communication of changes to all affected parties, such as purchasing, contractors, vendors, etc. As appropriate, activities that apply to internal operations are also applicable to vendors. Examples are disposition of in-process assemblies, use of revised drawings and/or procedures, and disposition of old documents.

Updating Documentation

The procedure must cover updating of primary and secondary documentation such as instruction manuals. Usually there are no problems with updating (revising) primary documentation—in fact, that is the major reason the given change order is being processed. In contrast, it is rather easy to forget that related secondary documents, such as component drawings and instruction manuals, must be revised if affected by a given change. The use of a good control form can alleviate this problem.

Documentation Distribution

Revised documentation must be distributed to persons responsible for the operations affected by the change and old documents removed and filed or discarded, as appropriate. Documentation must be accessible to company employees, as stressed in the preamble to the GMP and required by section 820.180. The revised documentation must be used and controlled as required also by 820.180. Distribution of new documents and disposition of old documents must be covered by the change procedure. Supervisors must be vigilant in overseeing the flow and use of documentation, especially if a change is being phased in, because both the old and revised documentation will exist in a given department during the transition period.

Disposition of In-Process Items

The procedure must list by name or job title the individuals designated as responsible for, and also cover the procedure to follow for the disposition of in-process devices, components, assemblies, and labeling. The written procedure and implementation of it must be adequate to prevent mixups of old and revised items.

Remedial Actions

Certain changes will require remedial action in the field or re-work of warehouse stock. Changes of this nature must be addressed in the change control procedure. It must outline the documentation and activities required for field remedial actions or re-work of warehouse stock. (Note that field remedial actions may be classified as recalls, depending on the nature of the change. Generally, re-work of warehouse stock that is under a firm's control does not involve a recall.)

Quality Assurance Review

After the change is implemented, resulting devices and components must be as specified in the revised DMR and Device History Record. This agreement, of course, is assured by the change control pro-

cedure and the remainder of a firm's quality assurance system.
Quality assurance or other designated personnel must make certain
that the agreement exists during routine production as required by
820.20(a), 820.160, and 820.184.   These GMP sections cover:

Review of production records
Approval of components, labels, materials, etc.
Assuring that quality assurance checks are appropriate and
    adequate for their purpose and are performed correctly
Finished device evaluation
Collection of history record data to demonstrate that the device
    is manufactured in accordance with the updated device master
    record.

The change procedure must cover these activities and must
specify that they be accomplished before the first lot of the changed
devices are released for distribution.

Regulatory Submissions

Decisions for modifications to devices or manufacturing processes as
required by regulations for premarket notifications [21 CFR 807.81(g)]
or premarket approval (PMA) supplements (21 CFR 814) must be made
and should be covered under the change control procedure or a regulatory submissions policy and procedure.   Also, by considering drug
and device GMP regulations and premarket requirements simultaneously, labor costs can be reduced and compliance enhanced.   The change
order form is a convenient document for reminding employees that
regulatory submissions must be considered.

Regulatory Background

Section 807.81 requires that a premarket notification submission
[i.e., 510(k)] be made to the FDA if a device or one of its components, or the intended use of either, is to be *significantly* changed
or modified.   Examples of significant changes or modifications cited
are those that could affect safety or effectiveness of the device, such
as those involving design, material, chemical composition, energy
source, or manufacturing process.
It is stated in comment 18 of the Preamble that precedes Part 807
in the *Federal Register,* August 23, 1977, that "under the Act, the
burden is on the manufacturer to determine whether a premarket
notification should be submitted for a change or modification in a
device.   The Commissioner believes that the manufacturer is the person *best qualified* to make this determination."   From the same preamble, "The Commissioner did *not* intend that the owner or operator
should submit a premarket notification for *every change* in design,
material, chemical composition, energy source, or manufacturing

process." Thus, it is clearly the manufacturer's responsibility to determine if a proposed change could significantly affect safety or effectiveness.

Changes in manufacturing, labels, packing, master record, etc., of a device are also subject to GMP requirements in sections 820.61, 820.100, 820.101, 820.115, 820.116, and 820.181. Compliance of most firms with these change control requirements is checked during comprehensive inspections by FDA investigators, who also challenge other quality assurance elements required by the GMP regulation. Firms may consider their degree of compliance with the GMP regulation as one factor, but not the sole factor, when making decisions about premarket notification submissions for modified devices or processes.

Premarket Notification Decisions

Premarket notification submissions are required for new or modified intended uses. Submissions are not required for marketing or convenience changes where safety or effectiveness could not be significantly affected. Establishment management must decide whether or not to submit a premarket notification for other changes as briefly described herein and detailed in the *Federal Register*, August 23, 1977. While waiting for an FDA review of the submission, a firm may continue to distribute the unchanged device for its original intended use.

Some manufacturers with highly qualified personnel and substantial experience may feel confident in performing various technical operations and analyzing results to determine that a particular change in a drug delivery device, component, or manufacturing process will not significantly affect safety or effectiveness of the device. After technical activities are completed and documented, the results should be reviewed by a design-review panel, change control board, or equivalent group. After reviewing changes, if you are confident— because of your design evaluation, change control procedures, equipment qualification, equipment calibration, process validation, personnel training, and routine manufacturing procedures—that the change(s) could not significantly affect safety or effectiveness of the device, then the intent of the regulation has been addressed and there is no need to submit a premarket notification for the modification.

After a thorough review of proposed changes, if a manufacturer is uncertain whether a change may significantly affect safety or effectiveness, or believes that a change will significantly affect safety and effectiveness, then a premarket notification must be submitted.

GMP Controls Always Required

Section 807.87(g) requires that a premarket notification submission "include appropriate supporting data to show that the manufacturer has considered what consequences and effects the change or modification or new use might have on the safety and effectiveness of the device." Regardless of whether or not a change is submitted under the 510(k) process, the change must be evaluated and the associated data *must be filed* for an appropriate period (820.180), because demonstration of process effectiveness and use of adequate quality assurance checks for finished-device release are GMP requirements. Change control is also necessary to assure that a modified device or process results in a device that meets company quality claims. Otherwise, the drug delivery device is adulterated according to section 501(c) of the FD&C Act.

The above information applies to changes contemplated for devices and associated processes that are subject to premarket notification requirements. If proposed device and process changes are for devices subject to investigational device exemption (IDE) or premarket approval (PMA) requirements, then FDA approval must be obtained, in advance, by submitting a supplemental IDE or PMA.

VI. COMPONENTS AND MATERIALS

A. Component Qualification

Manufacturers of drug delivery devices must maintain a consistent, systematic quality assurance program which, along with other quality assurance activities, must assure that all components and materials are acceptable for their intended use, that their quality is sufficient, and that adequate steps are taken to prevent mixups. This component control is a combination of component qualifications: data collection, analysis, and corrective action; component specifications; vendor qualification; identification and status labeling and/or quarantine; and operational procedures.

"Component" is defined in paragraph 820.3(c) of the Good Manufacturing Practices (GMP) regulation as "any material, substance, piece, part, or assembly used during device manufacture which is intended to be included in the finished device." For example, hardware, polymers, inactive ingredients, and labels are components. This definition excludes "manufacturing materials," which, by definition, are not intended to be included in the finished device. According to section 820.3(l), "manufacturing material" is any material such as a cleaning agent, mold-release agent, lubricating oil, or other substance used to facilitate a manufacturing process, which is not intended by the manufacturer to be included in the finished device. The GMP regulation, however, requires in 820.20(a) that both manufacturing materials and components be addressed by the quality assurance program and that each be approved or rejected. Thus, both must be controlled upon receipt using the requirements in Subpart E, Control of Components. Any inactive components within a drug compound must be evaluated to confirm whether or not they remain inactive within the delivery system.

If a component is manufactured in the same or proximal facility, and produced exclusively for use in finished medical devices, then the component is considered part of the production of the finished devices and subject to the applicable requirements of the GMP regulation. If the component is manufactured in a separate plant owned by the finished-device manufacturer, then the manufacturer has flexibility in handling the quality assurance activities related to the control of components. One satisfactory approach is to have the plant that builds the components operate in full GMP compliance. Under this arrangement, the plant that does the final device assembly would still be responsible for ascertaining that the quality and integrity of incoming components have not been damaged during shipment. Alternatively, the component manufacturing plant may not comply fully with GMP regulation. Then the plant that does final assembly must handle the acceptance of components with the same degree of control as if the components were purchased from an outside vendor.

The device GMP regulation also applies to component manufacturers who produce components or accessories ready to be used for health-related purposes. An accessory is viewed as any finished unit sold separately but intended to be attached to or used in conjunction with another finished device. Components and accessories ready to be used for health-related purposes and packaged or labeled for commercial distribution for such health-related purposes are considered finished devices. Therefore, manufacturers of accessories must meet all FDA regulations for a finished device. These regulations include 21 CFR Part 807 Subpart E, Premarket Notification; 21 CFR Part 807 Subparts B, C, and D, Registration and Listing; GMP; 21 CFR Parts 801, Labeling, etc.

Manufacturers of components sold only for further manufacturing are not required to comply with any of the requirements for finished devices. Many components of devices, such as transistors, containers, hardware, etc., are readily available in the marketplace and are not manufactured exclusively for use in devices. Many of these manufacturers supply only a fraction of their production to finished-device manufacturers. However, section 820.1 of the GMP regulation encourages component manufacturers to use the GMP elements as guidelines where appropriate.

Qualification of components is a very important step toward designing and producing a high-quality product. Qualification of components consists of verifying through documented testing that a com-

ponent will perform its function reliably in the intended application
and under the most adverse environmental conditions in which the
device is expected to be used. These conditions should consider
the user's expectations and must encompass the manufacturer's labeling claims for the device.

Components have to be carefully selected, using the requirements
of the product as a guide. Components should be chosen so that
they will not be overstressed and will be compatible with the internal device environment as well as the external environment that the
device is expected to encounter during manufacture, distribution,
and use. The components should then be appropriately tested,
alone and as part of the device, versus the specifications established
for the component and the device. This testing should include
parameter and life testing as well as compatibility testing for both
the internal and external environment. Well-known, industry-
standard components that are used in their normal application and
that are not overstressed will need only minor testing. A record of
the qualification testing must be maintained. This record should include the component identity, the testing methods that were used,
as well as the actual test data and results.

B. GMP Controls

After the drug delivery device has been properly qualified, component
quality is maintained through correct specifications, procurement, incoming acceptance, storage, handling, installation, and change control. Feedback from the quality assurance system is needed to monitor the adequacy of these activities and procedures, and make corrections if necessary.

Specifications

Component specifications are required to be part of the device master
record. The specifications must be well designed, achievable, and
acceptable to vendors. They must adequately describe the quality
characteristics, dimensions, design, materials, performance, and any
other feature necessary to assure receipt of the item desired. For
unusual, vital, new, or key components, the specification data is
derived primarily from the qualification data with minor details from
catalog data. For routine components, such as those that have been
used for a long time or have a known performance history, a catalog
designation may be adequate to describe a component and assure
purchase of the desired component. For some components such as
transistors, the catalog number also may be used to obtain complete
specifications from a reference manual. Specifications should reflect
both design requirements and quality/reliability needs. The quality
level for each component must be specified. Components usually are

available in several quality levels, such as reagent grade, military grade, etc. In some cases, a significant increase in component quality can be obtained for a modest increase in cost by specifying a higher grade, thus reducing the probability of future quality problems and possible significant costs associated with these quality problems.

Vendor Qualification

A major factor in obtaining high-quality components is the selection of vendors. Although a manufacturer's knowledge of vendor operations may be limited and information about the operations difficult to obtain, the GMP requirement that a manufacturer is responsible for quality remains undiminished. To the maximum extent feasible, selection and qualification of vendors by audits, performance analysis, etc., should be part of a quality assurance program. If the manufacturer does not have the capability to test components for conformance to specifications, then vendor test data or outside lab results are acceptable provided that components are tested and inspected in a statistically valid manner to show their acceptability for use in the finished device. Any outside test results should be accompanied by relevant raw data used for the test, so that judgments of authenticity may be made by the finished device manufacturer. Excluding a vendor whose components are unreliable from supplying components for a new design may help prevent problems with the final device and is certainly worthwhile as a cost-reduction effort.

It is important to remember that raw components acquire cumulative value as they are processed through receiving, assembly, test, inspection, and as they ultimately become part of the finished device. If a component fails during assembly, or as part of the device, additional costs will be incurred for fault isolation, removal, replacement, inspection, testing, etc. When field failures occur, the ultimate cost of the component becomes even higher, because replacement requires travel, trouble-shooting, and retrofit. In addition, customer dissatisfaction, user injury, product liability action, medical device reporting, or regulatory action may result. Usually, the initial cost of a component is relatively insignificant compared to the costs involved should the component prove to be defective or improper for the selected use. Many recalls occur because manufacturers fail to qualify components properly or to assure that a vendor's manufacturing methods and QA system are adequate.

Acceptance Procedures

In medium to large manufacturing operations, written instructions are usually necessary to assure that components and manufacturing materials are properly identified, processed, and stored when received. Written inspection and test procedures are necessary to prescribe the inspections and tests to be conducted, equipment to be used, test and inspection methods to be implemented, and data to be recorded. Prior to acceptance, all components must be either physically separated (quarantined) or clearly identified as not yet accepted. The decision to separate or tag not-yet-accepted components should be made based on the characteristics of the device, the potential for mixups, plant conditions, and manufacturing practices.

Although section 820.80 requires a written procedure for accepting components, the GMP regulation in 820.5 allows discretion in the QA program. Thus a very small firm, usually having 10 or fewer employees, may not need written acceptance procedures other than purchase orders and receiving tickets as noted above. As the size of the operation, the number of activities, and the number of people involved increase, the need for comprehensive written instructions generally increases.

Acceptance Criteria

Manufacturers must have specific acceptance criteria for components. Acceptance criteria are the attributes of a component that determine its acceptability, such as appearance, dimension, purity, performance characteristics, etc. Typically, acceptance criteria are made a part of the inspection/test procedure or may take other forms. For example, if component specifications or a drawing adequately describe the attributes needed in order for the component to perform in its intended manner, these may serve as the acceptance criteria. If components are noncritical and the suppliers of the components have a history of good performance, the components may be accepted for use after a visual check to assure they are the items intended and that they are not damaged or contaminated. Components that need only a visual inspection, particularly for a very small firm, may be accepted using the purchase order data as acceptance criteria. The purchase order and/or receiving ticket must at a minimum contain the following information for a noncritical device: name of vendor; description of component; and quantity shipped. For a standard component, the catalog number might serve as a description. QA personnel should determine whether use of any "abbreviated" criteria are adequate during their audit of production re-work, history records, complaint files, and service records.

Testing and Inspection of Components

The GMP regulation requires that all incoming components receive at least a visual inspection for contamination and/or damage and be identified as the component specified on the purchase order. A manufacturer of a noncritical component has the discretion to determine when and where components should be inspected, sampled, and tested for conformance to specifications. As appropriate, components may be tested and/or inspected at the vendor, as they are received, during manufacture of the device, or as part of the finished device. If components are tested as part of the finished device, the testing must be able to reveal failed *and* "out-of-spec" components. However, the GMP regulation requires a manufacturer to sample and test a component if deviations from component specifications could result in a noncritical device being unfit for its intended use.

Manufacturers who decide not to sample or test components must be able to justify that decision based on such factors as knowledge of the supplier's previous performance in providing high-quality components, the component performance history, and application of the components. Manufacturers may rely on component suppliers to conduct testing if the manufacturer specifies or is knowledgeable about the supplier's quality assurance program, particularly the inspection and test programs; and the supplier has specifications that properly define the manufacturer's acceptable limits for the component or material parameters. These specifications may meet the master record requirements for component specifications, if these accurately reflect the parameters, composition, and configuration required for the component to perform the function for which it was selected. Supplier specifications are usually adequate for standard components. However, a manufacturer who relies on supplier specifications usually has no control over changes in these and, therefore, must assure at an appropriate point in the manufacturing process that the components received meet the desired specifications. If components are tested by the vendor, acceptance of components can be based on certification and review of test data submitted by the vendor for the specific components supplied. Certification must accompany each lot of components. When certification is used, the manufacturer should periodically verify the validity of the certification through an audit of the vendor.

Where historical data shows that certain noncritical components have been substandard and repeatedly resulted in a device failing to meet specifications, or where performance history has not been established, specific steps must be taken to assure that components meet specifications. Typically, this task is accomplished by sampling and testing each lot of components to assure that the components meet specifications. Where appropriate, all complex components should be sampled and tested.

Another testing scheme allowed under 820.3(c) permits manufacturers to test entire assemblies of components rather than individual components. If, however, testing an assembly cannot assure fitness-for-use of components, components must be tested on an individual or lot basis, whichever is appropriate. For example, assemblies with an internal feedback circuit could have a very marginal component. Because of the circuit design, the condition of

the marginal component might not be detected by testing the entire
assembly. Therefore, the feedback loop in the assembly must be
opened during one of the tests, or the individual components must
be tested.

When using a contract laboratory to test production components
(not a design evaluation), the laboratory becomes an extension of
the device manufacturer's quality assurance program. The device
manufacturer is responsible for assuring that the contractor's test
and inspection procedures are acceptable. Typically, this assurance
is obtained by audits.

Inspection and testing will not improve the quality of components;
however, if the inspection and testing is appropriate and performed
adequately, these activities can be used to prevent or significantly
reduce the use of low-quality or defective components. Through
feedback into the overall QA program, data on components will help
identify basic causes of problems and lead to solutions. If problems
are found, actions such as design changes, tighter acceptance criteria, vendor audits, or change of vendors may be appropriate.

Acceptance and Rejection Records

Adequate records must be maintained to provide objective evidence
that components were inspected and accepted, or rejected. These
records are a part of the device history record and should be maintained in a format that facilitates review. The records, however,
are not required to be maintained in a single file with other production history records, and are typically filed in the receiving or quality control area according to part number or component nomenclature.
Small manufacturers can use purchase orders or packing slips to
record acceptance and rejection if they contain adequate information.

The GMP regulation specifies that a record of component acceptance and rejection be maintained. Typically, acceptance/rejection
records should indicate: the nature and number of observations;
number and type of deficiencies; quantities approved and rejected;
and nature of corrective action taken. As a minimum, the manufacturer must record the number of components accepted and rejected. In all situations a qualified individual(s) must be designated
as having the responsibility for accepting components.

Obsolete, Deteriorated, and Rejected Components

Obsolete, deteriorated, and rejected components must be identified
as such and placed in a separate quarantine area or specially identified area to prevent mixups. If practical, components should be
individually identified as rejects. Where it is not feasible to tag
each rejected component, as in the case of transistors, bolts, etc.,
the container or packages of rejected lots should be clearly marked

and otherwise appropriately segregated from accepted components. There is no specific GMP requirement for a written procedure for handling obsolete, deteriorated, or rejected components. Firms should determine the need for a written procedure for handling these components based on the size of the firm and the complexity of their devices and operations.

To assure that unacceptable components are not used, the GMP regulation requires that records be maintained of their disposition. These should state whether the components were returned, scraped, re-worked, etc. If it is unlikely that such components could be used because they would not fit, are obviously a reject, etc., records may not be necessary. Particularly in very small firms, disposition can be recorded directly onto the purchase order and/or receiving tickets. Small to medium-sized firms generally record disposition on the form used to receive components. Most large manufacturers record disposition of rejected components on standard forms such as Nonconforming Material Report (NMR).

When components and materials become obsolete, many manufacturers assign new identification numbers to the replacement components and materials. The obsolete items are retained for other uses, such as repair parts, engineering projects, etc. In these cases, the old and new items must be adequately segregated and/or identified to prevent inadvertent use of obsolete components in production.

Component Storage

Although not a direct GMP requirement, all raw materials and components used in the finished device should be received through a central control point. Centralized receiving leads to orderly storage, limits access to stored material, and aids a firm in meeting other GMP requirements. When components are not immediately processed, the GMP regulation requires that components be held in a quarantine area or identified upon receipt as not yet accepted. Components and raw materials must be identified or stored so that at all times it is obvious that a component or material has been accepted, rejected, or is awaiting a disposition decision. A quarantine area can be either a physically secure area or simply a limited-access area identified as a quarantine area. If special environmental storage conditions are required, such as for many biologically devived components, these conditions must be controlled and monitored, and the associated specifications included in the device master record.

If a drug delivery device is to be sterilized, consideration should be given to component storage conditions to prevent contamination of components by bacteria or filth. Also, temperatures must be controlled as necessary to prevent growth of bacteria. The higher bioburden (bacteria, etc.) levels may challenge the cycle to an extent greater than the capability established during validation and thereby result in a sterility assurance level that may not meet the finished-device specification. Aside from the hazard of increased bioburden levels, there is the danger that some of the viable bacteria may produce pyrogens. These fever-producing substances will not be destroyed by subsequent sterilization. Some components, particularly those used in the manufacture of in vitro diagnostic products, if not stored properly, may support growth of bacteria.

Critical Components

The GMP regulation contains additional requirements for critical components used in critical devices. A "critical device" is a device intended for surgical implant into the body or to support or sustain life and whose failure to perform when properly used in accordance with instructions for use provided in the labeling can be reasonably expected to result in a significant injury to the user. As a guideline, "significant injury" may be understood to include death, mutilation, amputation, dismemberment, loss of body function, disfigurement, long-term debilitation, or injury that requires extended hospitalization. A critical component is defined as "any component of a critical device whose failure to perform can be reasonably expected to cause the failure of a critical device or to affect its safety or effectiveness." "Failure to perform" can be defined as complete failure or variation from performance specifications to a degree that the component does not perform its intended function.

The FDA is concerned about the failure of components that would result in sudden or catastrophic device failure, such as no output from an implantable cardiac pacemaker; fracture of an implanted orthopedic implant; runaway in an implanted cardiac pacemaker; misfiring of a synchronized defibrillator; etc.; which can reasonably be expected to result in significant injury to the user.

The intent of the GMP requirements is to prevent the production of nonconforming product. Therefore, quality requirements cannot be relaxed on the basis that distributed devices are amenable to inspection, testing, and modification or that there will be backup devices or trained personnel available to relieve the result of failure. Although alarms and indicators may sometimes alert a user that a device is about to or has malfunctioned or failed, these features will not prevent a device from malfunctioning or failing. Therefore, repairs, backup devices, alarms, and indicators are not considered when identifying critical components.

The criteria for identifying a critical device should be restricted to the effect of its failure. Therefore, user error and the environment are not presently considered by the FDA when identifying critical devices. Identification of critical devices should be based on the health hazard presented should the device fail to meet its performance specifications when operated as intended. User error is not a performance failure, although it could be considered a result of inadequate directions for use or inadequate labeling. The environment could result in failure of a device, but it should not effect the result of failure of the device.

To identify a critical component, a manufacturer must know in detail how the device functions and the purpose of each component in the finished device. The effect that each component will have on finished-device performance, should the component fail to perform as intended, must be determined. Thus, manufacturers must carefully study the possible failure modes of their devices and decide which components are truly critical under the various modes. This determination may be time-consuming with respect to some devices, but it is necessary. It will, in the long run, save manufacturers liability, repair, and replacement costs. To make such a determination, manufacturers should conduct reliability tests and failure effects analyses, preferably during the design phase, in order to accurately identify critical components. The component under study can be considered a "critical component" if as a result of a failure, the performance, lack of performance, or effect on safety or effectiveness of the finished device could result in significant injury to the user when the device is properly used in accordance with instructions in the labeling.

The number of components that need to be considered as potential critical components can be reduced by considering the reliability of components and whether they "reasonably" can be expected to fail. For example, power cords, clamps, plugs, etc., seldom fail. Therefore, manufacturers may not need to consider these types of components when critical components are being identified. Also, manufacturers can consider a subassembly a component and thereby reduce recordkeeping.

If failsafe circuits can be designed into a device so that a component failure would not result in significant injury, then some components could be removed from consideration as critical components. However, the components that comprise the failsafe circuit then become critical components and could, depending on the design efficiency, actually increase rather than reduce the number of critical components.

Supplier agreements. Manufacturers of critical devices are required to obtain from critical component suppliers an agreement in which the supplier agrees to notify the manufacturer of any changes in the critical component or its manufacture. A manufacturer may not always find a supplier agreeable to such an arrangement. If unable to obtain an agreement, documentation of a good-faith attempt is sufficient in lieu of the written agreement. Copies of pertinent correspondence between the manufacturer and the supplier would be

considered acceptable evidence by the FDA of an attempt to secure
a supplier agreement.   If unable to obtain an agreement, the manufacturer must be vigilant in looking for gross and subtle changes in
materials, components, and their performance.

Rejected lots.   Records of critical component receipt must be in-
dexed by supplier name, and the percentage of lots that are rejected
must be recorded.   This data can be used by the finished-device
manufacturer to determine supplier performance.   If the raw acceptance data can be readily reviewed for this purpose, the GMP requirement to calculate and record percentages may be unnecessary.

Written test procedures.   A critical drug delivery device manufacturer must assure that all lots of critical components are accepted,
sampled, tested, and/or inspected using written procedures.   The
inspection/test procedure for each component must be dated and
approved.   The procedure also should specify the items to which it
applies, the component characteristics to be inspected/tested, accept-
ance/rejection criteria, data forms, sampling plans, and necessary
test inspection equipment and tools.

The GMP regulation does not require mandatory reserve sampling.
Although 820.81(a) includes a provision for maintaining reserve
samples of critical components, this requirement is discretionary per
GMP regulation preamble comment 76.

Sampling plans.   When seeking to assure that critical components
meet acceptance criteria, manufacturers may test either all critical
components or may test a portion of the components using a sampling
plan based on an acceptable statistical rationale.   A manufacturer
must be prepared to demonstrate the statistical rationale for any
sampling plan used.   Plans should be developed by qualified mathematicians or statisticians, or be taken from established standards such
as MIL-STD-105D or MIL-STD-414.   All sampling plans have a built-
in risk of accepting a bad lot.

This sampling risk is typically determined in quantitative terms
by deriving the "operating characteristic curve" for the selected
plan.   Each sampling plan has a characteristic curve.   Both MIL-
STD-105D and MIL-STD-414 contain operating characteristic curves
for sampling plans presented in the standards, and they can be used
to determine the risk a sampling plan presents.   A manufacturer
should be aware of the risks the chosen plan presents.   Operating
characteristic curves are a means of graphically showing the relationship between:

   The quality of lots submitted for sampling inspection, usually ex-
       pressed in percent defective, but may be expressed in defect
       per hundred units; and

The probability that the sampling plan will yield a decision to accept the lot, described as the "probability of acceptance."

Control numbers. Control numbers for component traceability are mandatory for critical components and "components" of in vitro diagnostic kits (21 CFR 809.10). Control numbers must be assigned to each lot or batch of critical components that were manufactured under similar conditions over the same time period, so that defects can be traced to the component manufacturer and the cause of the defects determined and corrected. If a subassembly is regarded as a critical component by the manufacturer, a control number for that critical subassembly must be shown in the device history record.

An example of a form that may be used for accepting, receiving, and inspecting components is shown in Exhibit 2. This example shows the types of information required by the GMP regulation. Procedures and forms for a particular situation may be more or less comprehensive than this, and may assume other formats or arrangements according to needs. This example is intended as an acceptance procedure that may be followed by a small to medium-size firm. The procedure has space for the number, revision level, and a blank for "ECN History." The history blank is for adding brief notes about changes that have been made to this procedure. Used as part of this procedure is a "Receiving History Log," which is a form where the purchase order number, lot number, date received, vendor, lot size, quantity accepted, quantity rejected, inspector, date, and comments are recorded.

Exhibit 2   Acceptance of Components

TITLE: ACCEPTANCE OF COMPONENTS

No. _____ Rev. _____ ECN History _____

Drafted by _____ App. by _____ Date _____

1.0   **SCOPE**

These procedures are to be followed in the receipt, inspection, and storage of materials, components, parts, raw materials, etc., used in the manufacture of the XYZ Stimulator, a noncritical device.

2.0   **RECEIVING**

2.1   All incoming shipments must be examined for external signs of damage. If the shipment is damaged, immediately notify Purchasing and move the shipment to the unloading Hold area until disposition is decided by Purchasing.

Exhibit 2 (Continued).

2.2   Upon receipt, check each shipment against the appropriate purchase order and verify identity and quantity.

2.3   Enter the appropriate data into the Received Goods Log for each shipment received.

2.4   After completing the data entry, attach a **yellow** "**HOLD**" tag to the components, etc., and move the components, etc., immediately to the receiving quarantine area. The pink copy of the purchase order must accompany the material.

2.5   Notify Quality Control when materials requiring inspection are received in the quarantine area. This information is obtained from the specification for the item ordered.

2.6   Quality control shall, after examining the components, etc., for damage and identity, move the components, etc., to be inspected to the Receiving Inspection area.

3.0   **INSPECTION**

3.1   Pull the inspection history file for the components, etc., to be inspected. This file contains the Receiving History form and inspection procedure. Enter the appropriate data from the purchase order onto the Receiving History form and perform the inspection per the procedure.

3.2   The QC manager shall assign a five digit lot number to each vendor lot received and enter the number on the Receiving History form.

3.3   After the inspection is completed, enter on the Receiving History form:
        a.   the quantity accepted and sent to stock;
        b.   the quantity rejected; and
        c.   your signature and the date.

4.0   **DISPOSITION**

4.1   Receiving and test data for each shipment are sent to the designated individual for review and the decision regarding the acceptability of the lot.

4.2   For accepted components, etc., enter the quantity accepted, date accepted, and lot number on a **green** "**ACCEPTED**" tag, attach the tag to the components, etc., and move them to the stockroom.

4.3   For rejected components, etc., attach a **red** "**REJECTED**" tag to the rejected components, etc., and complete a Rejected Material form. Place all rejected components, etc., in the rejected quarantine area and forward the Rejected Material form to Quality Engineering for disposition.

5.0   **STOCKROOM**

5.1   All items entering the stockroom must be accompanied by a **green** "**ACCEPTED**" tag.

5.2   Components and other materials shall be stored and issued per SOP 17320.

5.3   Components and other materials will be issued from the stockroom on a first-in, first-out basis. All materials with a limited shelf life or requiring controlled storage conditions will be stored appropriately per SOP 17321.

Note: Page 3, the receiving log is not reprinted here.

VII. PRODUCTION APPLICATIONS

A. Production and Process Control

The objective of production and process control is to assure that
the drug delivery device design is accurately transferred into
written specifications for the device and manufacturing processes.
Also, production processes must be adequate and controlled to the
extent necessary to assure that the finished device is manufactured
according to these specifications. Specifications describe the inten-
tion of the design, and processes are planned so that devices produced by them meet specifications. For a given design, note that
these specifications are the device-specific documents in the device
master record. Of course, general documents in the master record
are also used to manufacture a given device.

Specifications

Section 820.100(a)(1) requires manufacturers to establish procedures
to ensure that the approved design is accurately transferred into
written specifications; and that there are *sufficient* specifications
that accurately describe the device, its components, and packaging.
Typically, control of design transfer is accomplished through a
formal review process to verify that the design is adequately translated into specifications as is discussed in Section II. These specifications must be *adequate* to assure that design configuration and
performance requirements can be met if the device is manufactured
and assembled according to these specifications.

   If the design basis is not adequately translated into specifications,
as needed to procure components and materials, and manufacture
finished devices, the resulting product may be ineffective and unsafe.

   The need for a written procedure for this documentation and
transfer activity should be determined on the basis of need for communication, the complexity of the activity, etc. The GMP regulation
does not mandate a written procedure; however, many firms simply
use their change control procedure to introduce a new product into
production.

Specification Changes

Specification changes must be technically sound, acceptable, and
authorized before they are implemented. Specification changes may
be made using standard forms, such as Engineering Change Notices,
Drawing Change Notices, etc., or may use any other method that
will assure the history of the documentation is maintained and that
the change is properly reviewed, approved, and dated before implementation as described in Section VI. Change authorization must include the approval date and the date the change becomes effective.

Documentation of specification changes for the device, its labeling, and its packaging is necessary in order to control the device configuration and to determine configuration at any point in time. Such knowledge is essential when it becomes necessary to investigate a product defect or determine which devices must be recalled.

Processing Controls

Manufacturers must establish process controls to ensure that the device(s) is not adversely affected by the process and that the process will achieve its intended purpose. Process controls include standards, blueprints, first-piece evaluation, written instructions, operation certification, engineering drawings, inspection, testing, etc., as well as process validation. The need for written procedures to assure process control depends on the complexity of the process and the training of the operator(s). In some cases the success of the process depends almost entirely on the skill of the employee. In such cases, written instructions may not be needed. For example, written procedures are usually not needed in a routine soldering operation. Sometimes workmanship standards are made available to the employee and inspection is conducted to assure that the soldering is done correctly. For other processes, specifications or drawings may be used in lieu of written procedures. For example, a machinist may use a blueprint or engineering drawing for guidance.

Manufacturers must assure that all processes are conducted properly. This is assured through training, supervision, audits, inspection, testing, documentation, etc.

All changes to processes must be properly reviewed, validated, documented, and communicated in a timely manner. The methods used to obtain approval of and to control specification changes may be used to control and document process changes. Process validation is covered in Section II.

Critical Devices

In addition to the requirements in section 820.100, a manufacturer of critical devices must identify critical operations and establish additional controls for these operations.

A "critical operation" is an operation in the manufacture of a critical device that, if improperly performed, can reasonably be expected to cause the failure of a critical device or to affect its safety or effectiveness. Almost all manufacturing operations can have an impact on safety and effectiveness of the finished device, and therefore a reasonable approach should be taken when evaluating a critical device manufacturing process to identify critical operations. Answering the following "decision-tree" questions will help assist in establishing which manufacturing operations should be classified as critical.

1. Is this operation being performed on a critical component, assembly, or critical device?

>   If NO, this operation is not critical.
>   If YES, go to question 2.

2. Will improper performance of this manufacturing operation result in a serious hazard such as could be caused by the following events?

>   Toxic materials contacting the patient or operator
>   Unusual loss of blood
>   Air entering the bloodstream
>   Hemolysis
>   Asphyxiation
>   Infection in the patient or operator
>   Immediate and dangerous chemical imbalance in the patient
>   Electric shock (fibrillation or dangerous involuntary reaction)
>   Significant electrolysis (i.e., apply direct current)
>   Undermedication or overmedication
>   Mechanical, chemical, or thermal damage, or ionizing radiation
>   Operator or user confusion
>   Discontinued or inadequate treatment that is not detected
>   Nonfunctioning machine parameter that is not detected
>   (Other hazardous situations or events)

>   If NO, this operation is *not* critical.
>   If YES, the operation is critical.

In accordance with section 820.101, when a critical manufacturing operation is identified or designated by company management, it must be

>   Performed by a suitable (i.e., adequately trained) individual(s)
>   Conducted using suitable (i.e., adequately qualified) equipment
>   Verified
>   Recorded in the device history record

In the list immediately above, the main added requirement for critical devices is verification. The other elements are also required for noncritical devices. A critical operation may be verified by one or more methods such as:

>   Inspection or test of the characteristics added, removed, or
>   modified by the operation
>   The production process or assembly operation itself; that is, fur-
>   ther assembly operations that will reveal improperly formed
>   parts or assemblies

Controlling and monitoring production equipment or processes
used in manufacturing.

If physical examination, measurement, or test of in-process,
processed, or finished product is impossible or impractical, indirect
control by monitoring the processing method, equipment, and personnel may be used. Such processes must be validated.

The sterilization process used to sterilize a critical device is a
critical operation. The same process, however, is not, by definition,
a "critical" operation when the process is used to sterilize a noncritical device, because critical operations apply only to critical devices. In actuality, however, the process controls for sterilizing a
noncritical device are the same as for a critical device.

B. Reprocessing

If components, subassemblies, assemblies, in-process devices, or
finished drug delivery devices fail to meet specifications, they are
often reprocessed, repaired, re-worked, etc., to meet specification.
The GMP regulation reprocessing requirements apply to any activity
that involves recycling of the device or its components through any
part of the manufacturing process, including sterilization.

Section 820.115(a) states that "procedures" shall be established,
implemented, and controlled to assure that a reprocessed device
meets specifications. In this requirement, "procedures" refers to
actions or activities taken to assure that the reprocessed device
meets specifications. It does *not* necessarily mean a written procedure. When the GMP specifies that procedures shall be used,
but does not specify "written procedures," the manufacturer must
evaluate the controls in place and determine if they are adequate
without written procedures. If so, written procedures are not
required. Regardless of the decisions made, each manufacturer
should be prepared to provide a rationale for each decision. Medium
to large firms will tend to need written procedures for reprocessing,
particularly when the status of the in-process device cannot be determined by casual observation.

It is not always possible to predict in advance all types of reprocessing that might occur and, therefore, it is not feasible to
write a procedure that covers all occasions. For example, a manufacturer often finds it necessary to replace components. Although
this is technically reprocessing, it would be impractical to write a
procedure that would fit all situations where components are replaced.
If the manufacturer determines through observation of errors, defects, etc., that written procedures are necessary to assure that all
parts of an activity are performed, they should be written and implemented. In many cases, the reprocessing procedure can be

written into the original manufacturing procedure—separate reprocessing instructions generally do not need to be written if they simply duplicate another existing procedure.

Specifications for reprocessing should document the specific tests and processes to be repeated for each assembly or device and the limits on the amount of reprocessing permitted for a unit. These specifications should be based on studies to measure the effects of reprocessing operations. For example, if an electronic component is repeatedly replaced, the effect of repeated application of heat during soldering must be determined. If there is an effect such as separation of pad and conductors or degradation of insulation, limits should be set on the number of times a component may be replaced. On the other hand, replacing a defective printed circuit board (PCB) with a good one may only require marking the defective board, segregating it, and, after replacement with a good PCB, retesting the finished device. Procedures used in controlling such reprocessing need only be as detailed as deemed necessary to assure that the finished device or component meets the approved specifications.

For process-type industries, firms must evaluate the reprocessing to assure that devices will not be adversely affected. For example, following resterilization, devices must be inspected for characteristics that may have been altered. The following are examples of effects that might need consideration:

Temperature and moisture effects on steam-sterilized devices and packages
Vacuum and pressure effects and gas by-product residue levels for gas-sterilized devices
Package and device material degradation for radiation-sterilized devices

Devices and components to be reprocessed must be identified to distinguish them from acceptable devices and components. Depending on the degree of control needed, identification may be accomplished by tagging the individual devices or components, marking their containers, or marking the area in which they are held.

Retesting

Manufacturers must implement appropriate QA checks to assure that reprocessed devices meet specifications. When a finished device is reprocessed, the finished device must be subjected to reinspection, and/or testing, to the extent necessary to assure that the reprocessing was adequate and did not have an adverse effect on the performance of the device. In most cases the procedure used to inspect/test the original device is adequate for this purpose.

Returned Devices

Once a device is finished and distributed, the GMP reprocessing requirements do *not* apply. Therefore, when devices are returned for
repair or reconditioning due to failure or wear, the GMP reprocessing
requirements do not apply. If a product is returned due to a malfunction or defect, however, section 820.162, Failure Investigation,
applies. If the returned device is modified (updated), the GMP requirements also change, because modifying a device is manufacturing
and all the applicable requirements of the GMP regulation must be
met. These usually include revised processing or assembly documentation, test/inspection procedures, labeling, etc.

Critical Device Reprocessing

The GMP requires written procedures for reprocessing critical drug
delivery devices and components. Reprocessing instructions may be
included in the original process instructions, or separate procedures
may be used. However, there is some leeway, and the actual need
for written procedures should be determined beforehand based on the
degree of reprocessing that may be required. When procedures are
deemed necessary, they should prescribe the following elements.

> The equipment to be used need only be prescribed if it is differ-
> ent from that used during routine production.
> Any special QA methods or tests needed should be listed. If
> routine methods are used, these need only be referenced.

In addition, the activities listed below must be performed when
critical devices are expected to be or are reprocessed.

> The manufacturer must determine the effect of reprocessing on
> the finished device to make certain that it will not be adulter-
> ated or adversely affected. For example, when devices in-
> tended to be sterile are resterilized by heat, radiation, or
> ethylene oxide, the possibility of damage or residual con-
> taminants must be considered.
> The manufacturer must clearly identify those devices to be re-
> processed and separate them from those not requiring re-
> processing. When a device is reprocessed, this fact should
> be reflected in the history record of the reprocessed device.
> The individuals designated to approve changes must formally re-
> view and approve new reprocessing procedures or changes
> to these procedures. The change control procedures imple-
> mented by a manufacturer to meet the requirements of
> 820.100(a)(2), Specification Changes, can be used to meet
> this requirement.

The firm must generate written testing and sampling procedures to assure that reprocessed devices and components conform to approved specifications. The procedures used for routine inspection and test of the finished device may be used to meet this requirement, if appropriate.

C. Repacking/Relabeling of Delivery Devices

Repacking and relabeling are manufacturing operations and thus must be performed in accordance with applicable requirements of the GMP regulation as noted in Section 1. It is important to consider the flexibility allowed by section 820.5 of the GMP regulation when developing a quality assurance system for repacking and relabeling. Note the flexibility written into or implied by the following typical repacking process. For example, assembly drawings are usually not needed, and the quantity manufactured is not recorded—recording the quantity released for distribution is adequate to meet the flexible requirements.

Operation Control

Typically, a repacking and/or relabeling process involves kit assembly or reducing bulk amounts of material into smaller amounts. Written procedures have limited application but may contain such information as the packing order for complex kits, which is usually last-in, first-out (LIFO) in order of use. Other master record documents such as labels, package inserts, component lists, environmental control procedures, etc., are needed, as appropriate.

A typical kit assembly operation contains the following steps. These steps, however, are not mandatory. The applicable GMP controls are indicated for each step.

1. Using a work order or other manufacturing document, remove kit(s) items, labeling, packaging from stock following a first-in, first-out (FIFO) system as applicable. Examine labeling for identity and record [820.120(e)]. This record is a part of the history record and may be made on the work order or other appropriate document.
2. Clear the assembly area of prior kit items, labeling, etc. [820.120(c)]. Separate operations adequately to prevent mix-ups [820.120(b)].
3. Transfer kit items to the assembly area. Set up operations in a manner designed to assure conformance with kit specifications.
4. Verify that the kit items are the desired items by checking against work order, specifications, etc. Examine labeling for identity and record if not done as part of step 1. Record

lot number of kit items where required. Lot numbers are
required for critical devices or when specified by the kit
manufacturer. Lot numbers should be recorded in a manner
that will facilitate ready identification of all kits containing
items with the same lot number.

5. Assemble the kit(s). The work order, itemized list, pictorial
or actual model can be used as guidance in assembling the kit
in lieu of a written process procedure. Models, pictures, etc.,
used in lieu of master record documents must be approved
for use and kept current.

6. Visually inspect kit(s) to assure conformance to specifications,
including labeling requirements. The work order, itemized
lists, pictorial or model may be used as acceptance criteria.
If required, label the kit with the expiration date. Where
applicable, the expiration date of the overall kit should be
the same as the kit item with the shortest expiration date.

7. If specified, seal the finished kits and place them in cartons.
Label cartons if not preprinted. Inspect carton contents and
labeling to verify correct contents and labeling.

8. Record the dates of manufacture, quantity released for distribution, and any control number used. This date can be
recorded on the work order or on any other document that
will be retained. This record becomes part of the device
history record.

Reprocessing

Reprocessing at a repacker/relabeler typically involves only packaging
or labeling. However, in some cases a repacker/relabeler may reprocess a device that is damaged or contaminated.

When a repacker/relabeler elects to reprocess a device, the applicable GMP reprocessing requirements apply. When reprocessing
is necessary, the reprocessed device must meet the same quality
standards or specifications as the original device. The same controls used to determine the quality conformance of the original devices can usually be used to determine the quality of reprocessed
devices, and the additional GMP reprocessing requirements may not
be necessary. If processes other than simple packaging are used,
such as aseptic filling, sterilization, etc., additional GMP manufacturing and reprocessing controls may be necessary. In any case
the effect of the reprocessing on the device must be determined by
the repacker/relabeler.

D. Contract Sterilization

Production and contract sterilization of drug delivery devices must
be performed such that the device manufacturer and the contract

sterilizer meet the applicable parts of the Good Manufacturing Practices (GMP) regulation and the labeling requirements of 21 CFR 801, particularly 801.150(e). A contract as required by 801.150(e) is also helpful in meeting GMP requirements.

VIII. DEVICE EVALUATION

A. Finished Device Evaluation

Finished device inspection is typically a final test and review of safety, performance, and configuration characteristics to assure that these meet the specifications in the device master record. For many medical devices this assurance requires an analysis, electrical test, or mechanical test. For some simple devices, however, such as eyeglass frames, a visual or dimensional check may be sufficient to prove acceptability.

Manufacturers must have specifications or criteria for determining acceptability of the finished device as discussed in Sections II and V. It is important that the device characteristics to be evaluated are defined and also, where applicable, the equipment, environment, and handling procedure be defined and established. These are specified in a written procedure as required by section 820.160, which typically includes tests to be conducted, test equipment configuration, and any standards or reference materials to be used.

The GMP requirements for finished-device evaluation are covered in section 820.160, which requires written procedures for finished-device inspection to assure that device specifications are met. Before releasing devices for commercial distribution, manufacturers must assure that finished devices perform intended functions by checking or testing those characteristics that must meet device master record safety and performance specifications in order for the device to be fit for the intended use.

If a firm has adequate test and inspection procedures and these are used correctly by appropriately trained personnel, then there is a high probability that all devices released for distribution will meet the company device specification. Further, the data collected during in-process or finished-device evaluation are appropriate, complete, correct, and may be fed back into the quality assurance system to identify and solve real problems, and to help maintain and improve the quality assurance system.

Evaluation Specifications

A firm must decide which characteristics of a drug delivery device to test and/or inspect and to what detail or extent to test and/or inspect versus the device specifications in order to be assured that a device is fit for the intended use. For example, this decision is typically based on:

Intended use
Intended user
Nature of the device and its components
Intrinsic safety of the device
Reliability of the device
Overall process capability of the manufacturing operation
Characteristics of test and inspection equipment and procedures
Performance margin of the device versus the device specification

These evaluation decisions are made during the product and
process development phase; and final debugging is usually performed
during pilot production as discussed in Section II. At the start of
full-scale production, the test and inspections decisions must be
completed, documented as test/inspection procedures, and approved
for use. It is a violation of the GMP regulation to place inadequately
evaluated devices into commercial distribution. It is also a violation
of the GMP regulation to deliberately allow test and inspection procedures to evolve during production, except during a highly controlled pilot-production phase. Further, devices that are not adequately evaluated may not meet company written or unwritten quality
claims—firms cannot bypass their responsiblity by simply not writing
quality claims. Under section 501(c) of the Food, Drug and Cosmetic
Act, a device is adulterated if its purity or quality falls below that
which it purports or is represented to possess.

Device test and/or inspection specifications, and test and/or inspection procedures, must be carefully written and must cover all
appropriate points in the device specification, in order to improve
communications and reduce errors. Completeness is assured if each
appropriate and numbered paragraph in the device specification has
a corresponding numbered paragraph in the test and inspection procedure and numbered blank on the data form. Generally, each
numbered paragraph in the test and inspection procedure describes
the detailed process for evaluating a specific aspect of the device.
The data sheet or history record form has a blank with the same
unique paragraph number for recording the data obtained when
evaluating each characteristic of the device.

Thus, at the production phase, the device specifications are
supported by one or more test and inspection documents that form
part of the device master record. To reduce drafting, filing, re-
trieval, and copying costs, test and inspection specifications may
appear on process and assembly documents. Combination documents
are commonly used for the fabrication and inspection/testing of
subassemblies. There may be several test and inspection documents,
because evaluation may be performed at several in-process stages
and at the finished-device stage.

There are situations where a simple data sheet or blueprint that
lists the acceptance criteria can be used in lieu of a written proce-

dure. For example, the acceptance of a simple molded or machined device may be determined by using a checklist, blueprint, or specification that specifies finished dimensions, flash removal, etc. In machine-shop operations, a blueprint or engineering drawing may be used as acceptance criteria and to meet the GMP written procedure requirements.

Whether simple or complex, all manufacturing documentation, including data sheets, must be under formal change control. Likewise, the test equipment must be suitable, calibrated, and under a formal recalibration control program.

Simulated-Use Testing

Where practical, a finished device must be selected periodically and tested under conditions that simulate those under which the device is expected to operate reliably. These factors may include a specific environment, load, external interference, use with other devices, etc. Simulated use of implantable pacemakers could consist of submerging the pacemakers for a specified time in a 38°C saline solution with an electrical load applied to simulate the fluids, temperature, and electrical load presented by the body.

Many recalls could have been prevented if the manufacturer had adequately tested the device under simulated conditions before distribution. For example, blood tubing was recalled because it would not properly occlude when used in a blood pump. Testing under actual operating conditions would have detected this problem.

When a simulated test is used, the test specifications must be included in the device master record. These and all other test specifications must be designed for the intended use, and the adequacy of the resulting tests must be verified as discussed in Section II in order to help assure that finished devices meet quality claims [FD&C Act, section 501(c)].

Sampling Plans

Manufacturers may test all devices to assure that they meet acceptance criteria; or, if the manufacturing process is operating in a state-of-control, they may test a portion by using a sampling plan based on an acceptable statistical rationale. A manufacturer must be prepared to demonstrate the statistical rationale for any sampling plan used. Plans should be developed by qualified mathematicians or be selected from established standards such as MIL-STD-105d or MIL-STD-414.

All sampling plans have a built-in sampling risk. A sampling risk is the probability of shipping (or receiving, from the customer's viewpoint) a "bad" lot and is typically determined in quantiative terms by deriving the "operating characteristic curve" for the

selected plan. Each sampling plan has an operating characteristic
curve, which is a means of graphically showing the relationship
between quality of lots submitted for sampling inspection (usually
expressed in percent defective, but may also be expressed in defect
per hundred units) and the probability that the sampling plan will
yield a decision to ship the lot. MIL-STD-105d and MIL-STD-414
contain operating characteristic curves for sampling plans presented
in them; and these curves can be used to determine the risk each
sampling plan presents.

When sampling plans are used, a few defective devices will be
shipped to the user. Thus, manufacturers should be aware of the
risks a particular plan presents to the firm *and* to the user.
Questions such as those listed below should be considered before
selecting a sampling plan.

> Will the defect be obvious to the user? If not, what are the
>   consequences of using the defective device?
> What is the state-of-the-art technology for testing this device?
> Does the competition use sampling?
> What is the probability of a product liability suit?
> What are the regulatory consequences?
> Does the marketplace expect or accept devices that have been
>   sample-tested or inspected?

Acceptance of sample-tested devices is usually set by the price
the user is willing to pay—100% testing usually costs more than
sampling. Whether sample testing and inspection of a particular
family of devices is acceptable to the user also changes with
technology. Manufacturers should also recognize that straightforward logical answers to the listed questions are not always
suitable—political, litigious, and emotional climates should also be
considered when deciding which sampling plans to use or what
risks to take.

Labeling and Packaging Inspection

Before release, the finished device, its containers, and its packaging must be examined as applicable to assure that they are not
damaged or misbranded. That is, these must contain correct
labels, package inserts, or manuals. The packaging of sterile
devices must be examined after sterilization to make sure that
integrity, sealing, and labeling requirements are met.

Records

Section 820.160 is not specific regarding finished-device test and
inspection records for noncritical devices; however, these records
must be generated, as they must be included as part of the device

history record (820.184). A device history record is a compilation of records containing the complete production history of a finished device [830.3(h)]. The term "complete" is interpreted for each family of devices as allowed by 820.5. For many devices and manufacturing operations, the major documents in the device history record are the finished-device inspection and test records. The history record must be reviewed because these records are used to show that finished devices are manufactured in accordance with the device master record.

Product Release

Drug delivery device manufacturers must have sufficient controls to assure that only devices that have passed test and inspection are released as discussed in Section XI. To prevent mixups, devices that have been through final evaluation and accepted for release must be segregated from not-yet-accepted or rejected devices, or otherwise controlled, such as by location, boxing, or manifest tagging.

Production and inspection/test records should be reviewed before releasing each lot of finished devices. Section 820.20(a) makes the QA organization responsible for reviewing production records. This requirement does not specify when to review records. To meet GMP requirements, however, they must be reviewed often enough to assure that operations are in a state-of-control.

Additional Requirements for Critical Devices

If a critical device or critical component does not pass final inspection and/or testing, the cause of the failure must be determined and corrections must be made to prevent similar failures (820.101). The investigation, conclusions, and followup must be documented. When a critical or noncritical device fails testing, it should not be repeatedly retested until it passes without first determining the cause for failure. If a manufacturer's acceptance procedures allow acceptance after repeated testing and re work, there must be a valid basis for such an acceptance procedure. Failed devices must be identified and segregated from acceptable devices and from the flow of the production process.

Before critical devices are released for distribution, or released from control of the manufacturer, history records for the devices *must* be reviewed. The history record files should be in a minimum of locations in order to expedite reviews and increase the probability of maintaining a state-of-control. Reviews must be conducted to assure that all records and documentation required by the device master record are present, and that all operations required by the master record have been correctly completed. The responsibility for this function must be assigned to one or more designated individuals.

The GMP regulation does not mandate that all records be reviewed by a single individual at one time, although this is the preferred approach. The history records may be signed in stages by designated individuals. These individuals must authorize, by signature, the release of the device.

B. Failure Investigations

Device GMP sections 820.162 and 820.198 require investigations after a critical or noncritical finished device is released for distribution and fails or allegedly fails to meet performance specifications. Section 820.162 refers to analysis of *actual* failed devices, i.e., the determination of the failure mechanism, and whether it is design or manufacturing related. Section 820.198 is intended to apply to the investigation of complaints involving *possible* failure of a device, i.e., an investigation to determine if there actually is a failure.

After devices are distributed, if they fail to meet specifications, the failed devices must be investigated if the manufacturer has them or can obtain them. Failure to meet specifications also includes packaging and labeling integrity failures. Technically, all devices returned for repair or service due to failure to meet specifications are subject to 820.162. The FDA, however, will accept routine service and repair records in lieu of the written record of investigation required by 820.162 as long as manufacturers have a system for identifying failure trends [820.20(a)(3)] and investigating the cause of the trends.

The significance of the device and any hazard the defective device presents should be taken into consideration when determining compliance with failure investigation requirements. Analysis must be taken to the level necessary to determine the actual failure mechanism, e.g., defective component, incorrect raw material, erosion, composition, etc. The cause of failure is obvious in some cases, and a formal investigation may not be needed. A record of the investigation, follow-up, and conclusions must be made in accordance with GMP sections 820.162 and 820.20(a)(3).

Failure analysis should be conducted by experienced personnel using a written protocol to assure that handling and testing do not compromise determining the cause of failure. A written protocol, however, is not a GMP requirement. The cause of a failure is identified to the point of objective reality such that appropriate corrective action can be taken.

When a systematic failure has been diagnosed, manufacturers need not analyze every device with the same diagnosed symptoms. However, enough devices must be analyzed to clearly establish symptoms before any assumptions are made about the cause of failure or about corrective actions. When an investigation verifies that a particular device characteristic such as component, design, etc., is deficient, and that this deficiency may exist in other product lines, the investigation must extend to determining the effect on other product lines.

When a failure is determined to be related to documentation, assembly, processing, labeling, testing, packaging, or other manufacturing operations, the manufacturing deficiency must be determined, corrected, and documented. If the failure is design-related, the design must be corrected in order for the devices to meet company quality claims and be in compliance with FD&C Act section 501(c).

IX. LABELING

A. Labeling Regulations

Drug delivery devices in commercial distribution in the United States must be properly labeled according to laws and regulations enforced by the FDA. Specific labeling requirements for medical devices are contained in:

The Federal Food, Drug and Cosmetic (FD&C) Act.
The Fair Packaging and Labeling Act.
The Radiation Control for Health and Safety Act.
Title 21 of the U.S. Code of Federal Regulations, Part 801 for
    general devices, and Part 809 for in vitro diagnostic products.
Title 21 of the U.S. Code of Federal Regulations, Part 820 for
    manufacturing controls for labeling.
Title 21 of the U.S. Code of Federal Regulations, Part 1010—
    Performance Standards for Electronic Products. Also see Parts
    1020 and 1040.

Section 201(k) of the FD&C Act defines the term "label" as "a display of written, printed, or graphic matter on the immediate container of any article . . . ." The term "immediate container" does not include a package liner. Any word, statement, or other information appearing on the immediate container must also appear on the outside container or wrapper, if any, of the retail package or be easily legible through the outside container or wrapper. This labeling is not required on the shipping carton.

Section 201(m) of the FD&C Act defines the term "labeling" as all labels and other written, printed, or graphic matter: (1) on the device or any of its containers or wrappers, or (2) accompanying the device. The term applies any time the article is in interstate commerce, or being held for sale after shipment or delivery in interstate commerce. The term "accompanied" is interpreted liberally. It extends to posters, tags, pamphlets, circulars, booklets, direction sheets, fillers, etc., that may be displayed in proximity to the article or shipped to the user before or after shipment of the device.

The distinction between labeling and advertising, of which both draw attention to the article to be sold, is often nebulous or superficial. Both are forms of publicity and are used for an identical purpose. According to an appellate court decision: "Most, if not all, labeling is advertising. The term 'labeling' is defined in the Act [Section 201(k)] as including all printed matter accompanying any article. Congress did not, and we cannot, exclude from this definition printed matter which constitutes advertising."

Section 502(f)(1) and (2) of the FD&C Act requires that device labeling bear adequate directions for use, operating, and servicing instructions, and either adequate warnings against uses dangerous to health, or information necessary for the protection of users. All devices require directions for use unless specifically exempted by regulation. Conditions for exemption from this requirement are in 21 CFR 801, Subpart D.

Misbranding

Section 502 of the FD&C Act contains the misbranding provisions for drugs and devices. It states that a device is misbranded if:

Its labeling is false or misleading.

Its packaging does not bear a label containing the name and place of business of the manufacturer, packer, or distributer, and an accurate statement of the quantity of contents.

Words, statements, or other required information are not prominent on the labeling or are not stated clearly.

It is intended for human use, and the label fails to bear the name and quantity or proportion of any narcotic or habit-forming substance contained in the product, and fails to display the statement, "Warning: may be habit forming."

Its label does not contain adequate directions for use. These include warnings against use in certain pathological conditions; by children where its use may be dangerous to health; against unsafe dosage, methods, duration of administration or application unless exempt as unnecessary to protect the public health.

It is dangerous to health when used in the dosage or manner, or with the frequency or duration prescribed, recommended, or suggested in the labeling.

It does not comply with the color additive provisions listed under section 706 of the FD&C Act.

The Medical Device Amendments expanded the authority of the FD&C Act over misbranded medical devices. These amendments contain further circumstances under which a device is misbranded:

The device's established name, if it has one, name in an official compendium, or common or usual name, is not printed prominently in type at least half as large as used for any proprietary name.

The device is subject to a performance standard and it does not bear the labeling requirements prescribed in that standard.

There is a failure or refusal to comply with any requirement prescribed under section 518 on notification and other remedies; failure to furnish material or information requested by or under section 518; or failure to furnish any material or information requested by or under section 519 on records and reports.

The device is commercially distributed without FDA concurrence on a 510(k) premarket notification submission.

False or Misleading Labeling

Section 502(a) states that a drug or device is misbranded if its labeling proves false or misleading in any particular. It is not a necessary condition that the labeling should be flatly and baldly false for the FDA to take action. The word "misleading" in the FD&C Act means that labeling is deceptive if it creates or leads to a false impression in the mind of a reader. A "false impression" may result not only from a false or deceptive statement, but may be instilled in the mind of the purchaser by ambiguity and indirection. It might be caused by failure to inform the consumer of facts that are relevant to those statements actually made. In other words, the label that remains silent as to certain consequences may be as deceptive as the label that contains extravagant claims. Examples of misleading labeling include ambiguity; half-truths and trade puffery; expressions of opinion or subjective statements; and failure to reveal material facts, consequences that may result from use, or the existence of difference of opinion.

Objectionable labeling includes such practices as deceptive pictorial matter, misleading testimonials, misleading lists of parts or components, and brand or trade names instead of "established names" [see section 201(h), 502(e)(2), and 508 of the FD&C Act]. Examples of false representations are

Incorrect, inadequate, or incomplete identification
Unsubstantiated claims of therapeutic value
Inaccuracies concerning condition, state, treatment, size, shape, or style
Substitution of parts or material
Subjective or unsubstantiated quality or performance claims
Use of the prefex U.S. or other similar indication suggesting government or agency approval or endorsement of the product

Adequate Directions for Use

Title 21, CRF Part 801.5, defines "adequate directions for use" as "directions under which the layman can use a device safely and for the purpose for which it is intended." See Part 801.4 for a definition of "intended use."

Among other reasons, directions for use may be inadequate because there is partial or total omission or incorrect specification of one or more of the following items.

Statement of all conditions, purposes, or uses for which the device is intended. This includes conditions, purposes, or uses for which it is prescribed, recommended, or suggested in its oral, written, printed, or graphic advertisting. Also conditions, purposes, or uses for which the drug or device is commonly used; except that these statements shall not refer to conditions, uses, or purposes for which the drug or device can be used safely only under the supervision of a practitioner licensed by law and for which it is advertised solely to such practitioner.

Quantity of dose including usual quantities for each intended use and usual quantities for persons of different ages and physical conditions.

Frequency of administration or application.

Duration of administration or application.

Time of administration or application in relation to meals, onset of symptoms, or other time factors.

Preparation for use, adjustment of temperature, or other manipulation or process.

Prescription Devices

Labeling exemptions for prescription devices are in 21 CFR Part 801.109. These are devices that because of a potential for harmful effect, method of use, or the collateral measures necessary to use, are not safe except under the supervision of a practitioner licensed by law. Hence "adequate directions for use" cannot be prepared for these devices. They are exempt from section 502(f)(1) of the FD&C Act provided that all conditions specified in the labeling regulation are met.

These conditions state that the device must be in the possession of a person, or his or her agents, or employees regularly and lawfully engaged in the manufacture, transportation, storage, or wholesale distribution of prescription devices; or in the possession of a practitioner such as physician, dentist, or veterinarian licensed by law to use or order the use of these devices. These devices can be sold only to, on the prescription of, or order of such practitioner for use in the course of their professional practice.

The label of the prescription device other than instruments is required to bear:

The statement "Caution: Federal law restricts this device to sale by or on the order of a _____ ", the blank to be filled with the word "physician," "dentist," "veterinarian," or with the descriptive designation of any other practitioner licensed by the law of the state in which he or she practices to use or order the use of the device; and
The method for its application or use.

Labeling on or within the package from which the device is to be dispensed must also bear information for use under which practitioners licensed by law to administer the device can use the device safely and for the purposes for which it is advertised or represented. Labeling information on administration includes indications, effects, dosages, routes, methods, frequency, and duration. Safety labeling includes relevant information on hazards, contraindications, side effects, and precautions.

When a device is capable of producing serious injury, even when used by a person thoroughly familiar with its operation, the directions for use must provide detailed information. For example, the Food and Drug Administration has specific regulations on the labeling of intrauterine contraceptive devices, 21 CFR 801.427, and for diagnostic x-ray devices, 21 CFR 1020.30(h). In addition, the FDA has issued general guidelines for labeling certain devices, i.e., transcutaneous electrical nerve stimulators and electrical muscle stimulators.

Where appropriate, directions for use must be supplemented with adequate warnings against the use of the drug or device under certain conditions. Any caution statement, similar to the directions statement, may appear in the labeling of the product; it is not necessary that it be printed on the label. In each instance, the responsibility for the adequacy of the warning statement appearing on the labeling rests with the manufacturer or distributor. For some devices, there are national consensus standards that specify that certain caution statements be on the device.

Sterile Devices

Special attention should be given to the labeling of sterile drug delivery devices. Devices that are not sterile in their entirety (for example, sterility may be needed only for the lumen of certain devices) must be labeled to properly inform users what is actually intended to be "sterile" in the package. For example, a possible limiting statement might be: *"Caution:* Only the fluid path of the set is sterile and nonpyrogenic. Do not use in a sterile or aseptic area without proper precautions."

Some devices are intended to be sterilized by the user before use. In this situation, the labeling should provide adequate information as to the method of sterilization and any precautions or safeguards to be followed. For example, the labeling should describe any:

Special cleaning methods required

Changes in the physical characteristics of the device that may result from reprocessing that affect is safety, effectiveness, or performance

Limit on the number of times resterilization and reuse can be done without affecting the safety or effectiveness of the device

In the case of single-use sterile devices, many manufacturers include labeling to advise against resterilization and reuse. Some devices are simply not designed or constructed to be recleaned, and may not be capable of withstanding the necessary recleaning and resterilization procedures. Where reuse is common practice, manufacturers are encouraged to provide the information described in the above list.

The label of multidevice kits or packages containing a combination of sterile and nonsterile products must not state or imply that all contents are sterile.

The need for users to have instructions on how to open a sterile device package to avoid contamination of the device also needs to be evaluated, and when necessary, such instructions should be included in the labeling.

When the manufacturer modifies a device, the manufacturer must also review the labeling to ensure that it reflects current revisions and specifications. Some manufacturers identify labeling with a drawing number plus a revision code or date as an aid in identifying current labeling. The package insert or other labeling for in vitro diagnostic products is required to contain the revision data [21 CFR 809.10(b)(15)].

Shelf-life dating solely for package integrity and sterility is not usually required for general medical devices. There may be a need for expiration dating when a particular component of a device, such as a battery or diagnostic reagent, has a finite useful life. Labeling for in vitro diagnostic devices [809.10(a) and (b)] requires an expiration date or some other means by which users may be assured of quality at the time of use. This requirement applies to both sterile and nonsterile in vitro diagnostic devices.

Although not required by regulation, most manufacturers of complex devices and sterile devices voluntarily use lot or serial numbers for production control and, if the need arises, to expedite failure investigations, repairs, modifications, or recalls. Lot, batch, or other control numbers are required for:

Critical devices (820.121)
Some products subject to radiological health standards
In vitro diagnostic devices [809.10(a)(9)]

Adequate labeling for a medical device requires proper design and procurement of the labels and labeling. Design includes labeling content that meets the requirement of the GMP regulation as well as the needs of the customer. To achieve these goals a number of concepts must be kept in mind, such as writing to the reader, referring to the actual device in labeling, obvious identification of the controls used, etc. These concerns as well as others are discussed on the following pages.

B. Content Development and Approval

There are some basic guidelines, rules, and practices that can be used to immediately improve writing of labeling. The following paragraphs will discuss them, with emphasis on how they can be used to make labeling clear and comprehensible. Writers are also encouraged to obtain and use a standard college-level text on technical writing.

As an essential aid, writers are encourage to obtain a copy of *40,000 Words*, a similarly titled book by any of the reference book publishing companies. Most of these reference books have about four pages of punctuation rules. Using the four small pages of rules can immediately improve your writing. For example, you can avoid the common punctuation error of not using semicolons to replace commas when needed for clarity and as required by punctuation rules.

Write to the Reader

The most serious problem is that writers tend to write to themselves. Their material is clear to them—and they mistakenly think it is as clear to others. For example, the sensitivity control on an instrument is called "gain" control on page 1 of the instruction manual, "amplitude" control on page 2, and "level" control in the next section. Further, the photograph in the Introduction shows the same control with a call-out labeled "Signal Adjust." No wonder readers are confused! Yet the author of the example knew what he was trying to write about and, most certainly, he was writing to himself. In order to write to the reader, the author must refer to the actual configuration of the device, use obvious identification of controls, avoid distractions, be clear and concise, avoid gobbledygook, try the labeling, and know the reading level of the intended audience.

Refer to Actual Device

One simple way to reduce control identity confusion as described above, reduce other types of labeling errors, and increase clarity is for authors to keep a labeled drug delivery device kit or photograph(s) nearby and refer to it as they write. It is easier to write the truth when you know the truth. Make sure the terminology and descriptions in the labeling matches that on the device. Always use the same title for each given item or control throughout the manual, insert, label, or advertisement. Likewise, the same title should be used in charts, figures, or screen displays such as cathode-ray tubes, LCD panels, etc. Remember to:

Write to your intended readers.
Write with a labeled device or photographs in sight.
Use consistent titles.

Identify Controls

Because the titles of control items in screen displays and other labeling should be exactly the same as in the labels on delivery devices, accessories, etc., authors need to develop and use an appropriate correlation technique for corresponding titles in instruction manuals, package inserts, etc. One common technique is to use all capitals for titles of device controls in labeling. For example:

Flip the POWER switch to ON.
Now press the HEAT button to switch the heater on.
In about three seconds, the READY lamp will illuminate.

With this correlation technique, the words "on" and "off" are capitalized in the labeling only when they actually appear on the instrument control panel. Note that "ON" is capitalized in "POWER switch to ON," as the actual switch has "POWER," "ON," and "OFF" printed by it. In contrast, note that "on" is not capitalized in the example "to switch the heater on," as it is not a label of a control on the device. Also, be careful to use a simple correlation system that is readily apparent to the intended audience.

Don't Distract the Reader

Readers are very busy trying to learn how to use a new device. They should not be annoyed by unnecessary distractions such as:

Changes in format
Unusual typeface
Incorrect page numbers
Incorrect figure numbers

For a person trying to read in a hurry, a font or typestyle that
the author may consider to be routine, such as script, can be a major
distraction: therefore, don't use script, italics, or any other unusual
or hard-to-read typefaces. Remember, you have decided to write
for the benefit of the intended audience. Forget about your personal preferences and use only the most common fonts. Select a type
size that is readable at the intended distance. For example, labeling
displayed on the screen of a wall-mounted heart monitor must be
readable from several feet away. Also, use a consistent format
throughout the document. And, check the format and section titles
against information on the contents page. In some cases, the arrangement of information in the labeling may be dictated by a regulation.
Page numbers should not be referenced in instruction or service
manuals. It is too easy for the actual page numbers to be changed
during the original writing or when the manual is updated. It is
much better to refer to paragraph titles or paragraph numbers, as
they are less likely to change; and, if changed, titles are more
noticeable to writers and typists than are page numbers. Always
place figures close to the corresponding text. The use of correct
figure numbers is easy—just check them.

Be Short and to the Point

It is important to use sentence structure that will convey the intended message with a minimum of misinterpretation or need to
reread. Tests have been conducted to determine the ability of
readers to follow instructions in a sentence based on the number of
activities to be performed. The average person's ability to follow
instructions decreases rapidly when a sentence contains more than
two facts. (Keep in mind your own experiences in reading instructions.) Therefore, sentences in labeling need to be short and to
the point. Avoid long strings of adjectives, and be specific. In
many cases a *list* of activities to be performed is better than burying
the facts in long sentences. If it takes lots of words to get to the
point, the reader will probably miss the point! Short, choppy sentences are acceptable in instruction manuals and other labeling. You
are not trying to entertain readers with beautiful, flowing prose—
rather, you want to "shock" them into remembering key facts until
they correctly perform the specified instructions. Thus:

Use lists or short sentences.
Get to the point.
Be specific.

Try to be as specific as possible with your instructions. For example, "ambient" or "room temperature" generally should not be
used. Instead, specify the desired or necessary range of operating
conditions.

Avoid Gobbledygook

Another way to be more specific and shorten sentences is to avoid "gobbledygook." The following terms were collected from actual instruction manuals:

Original	Equivalent
Makes provisions for	*
Serves to	*
At the time of	When
In conjunction with	And
Carried out in	Perform
Comes up to	Reaches
Will also serve as a change to	May
Will be sure that will	Ensure
Available through the use of	*
Care should be used so as not to	Be careful
Be provided for positive determination	*
Causes power to be applied to	Switches power to

In most cases, the equivalent term in the list can replace the original term. For the asterisked items, the equivalent is simply a direct statement of what is intended. On the terms listed, the combinations most often used are "makes provision for" and "serves to." Simply eliminating these from labeling will result in an immediate improvement for readers.

Introduce Each Item

Always introduce each control, indicator, device, or subject before it is discussed in the text. The introductions should be brief and may be very brief. Keep in mind that the items will be described in more detail later. Abbreviations and new or uncommon terms must be defined. The introductions and definitions prevent readers from going into mental shock, breaking their train of thought, and asking: What is this? By then some readers have probably forgotten the last two or three facts read. Also, readers may wonder about any "cliff-hanging" item when they resume reading. This disturbance

may detract people from fully assimilating the next instructions being
read.   To avoid distractions and confusion, a writer of labeling
should always:

Introduce each item.
Define new or uncommon terms.

With respect to definitions, a writer should never give a new
meaning to an existing term.   For example, quality assurance personnel of medical device firms can no longer use the word "critical"
in their routine technical conversations, because "critical" was given
a specialized definition in the GMP regulation.   To avoid this dis-
service, coin a special term or code number such as Class C, Code
1, or Level 2.

Accent Key Terms

Whenever it is stated in instructions that something must be done,
then "must" should be underlined, set in bold type, or otherwise
delineated.   Likewise, caution and warning statements should be
delineated by underlining, boxing, bold type, etc.   Refer to regulations or standards for a specific product, if any, and use the
recommended or required caution statements.   When standard terminology exists, creating new caution statements is not the best way
for a writer to be creative.

Select Words Wisely

When large print is needed for reading at a distance or to attract
attention, signs, caution labels, screen prompts, and control labels
generally must be short in order to fit the available space.   This
situation places a burden on the writer to select terms that convey
the desired message.   Consider the following wording from two actual
highway signs:

PLANT TRAFFIC   NO FISHING
ENTERING HIGHWAY   OFF BRIDGE

Have you ever been run over by a pachysandra?   If you can't
fish off the bridge, does that mean you are allowed to fish only on
or from the bridge?   Better choices for the intended messages are
"Traffic entering highway" and "No fishing from bridge."

Try Labeling

Finally, always have people who are not familiar with the product
operate it *exactly* according to the draft instructions and screen
displays, if any.   People may need to be selected who have low

reading levels if the product is to be used at home. No coaching—
this is the "acid" test—good luck! During the trials, note any
significant problems and make appropriate corrections to the instructions, prompts, or other labeling.

Approval Policy and Procedure

Before release for use, labeling should be reviewed and approved
by product development, service, marketing, quality assurance, and
other appropriate managers. Firms need to have a policy/procedure
that covers the drafting, review, and approval of labeling. Approval
forms are generally used in conjunction with such a policy/procedure.
A sample approval form and procedure, Exhibit 3, are presented
later in this section. Other procedures and forms such as "Change
Control" are referenced in this procedure. Note that this procedure
also covers some GMP elements such as a correct master record, correct transfer of labels into production, lot control, change control,
etc.

C. GMP Control of Labeling

Drug delivery device manufacturers must incorporate in their QA
program several elements that relate to labeling in order to meet
the requirements of the GMP regulation. The QA program must be
adequate to assure that labeling meets the device master record requirements with respect to legibility, adhesion, etc., and assure
that labeling operations are controlled so that the correct labeling
is always issued and used.

Because several activities must be performed and controlled
during the development and use of labeling, Table 4 is presented
as a guideline or checklist. It contains a typical sequence of events
required to develop and control labeling.

Labeling includes equipment labels, control labels, package labels,
directions for use, maintenance manuals, etc. The displays on
CRTs and other electronic message panels are considered labeling
if instructions and parameter identification information are given.

Various sections of the GMP regulation have an impact on labeling:
Section 820.20(a)(2) requires approval or rejection of packaging
materials and labeling; and section 820.40 requires building to be
of suitable design and to have sufficient space for packaging and labeling operations. Section 820.120 deals with specific requirements for
the design and control of labeling. It applies to the physical design
application of labeling to assure legibility under normal conditions
of use over the expected life of the device, and also to inspection,
handling, storage, and distribution of labeling. The FDA considers
a device to be adulterated if these requirements are not met. These
requirements do not apply to the adequacy of labeling content, except to ensure that the content meets the labeling specifications con-

Table 4 Typical Sequence of the GMP Control of Labels

Phase	GMP device type[a]		Section[b]	Control activity
	NC	C		
1. Development	NC	C	.120 & .100	Text review. Quality of mounting (rivets, adhesives, etc.). Quality of ink, anodize, etc. Content per 21 CFR 801, 807, 809, company claims and standards.
2. Evaluation	NC	C	.120	Simulated or actual processing (e.g., sterilization), shipping tests, etc.
3. Documentation	NC	C	.181	Approve, date, and change control label drawings.
		C	.121a	A key label must contain control number of finished device.
4. File sample		C	.182b	Copy of actual label or artwork in the master record. See .181.
5. Procurement	NC	C	.120a	Proofread before release to inventory stock.
		C	.121b	Record signature of proofreader and date.
6. Storage	NC	C	.120d	Store labels so as to prevent mixups.
		C	.121c	Restrict access to labels to authorized persons.

Table 4 (Continued).

Phase	GMP device type[a]		Section[b]	Control activity
7. Separate operations	NC	C	.120b	Separate multiple operations to prevent mixups.
8. Area inspection	NC	C	.120c	Before beginning labeling operations, designee to inspect area and remove extraneous devices and labels.
9. Issuance	NC	C	.120e	Examine for identity and, where appropriate, expiration date and control number. Record date and person examining labels.
10. Inspection	NC	C	.160	Inspect finished device per written procedure.
		C	.161	Designee must check all acceptance records and test results and see that records are present and complete.

[a]NC = noncritical; C = critical.
[b]Numbers refer to Part 820, e.g., .120 is 820.120.

tained in the device master record. However, failure to comply with GMP requirements such as proofreading and change control could result in content errors. In such cases, the device is misbranded and adulterated.

Specifications are required in the device master record for the content and physical design parameters of labels. (See Section V.) Labeling specifications are the engineering drawing and/or artwork for each label, appropriate inspection or control procedures, and appropriate procedures for attaching the labels. All procedures, drawings, and artwork must have the name of the preparer, an approval signature, and a date. The approval signature, date, etc., may be on the back side of artwork or on a label approval form. Further, artwork may contain only an identification code or title if the "content" of the artwork is duplicated on approved engineering drawings or adequately identified (cross-referenced) with respect to the label approval form.

Hard-copy labels, package inserts, and similar labeling are specified and purchased as components. (See Section VIII.) For correct purchase and use of labeling, specifications are usually stated on engineering drawings and/or purchase specifications. Thus, artwork or "copy" alone will not fulfill the device master record requirements for labeling except for the most simplistic labeling such as brief errata sheets.

The engineering drawings or purchase specifications must specify, as appropriate, the label substrate, dimensions, ink, finish, mounting method, etc., so that the purchased label will remain attached and legible during the customary conditions of processing, storage, handling, distribution, and use.

Front panels, other instrument panels, meters, fuses, pushbuttons, and the like often either are labels or contain labels and thus must, as appropriate, meet GMP master record and control requirements. Component specifications, assembly drawings, and test/inspection procedures are appropriate GMP controls to prevent mixup of meters, pushbuttons, and other labeled instrument controls. Controls to prevent mixups are generally not needed for front and other panels.

Whether a firm considers a software-driven display to be labeling or data makes little difference under the GMP regulation, because, either way, the finished device labeling or data must meet the device master record specifications. When firms develop and validate software, they should also review these electronic displays to see that the "labeling" meets all applicable requirements, such as adherence to specifications in the master record, correct parameter identification, agreement with the instruction manual, and, of course, correct display of performance data.

When reviewing or auditing labeling operations, it is wise to keep in mind that the GMP regulation is a flexible quality assurance pro-

gram. The degree of labeling control needed to satisfy the GMP
regulation varies considerably for different devices and operations.
In order to avoid wasting money and increasing the cost of health
care, manufacturers need to give considerable and prudent thought
to the appropriate level of control needed for their operations as
allowed by section 820.5. Information and guidelines presented in
this chapter should aid manufacturers in making these decisions.
The level of control needed should be reconsidered when products
are changed. Likewise, the controls needed and success of the
existing control program must be reviewed during QA system audits.
(See Section XIII.)

Label Integrity

All labels must be designed and applied to devices and containers
so that the labels will remain in place and legible during the customary conditions of distribution, storage, and use. Likewise, other
labeling such as user instructions should remain legible during customary storage and use. Note that 820.120(a), which states,
"Labels shall be designed, printed, and applied so as to remain
legible . . . ." refers to the actual design of the label and mounting method—not just testing or inspection of these to show that
design requirements have been met. [Inspection is covered by the
second sentence of 820.120(a), and by 820.120(e), 820.20(a),
820.80, and 820.160.] For example, labeling printed by machines
onto plastic plates is often smeared and thus in inadequate [FD&C Act,
502(f)]. The manufacturers of such items must assure that the
print is legible and will remain legible until used.
    Labels may be mounted by adhesives, screws, rivets, drive
screws, etc., or printed or etched onto panels and/or onto controls.
The labels should be located so that they will be seen but not be
abraded during use. (All of us have seen the cases where safety
labels on ladders and riding lawnmowers were placed in the foot rest
areas. Of course, they were worn off after a few uses!)

Receipt and Inspection

Upon receipt, all packaging and labeling materials, including preprinted containers, inserts, and preprinted packaging materials, must
be examined and, if deemed necessary by the company, tested to assure conformance with specifications as discussed in Section VI.
Also, samples of labels must be proofread by a designated individu-
al(s). After being accepted by a responsible individual, these components may be placed into inventory or into production. These inspections must be recorded in the device history record as required
by 820.80(a) and 820.120 to show that inspection and proofreading
were performed. The inspection record for device labeling should
be kept simple.

Area Separation and Inspection

All labeling and packaging operations should be separated to the
degree necessary (820.5 and 820.40) to assure that there are no
mixups between similar products or labels. Separation may be either
a physical or spatial separation or by performing the labeling and
packaging at different times for different devices. Separation is not
required when mixups are impossible, such as in the case of labeled
front panels that fit only the intended family of instruments (devices).

The likelihood of a labeling mixup determines how stringent production area controls should be. For example, label control need
not be stringent if only dissimilar products and labeling are processed. Before beginning any packaging and labeling operation in
which mixup could occur, the production area and equipment for the
operation must be thoroughly examined to ensure that any devices
and labeling materials remaining from previous operations have been
removed. It is important to make certain that the surrounding area,
tables, packaging lines, printing machines, and other equipment are
cleared of labels and other materials used in the previous operation.

Unused labeling that contains precoded serial numbers, manufacturing date, expiration date, control number, etc., should be destroyed and not returned to the label storage area. The GMP regulation does not require reconciliation of the number of labels used
versus the number issued, although this control is recommended for
some devices, such as when different sizes of the same product are
being packaged or otherwise labeled.

Storage

All printed packaging and labeling materials, including preprinted
containers, inserts, and preprinted packaging materials, must be
stored in an area and manner suitable to prevent mixups (820.40,
820.120). Labeling should be identified and segregated to the degree
necessary to prevent mixing of similar labeling. Access to labeling
should be limited to authorized personnel.

Storage control should be appropriate for the number and kind of
devices. For example, a firm that manufactures only one product
with one label does not need an elaborately controlled storage area.
Similarly, a firm with only a few types of devices having dissimilar
labeling would not normally require stringent control.

One case that requires dedicated attention to storage and control
is prelabeled "sterile" but not-yet-sterilized devices. Firms must
make absolutely certain that mixups cannot occur. Also, *make certain* that all such samples, if used for market promotion, are sterile
or stamped with a manifest caution statement, because a packaged
and labeled market-promotion sample might be used by the recipient.

Quality awareness training is required by section 820.25, and
marketing personnel must be informed of labeling control requirements and the consequences of a violation.

Label Check and Record

When issued for use, labeling must be carefully examined to assure
that the contents of the labeling comply with the labeling specifications in the device master record. This examination must include
any control numbers or expiration dates used on the labels. A
record of this issuance check, including the date and name of the
person performing the examination, must be made in the device
history record.

If expiration dates are used, they must reflect the time after final
packaging during which the device is fit for its intended use when
stored and used per its labeling. The manufacturer should have
stability test data that establishes the interval during which the device remains fit for use.

If label mixups *cannot* occur—for example, a firm makes only one
device or uses only one label—and there are no control numbers or
expiration dates, the original inspection when the labeling is placed
into inventory is an adequate check for compliance with the master
record specifications. A second check need not be performed because it serves no purpose (820.5). If, however, there is any possibility that incorrect labeling can be used, a second check must
be made when the labeling is issued for application, packaging, or
shipping.

Critical Device Labeling

Labeling for critical devices must meet the noncritical device labeling
requirements and must also meet the three additional requirements
in section 820.121 as covered below.

Control number. Critical device labeling must contain a control
number, serial number, letters, etc., for traceability. This means
a control number for the finished device, and not the label itself.
Most labeling, however, also contains another number, such as a
drawing number, for control of labeling configuration and procurement.

The control number for traceability need not be on every label
on the device; however, the control number must appear on the
unit label that goes to the ultimate user. The label on a shipping
carton does not meet this requirement, because bulk items may go
to a central distribution point in the user facility and the shipping
carton will most likely be discarded. In order to meet this traceability requirement, a label that will most likely reach the nurse
or other user station must have the control number.

Proofreader's signature. Before releasing labeling for critical devices to inventory, samples of labeling must be proofread as required for noncritical devices. In addition, the signature of the proofreader and the date of the proofreading must be recorded in the device history record.

Access restriction. Access to labeling must be restricted to authorized personnel. Labeling also should be stored in an adequately segregated area to minimize the change of mixups. Although the access requirement applies to labeling for critical devices, it is also recommended for labeling for noncritical devices because it increases the control over the label storage area with no significant increase in cost.

D. Revisions

Labeling is part of the device master record; therefore, all changes to labeling must be made under a formal change control system similar to that required for specifications [820.100(a)(2)]. Any changes to labeling must be formally reviewed and authorized before implementation as discussed in Section V.

When making changes to primary aspects of a device and to primary documentation, the review group must determine if any secondary items such as labels or instructions are affected and also need changing. There should be a checkoff block on change order forms for recording that the effect of the primary change on labeling was considered and appropriate action was taken.

Shipping for Processing

Drug delivery devices that have been sterilized and shipped to the manufacturer's warehouse or other *controlled* distribution point before final release must be properly labeled. The pallets, or designated unit, must be marked to indicate the status of the device, such as "nonsterile," "sterilized: awaiting test results," or an equivalent statement. The company must be able to show that it has control of the devices until final release and, if necessary, could have them destroyed or returned for reprocessing. For this reason, a distributor's warehouse or facility is not considered a controlled distribution point. For regulations on distribution, see 21 CFR 801, Subparts A and E; and sections 820.150, 820.160, and 820.161.

The drafting and approval procedure shown in Exhibit 3 is used to establish a uniform system for controlling the content of labeling and for approving labeling. This procedure is adaptable to use by any size firm.

Exhibit 3 Drafting and Approval of Labeling

POLICY/PROCEDURE TITLE: **Drafting and Approval of Labeling**

Procedure Number _____   Revision Level _____

Prepared By _____ App. By _____ Date _____

ECN History _____

1.0 PURPOSE

To establish a uniform procedure for controlling the content of labels and obtaining label approval.

To assure compliance with GMP requirements and with company policy directives.

2.0 SCOPE

Applies to all devices including those used for market research or clinical investigations.

Promotional material is excluded from this SOP. It is covered by SOP #___, "Promotional Material Control and Approval."

3.0 REFERENCE DOCUMENTS

3.1   Food and Drug Administration GMP requirements
3.2   SOP #___, "Promotional Material Control and Approval"
3.3   SOP #___, "Change Control System"

4.0 FORMS

4.1   Form SOP #___, Labeling Approval Form
4.2   Form SOP #___, Engineering Change Order Form

5.0 DEFINITIONS

5.1   Labeling is all labels and other written, printed or graphic matter accompanying or attached to the device or its container.

6.0 PROCEDURE

6.1 **Preparation and Approval**

6.1.1   The need for a label or labeling is determined by an operating department such as Engineering, Marketing, Manufacturing, or Quality Assurance.

6.1.2   The Engineering Department prepares a manuscript complete with illustrations or prepares a drawing(s) of the label showing the wording, label use, and/or location.

6.1.3   The Engineering Services Department then prepares form SOP #___, "Labeling Approval Form", and circulates it to the originating department, Training and Education, Marketing, and Quality Assurance for approval. (See the following approval form in this manual.)

6.1.4   Engineering Services will coordinate and keep track of all label approvals and approval forms.

Exhibit 3 (Continued).

    6.1.5 When approval is received, the label or manuscript is assigned a drawing number and is released and added to the product structure (DMR Index) following the Engineering Change Control System (SOP #___).

    6.2 **Implementation and Control**

    6.2.1 When the labels or labeling (printed material) are produced. Quality Control must proofread the material and verify that it is correct and so indicate by signing an appropriate document (first article inspection.)

    6.2.2 All labels and labeling will be reviewed for criticality and lot control requirements. Each document will be marked to indicate the level of control required. At least one label on each critical device must have a lot, serial, or other control number.

7.0 **EXPERIMENTAL DEVICES**

    7.1 Labels and labeling for experimental devices is required.

    7.2 The documentation need not be as complete as for production labels and labeling; but, it must be adequate to allow procurement of the labels or labeling and adequate for the intended use.

8.0 **CHANGES**

    8.1 Any changes to labels or labeling are accomplished by SOP #___. "Change Control System".

9.0 **SCHEDULES**

    9.1 Drafts must be generated according to a schedule that allows a normal approval procedure. While urgent copy approval is occasionally necessary, it should not become standard operating procedure.

X. PACKAGING

A. Packaging Design and Materials

Manufacturers of drug delivery devices should integrate the design of the device, packaging, and manufacturing processes; and they should consider the needs of the user. They must document these designs in the device master record; then, procure, handle, store, and use the specified materials according to the master record.

Packaging and sealing machines must be set up according to a written procedure based on the known process capability of the packaging and sealing system. Process capability must be determined by validation. The results must be documented.

Finally, manufacturers must perform quality assurance tests on the finished packages and, if sterilized, repeat the tests after sterilization. The results of testing and/or inspection must be recorded in the device history records. Performing these activities correctly can prevent product liability actions and recalls.

An effective primary package for a medical device should be designed and developed along with the product as discussed in Section II. In fact, the total device and package system should be considered with respect to device characteristics, sterilization process, bonding, labeling, secondary packaging, shipping, environment, end use, and federal regulations. Defective packaging and seals have been a major cause of medical device recalls—recalls that can be eliminated by correct design of the device and package system; correct design and validation of packaging and sealing processes; and subsequent production, packaging, and sealing of the device under an adequate quality assurance system.

During development, if design tests and analysis point toward limited reliability, changes in the device, packaging, sealing method, and manufacturing processes should be made before production starts in order to minimize cost and liability. Package redesign, change of sterilization process, even device redesign during the development states, might prevent needless patient risk and save dollars that might be spent later in replacing damaged or contaminated goods and, of course, the belated redesign will cost the same or more than if it had been performed before production started.

The package and device should be designed together so that all factors in the product and package system can be considered, such as device sharp edges and severe vacuum stresses. Some factors to consider are

End use	Sterilization process
Temperature	Adhesives
Moisture resistance	Package porosity
Thermal capacity	Cling resistance
Device composition	Pressure
Device size and shape	Vacuum

It is important to be aware of the state-of-the-art in sealing methods and packaging materials, including their physical, chemical, biological, and compatibility characteristics and, of course, cost. If necessary, obtain guidance from suppliers, technical literature, and consultants.

FDA regulations are compatible with this total system approach to device, package, and process design. To assure the integrity and appropriate sterility assurance level of sterile medical devices, the FDA regulates devices, their processing, and their packaging. The FDA assures that adequate device packaging is used mainly by implementing the Good Manufacturing Practice regulation. Also, the quality of packaging must be appropriately considered in relation to the 21 CFR Part 812, investigational device exemptions (IDEs) for clinical evaluations; Part 814, premarket approval (PMA) applications;

Part 807, premarket notification [510(k)] submissions, and, of course, customer requirements.

Requirements for components, device master records, environmental control, etc., that affect the selection and use of packaging appear throughout the GMP regulation. The specific requirements for packaging are in section 820.130; and the closely related label integrity requirements are in section 820.120. The packaging requirement in the GMP regulation is not lengthy; however, it is far-reaching. For example, packaging is one of the few areas in the GMP regulation where design is addressed directly. Section 820.130 states that: "The device package and any shipping container for a device shall be designed and constructed to protect the device from alteration or damage during the customary conditions of processing, storage, handling, and distribution."

As can be seen from the regulation, the primary package and the secondary package or shipping container must adequately protect the device under all reasonable conditions from packaging to ultimate use. Failure to meet this requirement renders a device adulterated and has resulted in recalls of sterile devices.

Sterile devices and their packages must be designed to meet the requirements of the sterilization process, package sealing method, and intended use. For example, radiation sterilization may discolor packaging and sealing materials, or modify their functional capabilities. All plastics are somewhat affected by radiation sterilization, and consideration should be given to the effect produced and the radiation dose needed to produce an effect. In some materials, parameters are improved, whereas in others, they are degraded by radiation. Complete storage and stability data should be compiled for sterilization packaging or obtained from the vendor.

In addition to the GMP requirements, manufacturers should al ways study current packaging practices for products similar to theirs to determine current favorable practices and to prevent packaging problems. For example, customary use may dictate the use of double primary packaging for some sterile devices.

The design and processing factors noted above must be considered when selecting packaging, adhesives, and sealing method. Finally, any packaging used for medical devices must satisfy the end user as well as GMP requirements—a key point to be considered during the design phrase.

B. Procurement, Acceptance, and Storage

The device master record (820.181) must contain appropriate specifications such that the desired packaging components may be purchased, properly stored, and properly used. A manufacturer must have adequate procedures for approval or rejection of all incoming

packaging components, such as adhesives, pouches, and cartons
(see 820.80 and Section VI). The supplier might test these components and provide the manufacturer with a protocol for testing
and the test results for each batch (i.e., certificate of conformance
to purchase specifications). The manufacturer could accept this
specific data as sufficient certification or order his own testing.

At a minimum, incoming components must be examined visually for
damage and identity before being used. Thereafter, primary packaging must be handled and stored in such a way that it is kept clean
and safe from damage. Primary packaging and devices to be sterilized must be kept especially clean before sterilization. For implant,
indwelling, and infusion devices, the firm must carefully and appropriately control the environment to which the associated packaging
materials are exposed in order to control bioburden and bacteria
cellular debris. Pyrogens arise primarily from cellular debris of
gram-negative bacteria.

C. Packaging Process

The packaging operation is a manufacturing process, and GMP sections 820.80, Components, 820.100(b), Processing Controls, and
820.160, Finished Device Inspection; apply to packaging. These
sections require adequate controls for components, processing, and
test/inspection. The controls necessary for all devices must assure
that:

> Labeling (separate label or printed on the package) properly re-
> flects the package contents.
> Only devices approved for release are packaged and released.

The controls required will vary with the type of device packaged.
For example, when a sterile device is packaged, a manufacturer's
considerations must include:

> Environmental and personnel hygiene control
> Validated operating procedures for sealing equipment
> Inspection to assure package integrity and sanitation
> Control of devices marked "sterile" but not yet sterilized

For a product to be sterilized in-house, either a physical quarantine area or label control must be used to prevent shipment of
devices that are marked sterile but not yet sterilized. The required
level of control is relatively high. The control extends to giveaway
samples: Samples *must* be sterile if so labeled, because they might
be used.

If the labeled product is to be shipped to a contract sterilizer, the shipping, handling, and processing must be controlled as required by the GMP regulation and section 801.150(e) of the labeling regulation. For all cases, the FDA recommends a contract as required by 801.150(e) for interstate shipping.

Section 820.181(d) requires that the device master record include packaging methods and processes. Written instructions should be provided to assure that the necessary controls are understood and consistently implemented. The need for and extent of written instructions should be determined based on the complexity of the operation and the nature of the product. Some products, such as radioimmunoassay test kits, can deteriorate during packaging if the process is not timed properly. In such cases, written instructions should describe how the device(s) should be handled and expedited during packaging in order to prevent delays and thus deterioration.

The process capability of packaging and sealing equipment should be determined by process validation and documented. Process validation must be performed for sealing systems for sterile devices. Then a sealing cycle is selected, verified, and written into a setup and operations procedure to be used for routine packaging and sealing of the device with the selected packaging materials.

The procedure for test and/or inspection of finished packages must be written (820.160). To the extent feasible, the testing of finished packages should be quantitative. The packaging of sterile devices should be tested and/or inspected before and after sterilization and is usually done on a sampling basis.

The results of test and/or inspection must be appropriately recorded in the device history record along with control (lot) numbers, if any. The use of lot numbers for sterile products is common practice. Control numbers are required for critical devices (820.121) and in vitro diagnostic products (820.10).

The test and/or inspection procedures must include any sampling plan(s) to be used when large quantities of devices are being produced or when the testing is destructive. Sampling plans are valid only when a process is in a state of control; therefore, the device must be manufactured and packaged using a quality assurance system as described in this chapter.

XI. DISTRIBUTION

A. Holding and Distribution Procedures

The device Good Manufacturing Practices (GMP) regulation covers the manufacture, distribution (820.150), and installation (820.152) of finished devices. Distribution is important from a quality assurance standpoint. After a product is distributed, a firm no longer has direct control over the product or how it is used. It is important that controls be in place to assure that only correctly labeled and approved finished drug delivery devices are distributed.

The GMP regulation requires that written procedures be provided for warehouse control and distribution of finished devices. The purpose of this requirement is to assure that only approved devices are distributed. Each manufacturer should determine whether written procedures will contribute to assuring that only "approved for release" devices are distributed from their firm. This flexibility is allowed by section 820.5 of the GMP regulation.

Many manufacturers mark their released finished devices or identify them by location or packaging so that a simple visual check is sufficient to indicate whether the product is acceptable for release for distribution. For example, for radiation-emitting electronic products subject to a performance standard, the application of the certification label is often the last step in approving product release for distribution; and the label is used to distinguish such devices. This type of operation may preclude the need for a written procedure.

For interstate contract sterilization, section 801.150(e) of the labeling regulations requires a written procedure to help prevent the erroneous release of packaged and labeled "sterile" but not yet sterilized devices that appear to be but are not ready for release. Regardless of whether 801.150(e) applies, the GMP regulation requires controls as necessary to prevent mixups in complex situations such as contract sterilization. For consistency, a contract as described by 801.150(e) is commonly used by manufacturers for interstate and intrastate contracts. Such a contract and compliance with it satisfies the applicable GMP requirements.

Sometimes manufacturers need to ship "finished devices" that have not been officially released because the final test data is not yet available. The most common example occurs when a firm is waiting for the results from biological indicator tests. Manufacturers may ship such devices to their own *controlled* warehouses or to other finished-device manufacturers, where the devices may be readily recalled if the need arises. Firms are *not* allowed to ship nonreleased devices to routine distributors. Nonreleased products or products on "hold" for any quality reason must be controlled to prevent release. A suitable control is quarantine or a label on the units, pallets, etc., to indicate the status.

Warehouse Storage

Storage should always take place under systematic, orderly conditions (820.40). Manufacturers must use a first-in, first-out (FIFO) distribution system when fitness for use of a device deteriorates over time (820.150).

When a controlled environment is necessary to prevent abnormal deterioration, the environment must be specified, controlled, and monitored according to sections 820.46 and 820.60 (see Section III). Environmental specifications, such as storage temperature, must be included in the device master record.

A designated person(s) should be responsible for storage and handling of devices to be distributed (820.25). These activities may be extensive. For example, damaged, recalled, or returned devices must be suitably marked and segregated from devices acceptable for release. Also, note that returned defective devices must be formally investigated according to 820.162 and any associated complaints investigated according to 820.198. Therefore, firms will need controls to assure that returned defective devices do not dead-end in the warehouse, but are expeditiously routed to the appropriate department for investigation, conclusions, and followup.

Distribution Records

GMP section 820.184, Device History Record, requires manufacturers of noncritical devices to maintain basic distribution records for the quantity distributed, and any control number used. These may be the same as, or part of, the normal business records. Generation of a separate record is not required unless the business records are not readily available, e.g., not maintained at the same establishment as the device history record. For purposes of recall, repairs, etc., a firm may elect to keep more records than specified by the GMP regulation, such as the date shipped and consignee information.

In addition to the requirements for noncritical devices, manufacturers of critical devices must maintain distribution records that contain:

Consignee name
Consignee address
Quantity shipped
Date shipped
Control number

Many firms, regardless of whether their devices are critical, keep distribution records containing the detailed information listed above for billing and market survey purposes.

Manufacturers of radiological electronic products listed in 21 CFR 1002.61 must maintain distribution records that will enable them to trace specific products or production lots to distributors, or to dealers in those instances in which the manufacturer distributes directly to dealers (see 21 CFR 1002.30, Records to be Maintained by Manufacturers).

Distribution records must be kept for a period of time equivalent to the design life and expected life of the device, but in no case less than two years from the date of release for commercial distribution by the manufacturer. The intent of this requirement is support for potential repairs, corrective actions, and recalls. The intent of the regulation is not to require the retention of distribution records for the entire life of devices such as stretchers. Thus, after two years, each manufacturer must make a prudent decision whether to discard records or keep them for a longer period. When requested, distribution records must be made available to FDA investigators for review and copying during normal business hours.

B. Device Installation

Section 820.152, Installation, applies to medical device systems and complex devices that must be set up and adjusted at the location where they are to be used. For example, before a diagnostic x-ray machine can be used, it must be installed, adjusted, and the performance checked. Cardiopulmonary bypass machines must be set up and adjusted at the user location. Manufacturers of such devices must:

Install the device, or have it installed by a representative;
Inspect the device after installation to assure that the device will perform as intended; or
Provide adequate instructions and procedures for proper installation.

These instructions and procedures for proper installation by the firm's representative, user, or third party (820.152) must include an appropriate means for an instructions on how to determine that the installed device is safe, performing satisfactorily, and ready for use. Such procedures and instructions are part of the device master record and generally include a checklist for the installer to make certain that all necessary installation and checkout activities have been performed correctly. If available to the manufacturer, the filled-in checklist or other installation records are part of the device history record.

Safety checks at this stage refer to safety aspects related directly to the installation and setup activities and not to intrinsic safety features that have already been checked during final testing at the factory.

XII. COMPLAINTS AND FAILURE INVESTIGATIONS

A. Multifaceted Processing

All drug delivery device manufacturers are subject to the complaint requirements in 21 CFR Part 820, Good Manufacturing Practices

(GMP) regulation, and to the reporting requirements in 21 CFR Part 803, Medical Device Reporting (MDR) regulation. As defined in GMP section 820.198(a), a complaint, whether written or oral, is an expression of dissatisfaction regarding the identity, quality, durability, reliability, safety, effectiveness, or performance of a device.

Manufacturers are required to review and investigate any complaints received, establish ways to perform these activities, and designate someone to perform these tasks. Complaints concerning death or serious injury, as defined in the MDR regulation, must be reported to the FDA as discussed later. Manufacturers of any class of medical devices are never exempted from the GMP complaint requirements (820.198), nor the general record requirements (810.180) that allow the FDA to review and copy records. Complaint file requirements are necessary to ensure that manufacturers have adequate systems for investigating complaints and taking corrective action. Access to complaint files, device-related injury reports, and complaints about product defects enables the FDA to determine if a manufacturer's quality assurance system and corrective actions are adequate.

Manufacturers can identify problems with device and component quality by several methods. To be adequate, these should include a review and investigation of complaints, failed devices, and service requests. Complaints and service requests are important sources of feedback information for the quality assurance system. This data, in conjunction with product audits, systems audits, operational analyses, inspection and test data, etc., are used by the quality assurance organization to:

Identify poor performance in the overall quality assurance system, particularly faulty manufacturing processes and design of devices

Aid in implementing solutions to these quality problems

Verify confidence in, and improve the performance of, the quality assurance system

Improve the safety and performance of devices

Reduce medical device reporting

Reduce costs

Improve customer relations by reducing the frequency of problems, complaints, and recalls

Assure compliance with device regulations and consensus standards.

Thus, a complaint handling system is one of the best sources available for use-related information about product performance, safety, durability, and changing customer preferences.

Complaint Handling System

The GMP regulation requires in section 820.20 that each manufacturer have a formally established and documented quality assurance
program of which complaint handling is an important element. Even
if manufacturers have never received complaints, they must be prepared to receive and process them. Using written procedures for
handling complaints increases confidence that all complaints will be
handled properly. Manufacturers should determine the need for
procedures for processing complaints the same way as they determine
the need for procedures for any other operation: Is there a reasonable probability that these written procedures will solve or prevent quality problems? Written procedures usually are provided to
employees to facilitate communication, maintain consistency, and reduce quality problems. The GMP requirements for complaint handling
are extensive and normally require a written procedure specifying
authority, responsibilities, and the process to follow in receiving,
reviewing, and investigating complaints. However, for very small
firms where division of work is minimal, and authorities and responsibilities are obvious, the GMP requirements as detailed in
820.198 in conjunction with appropriate forms may be sufficient as a
protocol for handling complaints.

    Although the FDA does not specify a standard complaint handling
system, the GMP regulation does specify certain required actions
that must be included in any system. Manufacturers must:

    Review, evaluate, and file all complaints
    Formally designate a unit or individual to perform these activities
    Determine if an investigation is necessary
    Record the reason if no investigation is made
    Assign responsibility for deciding when not to investigate

Complaint Responsibility

Drug delivery device manufacturers must formally assign responsibility for maintaining complaint files and conducting complaint investigations to individuals or an organizational unit. Regardless of the
approach used, the duties of those responsible must be clearly delineated and thoroughly understood by them. These employees must
have the proper education and training to process complaints. Any
difficulty noted in employees performing required tasks for proper
complaint handling may be an indication that additional training is
needed. Any training programs must be documented (820.25).
    The person(s) assigned to review complaints should have a
thorough knowledge of the product line in order to make an informed, reasonable decision as to the severity and significance of a
complaint and to decide whether an investigation is necessary. If it
is decided that an investigation is not necessary, a record must be
made of the rationale used to arrive at this decision.

Death and Injury Complaints

Section 820.198(b) specifically requires that any complaint involving the possible failure of a device to meet its performance specifications must be reviewed, evaluated, and investigated. Also, section 820.198(b) further specifies that any complaint pertaining to injury, death, or any hazard to safety shall be immediately reviewed, evaluated, and investigated by a designated individual(s), and shall be maintained in a separate portion of the complaint file. However, for trend analysis by product, a firm should duplicate these serious complaints in the regular complaint file. Trend analysis is a means of identifying quality problems as required by section 820.20(a).

Complaint Records

The FDA does not specify a standard method for recording or retrieving complaint information. Each manufacturer should develop a method for maintaining records of complaints and investigations that is easy to use and economical, and that meets company needs and requirements of the GMP regulation. A form, usually two sided if a hardcopy, is commonly used to help process complaints. One side or page is used to record complaint information, such as sequential number of the complaint; origin of the complaint; customer information; product information; any corrective actions already taken; details of the complaint; and dates, signatures, assignments, etc. The other is used to record instructions; investigations; analyses; conclusions; corrective action with respect to the product and to the customer; and dates, signatures, etc. The completed forms are stored in the complaint file which may be a physical or electronic location.

Investigation Records

The designated unit or person(s) responsible for maintaining the complaint file(s) must prepare a written record of any investigations. The record of investigation must include:

> The device name
> Control number, if any
> Name of complainant
> Nature of complaint
> Reply to complaint

For convenience, these files would usually include dates, phone number, user location, etc.

File Accessibility and Location

Complaint files must be reasonably accessible to the FDA for review
and copying. Written records of investigation must be maintained in
the complaint file and be readily available at the manufacturing site.
The FDA has clear authority under section 704(e) of the Food, Drug
and Cosmetic Act to inspect and copy all records required under
section 519 or 520(g). Because the GMP regulation was promulgated
under the authority of sections 519 and 520(g), the regulation provides the FDA with authority to inspect, review, and copy any complaints on devices manufactured on or after December 18, 1978. The
GMP regulation requires that complaint files be located with a formally
designated unit; if the unit is at a different site, a copy of the
record of investigation must be maintained at the actual manufacturing site.

If the unit or individual(s) designated as responsible for investigating complaints is located away from the actual manufacturing
site, copies of records of investigations and, of course, copies of
the related complaints must be transmitted to and maintained in a
complaint file at the actual manufacturing site. Records of nonvalid
or other complaints that are not investigated need not be sent to the
actual manufacturing site. In a corporate or multiplant setting,
complaint files may be maintained at the home office or headquarters,
if copies of complaints and related investigations can be retrieved
at the manufacturing site using electronic mail or other high-speed
data transfer system.

When devices are produced for a firm by a contract manufacturer,
the firm must forward to the contractor copies of complaints and
investigations that pertain to operations performed by the contractor. The contractor must maintain a complaint file as discussed
herein for the primary manufacturer. Relabelers, importers, and
others who distribute under their own name must forward complaints
to the actual manufacturer, because the GMP regulation requires
that copies of complaints be located at the manufacturing site.

Nonmedical Complaints

If a manufactured product is used as a medical device and also for
nonmedical uses, complaints received from the nonmedical users do
not necessarily have to be included in the complaint files. However,
the person receiving such complaints must be trained (820.25) to
identify complaints that also affect those units used as medical devices. This action would assure compliance with 820.20(a)(3), which
requires identifying, recommending, or providing solutions for quality assurance problems and verifying the implementation of such
solutions. Nondevice or nonmedical complaints should not be maintained in medical device complaint files.

Trend Analysis

To facilitate detection of failure or defect trends, complaint files should be arranged in a manner that permits correlating present and past complaints for a particular product or product line. Thus, files are usually organized according to product or product lines. Manufacturers who do not organize complaint files by product or product line must search several files to find similar complaints or indications to identify problem trends. Complaints may be maintained in a computer so that complaint data on a specific device or type of complaint can be readily accessed and analyzed. If a manufacturer cannot readily identify defect trends, the firm's management is not complying with the intent of 820.198 and 820.20(a)(3) and (4).

GMP Sections Related to Complaints

Following are excerpts from several sections of the Good Manufacturing Practices regulation that deal directly or indirectly with complaint files.

820.5   Quality Assurance Program: "Every finished device manufacturer shall prepare and implement a quality assurance program . . . ." This topic is discussed in Section I.

820.20   Organization: "Each manufacturer shall have in place an adequate organizational structure and sufficient personnel to assure the following functions are performed: . . . identifying, recommending, or providing solutions for quality assurance problems . . . ." See Section 1.

820.25   Personnel: "Each manufacturer shall have sufficient personnel with the necessary education, background, training, and experience . . . ." See Section 1.

820.162 Failure Investigation: "After a device has been released for distribution, any failure of that device or any of its components to meet performance specifications shall be investigated." Discussed in this section.

820.198 Complaint Files: "Written and oral complaints relative to the identity, quality, . . . of a device shall be reviewed, evaluated, and maintained by a formally designated unit."

Note that there is a close relationship between the sections of
the GMP regulation that deal specifically with complaints and those
that deal with the prevention or solution of quality problems. Complaints often arise from real quality problems, and, therefore, must
be adequately analyzed and resolved to meet the requirements of the
company, the customer, the Food, Drug and Cosmetic Act, and
GMP sections 820.198, 820.162, and 820.20. In addition to the
direct requirements in 820.198, Complaint Files, and 820.162, Failure
Investigation, the general quality assurance program in 820.20(a)(3)
contains a fundamental and important requirement for identifying,
recommending, or providing solutions for quality assurance problems.
The evidence that a problem exists and the information to identify it
may arise through a complaint and the resulting investigations of the
complaint and failed device.

Device Failure Analysis

Section 820.198(b) of the complaint file requirements applies to the
investigation of complaints involving the *possible* failure of a device
to meet performance specifications, to determine if there actually is
a device failure. This requirement to investigate the possible failure
of a device to meet specifications is similar to requirements in section
820.162, Failure Investigation, which requires that after a device has
been released for distribution, any *actual* failure of the device or its
components to meet performance specifications shall be investigated
and any followup and conclusions recorded. Thus, section 820.162
refers to actual failure analysis, i.e., the determination of the device
failure mechanism, and whether it is related to design or manufacturing. The significance of the device and the hazard the device presents, if defective, should be considered when determining compliance
with this requirement. When the cause of device failure is obvious,
a formal investigation generally is not needed.

Failure analysis should be conducted by appropriately trained
and experienced personnel. They should use a written protocol to
assure that the process of device handling and analysis will not
compromise the determination of the cause of the device failure. A
written protocol, however, is not a specific GMP requirement. The
failure investigation and analysis must determine the actual failure
mechanism to the objective level necessary to correct the problem.
When systematic failure has been diagnosed and corrective action
established, a manufacturer need not analyze all additional devices
that are returned with the same symptoms.

If a failure is determined to be related to manufacturing, the
manufacturing deficiency must be determined, corrected, and documented. If an investigation verifies a particular device deficiency
and that this deficiency may exist in other products, the investiga-

tion must extend to determining the effect on other medical products.

B. Feedback for QA System

In order for a quality assurance system to be dynamic or self-correcting, data on quality problems from all sources must be fed back into the system. Complaints are a valuable source of data that can point to corrective actions. The more comprehensive a QA system is, the lower the probability of receiving complaints. As noted in Section I, a QA system, to be effective, must, at the minimum, include all the GMP requirements. Besides the GMP requirements covering packaging and label design, design transfer, manufacturing control, packaging, labeling, installation, complaints and failure analysis, a truly satisfactory QA system should also cover customer needs, design, design evaluation, and all aspects of repairs.

Feedback data should flow into all operations that could be affected by the data and should be used to aid in device and process design evaluation and/or redesign, and to aid in improving the overall quality assurance program.

Regardless of the size of the formal QA system, the feedback data path in any company should be the same; that is, the data should flow into all affected operations even if some of these are not covered by the formal QA system.

Because feedback is an important element in a quality assurance system, and because the GMP requirements for complaints are versatile in that the degree of investigation may be varied to fit the nature of the complaint, some firms actively solicit feedback information on minor quality problems from their customers by shipping customer feedback data cards with finished devices. Customer feedback cards are also a valuable public relations tool. Although the use of the forms is optional, complaints received by the feedback forms should be processed according to a complaint handling procedure that meets the requirements of 820.198 and any additional company requirements.

C. Complaint Sources

Complaints that must be processed according to the GMP requirements may be received from:

Customers by letter, credit memo, returned goods form, or phone
A firm's representative, or other employee
Journal articles
A service request
The FDA

All must be equally addressed by and be processed according to the company complaint policy and procedure. The company must make certain that marketing, sales, engineering, manufacturing, regulatory, installation, and service personnel report complaints. These employees must be made aware of this requirement according to section 820.25(a). It bears repeating: All complaints from all sources must be processed; and it is best if they are all processed according to the same procedure.

Repairs

Routine service requests for maintenance, adjustment, or repair of damage or failure resulting from long use, misuse, or accident usually do not need to be considered as complaints. However, all repair or service requests resulting from failure of a device to perform its intended function due to inadequate design, design defects, unanticipated component failure, or other causes of a nonroutine nature must be evaluated as candidates for the complaint file.

All devices that are serviced or repaired because they no longer perform as intended, i.e., they fail to meet specifications, are subject to the requirements of 820.162, Failure Investigations. Also, some service and repair requests may meet the definition of a complaint in 820.198, i.e., a written or oral expression of dissatisfaction relative to the identity, quality, durability, reliability, safety, effectiveness, or performance of a device. Technically, therefore, all service and repair requests must be screened for complaints and failure investigations. For those selected, that is, devices that are serviced or repaired due to failure to meet specifications, investigations must be conducted; and a written record of the investigation, including conclusions and followup, must be made.

The FDA has not, however, required manufacturers who service and repair devices to investigate each request for service or maintain complaint records in order to meet the record-keeping requirements of 820.162 and 820.198 as long as manufacturers:

Maintain service and repair records
Allow the FDA to review and copy such records
Have a program for evaluating service/repair information for
    trends
Per the requirements of section 820.162, investigate the cause
    of trends when they develop

As mentioned, manufacturers should maintain records of repairs and include the repair data when performing trend analysis and calculating reliability.

Parts Shipping Trends

Where feasible, manufacturers should periodically (e.g., monthly) examine shipping records for repair parts. Any increase in shipment of specific parts due to unknown reasons should be analyzed to determine if a significant failure problem exists. Such increases may be an "automatic trend analysis." Manufacturers have identified quality problems by this low-cost technique.

D. Medical Device Reporting

In addition to the GMP requirements covering complaint handling and failure investigations, device firms must also comply with the Medical Device Reporting (MDR) regulation, 21 CFR Part 803.

Who Should Report

The MDR regulation requires that manufacturers and importers of drug delivery devices notify the FDA when they become aware of a death or serious injury that may have been caused by one of their marketed devices and/or any malfunction in one of their devices which, if it were to recur, could reasonably be expected to cause a death or serious injury. These are essentially the same complaints that the GMP regulation requires a firm to place in a special file— the death/injury/hazardous complaint file [820.198(b)]. The MDR regulation is intended to supplement the GMP regulation—it is not meant to replace the GMP complaint and failure investigation requirements.

When to Report

There are specific time limits within which the MDR reports must be made. Any report of a death or serious injury must be made by phone no later than 5 *calendar* days from the initial receipt of the information. Malfunction reports must be made by phone or letter no later than 15 *working* days from the initial receipt of the information. In all cases a phone report must be followed by a written report within 15 *working* days from the initial receipt of the information by the firm. To meet these requirements, firms must have an information handling system to assure that data are screened to determine what must be reported to the FDA. This system must also be able to follow up this information quickly and accurately in order to comply with the MDR regulation. Firms that have a good system for processing complaint and failure investigations such as described in this chapter will have the organization and data processing capabilities to meet the MDR requirements.

XIII.   QA SYSTEM AUDITS

A.   Company Audit Requirements

Section 820.5 of the Good Manufacturing Practices (GMP) regulation
requires that "every finished device manufacturer shall prepare and
implement a quality assurance program that is appropriate to the
specific device manufactured and meets the requirement of this part."
Section 820.20 outlines the quality assurance requirements of the
GMP regulation. As discussed in Section I, every quality assurance
(QA) system should include: management policies; objectives; an
organization; documentation; performance of tasks according to
policies; and monitoring of the system (feedback). Section 820.20(b)
requires that the QA system be monitored through audits. The
analysis and use of feedback data from audits, complaints, and other
sources is a necessary part of a QA program in order for a QA system to be self-correcting. Thus, the quality audit of a QA system
is one of the most important requirements of the GMP regulation.

A quality audit is a independent inspection and review of all
aspects of a QA system. The audit is performed in accordance with
written procedures on a periodic basis and the findings are documented. The objective is to verify, by examination and evaluation of
objective evidence, the degree of compliance with those elements of
the quality assurance program under review. These audits are an
essential part of every medical device manufacturer's effort to assure
safe and effective devices. Regardless of how well a quality assurance program is planned, monitoring of the program is necessary if
the QA program is to be effective in assuring that finished devices
meet specifications. Manufacturers who do not have an adequate
quality audit system usually do not have adequate QA programs.

The GMP regulation requires that planned and periodic audits of
the quality assurance program shall be implemented to verify compliance with the quality assurance program requirements. The
audits are to be performed in accordance with written procedures by
appropriately trained individuals who do not have direct responsibility for the matters being audited. Audit results shall be documented
in written audit reports, which must be reviewed by management
personnel who have responsibility for the matters audited. Followup corrective action, including re-audit of deficient matters, shall
be taken when indicated. Upon request of a designated FDA employee, a responsible official of the manufacturer shall certify in
writing that the audits have been performed and documented and
that any required corrective action has been taken.

To assure that company quality goals will be routinely met and
to comply with the GMP regulations, quality assurance system audits
should measure the effectiveness of the quality assurance program;
provide objective evidence that adequate controls are in place; and
assure that products and processes conform to specifications.

Where practical, drug delivery device manufacturers should include audits of their vendors, calibration laboratories, and contractors as part of a QA audit. Manufacturers should audit vendors to assure that they have adequate QA controls for components received by the manufacturers under certification (certificate of compliance with specifications) by vendors.

Procedure

All manufacturers must have a written quality audit procedure, although the details will vary with the firm size and nature of the manufacturing operations. An audit procedure should include:

An objective
Audit scope
An audit schedule
Assignment of responsibilities
Evaluation criteria

One example of a quality assurance audit procedure is shown in Exhibit 4.

Before writing their audit procedure, some firms may find it helpful to rearrange the key device GMP requirements, for an audit in a structured format as shown below:

Who?	Designee
What?	QA system
When?	X months
How?	Per checklist
Results?	Report/review
Actions?	Corrective

This format helps lead authors into covering key requirements and "getting straight to the point when writing procedures." Thus, this format tends to reduce the length of procedures and increase the clarity.

Formal procedures should start with an objective. In this case, the audit objective was discussed in the opening paragraphs of this section: to monitor the complete QA system. The audit scope must include *all* functions that significantly impact on whether products will meet specifications. These functions include personnel training, facilities, environment, device master and history records, equipment calibration, vendors, label control, validation, complaint files, data feedback, preparation for FDA GMP inspections, etc. Firms that have a product assurance or total QA system should audit the entire system; otherwise, it is no longer a total QA system! Audits should cover all buildings and operations as necessary to made certain that

Exhibit 4   Quality Assurance Audit Procedure

QUALITY ASSURANCE AUDIT PROCEDURE

Sheet 1 of 2

No. _____   Rev. ___   Approved _____ Date _____

ECN History _____

POLICY: Periodic and planned audits of systems, processes, and product flow shall be performed to assure compliance with regulatory and company requirements for current Good Manufacturing Practices (QA system).

SCOPE: All facilities, operations, and product lines.

PROCEDURAL GUIDE: Routine quality audits of selected areas shall be conducted each month. The entire operation shall be covered during a 12-month cycle. An area may be audited more than once. An "Action Audit" may be initiated by the Manager of Quality Assurance at any time if a special problem arises.

The teamwork approach shall be utilized to identify and correct deficiencies.

The audit team shall consist of the Senior Quality Auditor (team leader) plus one or more individuals from other disciplines who have no direct responsibility for the area being audited. A team auditing an Operations unit should include an R&D representative. A team auditing a Quality Control unit should include an Operations representative.

The Manager of Quality Assurance selects the team member in consultation with the Department Managers.

A. **AUDIT PREPARATION** - The Quality Auditor (team leader) reviews standard manufacturing procedures, device histories, complaint history, device labels and inserts, previous audits with results, followup audits, plus any other document relative to the audit.

B. **AUDIT INITIATION** - The Quality Auditor prepares an audit checklist for systematic examination of the area to be audited, informs the Manager of the department being audited at the start of the audit, and reviews observations with the Department Manager.

C. **AUDIT ANALYSIS** - The Quality Auditor reviews the data gathered, verifies important details, and writes an audit report according to the format delineated in the attached audit report outline.

D. **ISSUANCE OF AUDIT REPORT** - The Quality Auditor issues the written audit report to the President and Department managers within 3 working days following completion of the audit. If conditions are critical, the Director of Quality Assurance shall verbally brief appropriate staff members within 12 hours following audit completion. Audit reports shall be stamped "Confidential".

E. **CORRECTIVE ACTION** - The appropriate Management staff member shall be responsible for developing a schedule for correcting deficiencies cited in the audit report and submitting same within 5 working days to the Quality Assurance Manager. Included in the correction schedule shall be the responsible individual, and the date when corrective action is to be effected. The Manager of Quality Assurance shall act as arbiter, if necessary, to judge validity of the deficiency, responsible individual, and reasonable date to complete the corrective action.

Exhibit 4 (Continued).

F. **AUDIT FOLLOWUP** - The Quality Auditor maintains a log listing deficiencies, responsible individual, target date for corrective action, and actual date of correction. If the same deficiency occurs on a second followup audit, the President shall be notified in writing by the Quality Assurance Manager.

G. **LOG OF AUDITS AND FOLLOWUP AUDITS** - The master log shall be maintained by the Senior Quality Auditor. The audit log file shall include a copy of current audits, list of areas to be audited during the 12-month period, and list of areas audited to date (i.e., part of the Master Log).

H. **REPORT NUMBERS** - Audit numbers shall be composed of the date followed by the sequential number of the audit being reported (e.g., 88-4 for the 4th audit during 1988).

AUDIT REPORT COVER DATA

Area Audited _____ Audit No. _____ Date: _____

Audit Team Members: _____

_____

_____

Sr. Auditor's Sign: _____
(Team Leader)

REPORT OUTLINE

1. **PURPOSE AND AREA DESCRIPTION** - Describe initiating factors for the audit, limitations of audit, and area being audited

2. **MAJOR FACTS** - Summarize for management review the most undesirable conditions and practices in order of their relative importance.

3. **OBSERVATIONS AND FACTUAL DETAILS** - Give a detailed account of the current practices and the deficiencies listed in 4 below.

4. **DEFICIENCIES** - List deficiencies in procedures, standards, documentation, safety, etc., along with Identity of relevant regulation, SMP, SOP, etc.

5. **FOLLOWUP** - State plans for followup review to establish individual responsibilities and completion dates.

---

the desired or required quality assurance program is properly implemented.

The quality audit required by the GMP regulation is not intended to be a product audit. However, the adequacy of procedures used to determine product acceptability msut be reviewed (audited) periodically. Product audits and review of the master record are desirable as independent evaluations of product quality to determine the product's fitness for use and conformance to specification; and, these may be acceptable in satisfying most quality audit requirements when product and process are very simple. As products and processes become more complex, evidence from inspection and testing of products no longer provides full assurance that the manufacturing system will consistently produce quality products. Instead, full GMP/QA system audits are required to ensure that the established QA system is adequate for producing devices that consistently meet the master record requirements and that all system requirements are being met.

Audit Schedule

Manufacturers are responsible for deciding the frequency of audits. The frequency should depend on previous audit findings, any indications of problems, and known stability of the manufacturing process. If an audit reveals no problems, the audit intervals may be lengthened; if problems are identified, audits may need to be conducted more often. Audits are usually conducted every 6 to 12 months, but the interval should not exceed 12 months. Some companies split their audit into parts and perform one or more parts per month or quarter, or audit one or more operations per month or quarter. This approach is valuable because it tends to direct attention toward problems that can be resolved within reasonable time limits and existing budgets. However, such segmented audits may fail to identify company-wide problems. Thus, reviewers of segmented audit reports should look for indications of company-wide problems.

Independent Auditor

The GMP regulation requires that QA system audits be conducted by individuals not having direct responsibility for the matters being audited. This requirement may be satisfied by an audit team consisting of persons representing product development and manufacturing. Then, when the product development area is being audited, the manufacturing persons should have the lead responsibility and vice versa. For any element of the quality assurance system being audited, at least one member of the team should *not* have direct responsibility for the element being audited. Management should designate one member as team leader for a given audit in order to support consistency, timeliness, completeness, and uniform response. Of course, a consultant, corporate, or other independent auditor may be used.

The requirement for an independent audit must generally be met; however, if a very small manufacturer, particularly one in which everyone is directly involved in daily production activities, concludes that independent audits would be unduly burdensome or impractical, the requirement for independence may be waived. However, if the FDA finds, as a result of inspection or other means, that this waiver has compromised the quality assurance program, the FDA may require an independent audit, increase the frequency of FDA GMP inspections, or take other appropriate regulatory action.

Employee Training

Individual(s) responsible for conducting audits must be sufficiently trained and experienced to detect variations and problems in the quality assurance system [820.20(b), 820.25]. An auditor is expected to objectively compare existing manufacturing processes, records, test/inspection activities, label control systems, feedback, etc., against what they should be. To do this, the individual(s) must have a working knowledge of:

How the product are made
The manufacturing processes
Quality assurance principles that apply
The human relations aspect of auditing

As with any GMP training, a record should be maintained of the training given each employee.

Because the GMP requires a written audit report, auditors must have sufficient writing skills to communicate findings and recommendations effectively.

Evaluation Criteria

Each firm must determine the criteria to be used for conducting the audit. In general, medium to large firms will need extensive documentation outlining the areas to be audited and the acceptable criteria for each of these areas. The GMP requirements can form a basis for the evaluation criteria; however, because the GMP regulation is broad, each firm must tailor the criteria to the operations they are actually performing. Small manufacturers may need only minimal documentation, and this may consist of a checklist with appropriate ancillary instructions to assure that all aspects of the QA system are covered.

An audit checklist may be a series of questions, phrases, trigger words, or any combination of these that will prompt auditors to cover the entire quality assurance system. Checklists should cover requirements of the GMP regulation applicable to company products, operations, and other areas that company management has decided are included in their total quality assurance system. If operations or devices change, evaluation criteria and checklists must be updated appropriately.

Results and Corrective Actions

A QA system audit program that has been established in accordance with the GMP regulation and implemented in sufficient depth can detect undesirable variations and trends in operating procedures. Management awareness of these undesirable variations should lead to corrections and help prevent production of unsafe, unreliable, or ineffective devices.

The GMP regulation requires follow-up corrective action, including re-audit. When indicated, audit results must be given to individuals responsible for each of the operations audited, especially if deficiencies are found. Audit results must be reviewed by all key management personnel, especially those responsible for the matters audited.

An audit should never be used as a disciplinary tool. This use will lead to ineffective audits because employees may become reluctant to reveal any possible problems for fear of retribution.

If conducted properly, a quality audit can detect QA program defects. Identification of unsatisfactory trends and correction of factors that cause defective products prevent the production of unsafe or nonconforming devices. Without an effective quality audit function, the quality assurance program is incomplete—there is no assurance that a manufacturer is consistently in a state-of-control. In addition, the proper implementation of a QA audit system can result in cost savings by identifying and correcting problem areas. Without an audit, the quality assurance system becomes an open loop with no feedback to management. Without management support, the QA program will eventually become ineffective and ignored.

Audit Certification

The FDA has authority to review and copy all records required by the GMP regulation; however, the FDA has elected not to routinely review audit reports. The one exception to the FDA's policy of not seeking access to reports of audits of quality assurance programs is that the FDA may seek production of these reports in litigation under applicable procedural rules, as for other otherwise confidential documents. Thus, a copy of the current audit report should be maintained by the firm. FDA policy was established because the agency does not wish to prejudice audits by having auditors concerned that their comments will be reviewed by FDA investigators. Although FDA investigators do not have routine access to audit reports, they can request manufacturers to certify that audits have been conducted and the results documented; however, investigators do not routinely request certification. If requested, a responsible official of the firm must certify, in writing, that the firm has complied with the audit requirements of the GMP regulation. Investigators usually will ask questions regarding the audit report, such as who prepared the report, when was the report written, who reviewed the report, was corrective action taken based on the audit result, etc. If investigators suspect audits are not being conducted, questions to determine consistency in answers may be addressed to those individuals who should have reviewed these reports. FDA investigators will routinely review audit procedures and audit checklists.

B. FDA Factory Inspections

The FDA determines compliance with the GMP regulation primarily by factory inspections. An FDA inspection of an establishment, however, can be initiated for a number of reasons. The reasons may be general, such as routine scheduling or a need to obtain data on industries new to the FDA; or the reasons may be specific, such as investigation of a consumer or trade complaint, a product defect report, an adverse reaction, or a death. The FDA also conducts inspections under the Government-Wide Quality Assurance Program (GWQAP) on behalf of the Veterans Administration (VA), Department of Defense (DOD), and Health Resources and Services Administration (HRSA). Upon arrival, the investigator presents his or her credentials and issues a Notice of Inspection form FDA 482. During the inspection, observations are recorded on FDA 483. List of observations are discussed with the firm's management. Later the investigator will write an Establishment Inspection Report (EIR), which is a detailed record of the inspection and findings.

Authority and Coverage

Section 704(a) of the Food, Drug and Cosmetic Act gives the FDA the authority to conduct GMP inspections of medical product manufacturers. During these inspections, facilities, manufacturing processes, records, and corrective action programs are examined by an FDA investigator. The results provide information necessary to evaluate a firm's compliance with the GMP regulations (21 CFR 210 and 820).

Anyone who manufactures, labels, packages, imports, or stores medical products can be inspected. A manufacturer is any person, including a repackager or relabeler, who writes specifications for, manufactures, fabricates, assembles, or processes a medical product.

Inspection Plan

This section offers ideas on ways that a firm might prepare for, undergo, and respond to an FDA inspection. First and foremost, it is important to plan ahead! Before being visited by an FDA investigator, a firm should have in place an inspection procedure that takes into account, and prepares a firm for, any eventuality. It should detail company policy regarding such an inspection; and, very important, designate those individual(s) who are to work with the FDA investigator. Try to anticipate situations and have written procedures covering them. These procedures will provide continuity from one inspection to another and help assure that corporate policies are followed by employees receiving and accompanying the investigator.

Each person designated as an FDA contact should be chosen carefully and be thoroughly familiar with the inspection procedure and
company operations. An inspection will take longer if the contact
person cannot answer questions without continually referring to the
written procedures. The contact should be familiar with FDA regulations and practices and be able to anticipate problems or requests.
FDA contacts must be knowledgeable about plant operations, and able
to answer or obtain answers to the investigator's questions. Other
individuals, with similar qualifications, should be designated to fill
in during absences of the primary contact. A firm might want a
secondary contact to accompany the FDA investigator even when the
primary contact is present in order for the secondary contact to become familiar with FDA methods and procedures.

Along with the designated contact, the firm may want operations
managers to accompany the investigator, such as the production
manager, QA manager, etc. These individuals must be familiar with
the plant operations and company policy, and be able to answer questions about procedures and processes. However, a firm should keep
the number of individuals accompanying the investigator to a minimum
to prevent problems such as contradictory statements.

Receptionists should be informed that an FDA investigator will
eventually visit and have procedures to follow when they arrive.
These procedures should include instructions to call the FDA contact
person and what to do or whom to contact when that person is not
available.

Inspection Refusals

As noted above, section 704(a) of the FD&C Act gives the FDA clear
authority to conduct inspections. It is bad policy to refuse an inspection, because this sets up an adversarial situation and arouses
an investigator's suspicions regarding the firm's compliance with the
GMP regulation. If a firm refuses an inspection without a valid
reason, the FDA usually obtains a warrant that grants entry for an
inspection. Refusal is noted in the firm's file maintained by the
FDA and may be interpreted as a lack of cooperation.

There may be instances, however, when a firm needs to ask the
investigator to return at a later time to conduct the inspection. Explain why it is best that an inspection be done at a later time. For
instance, if the FDA contact person(s) is not in the factory and no
one knowledgeable about the firm's overall operations is available,
ask the investigator to come back. However, FDA investigators do
expect to be admitted if a device factory is operating. The rationale is that if a factory is operating, someone must be in charge and
that individual should understand factory operations and procedures.
If the factory is not in operation or if it is not yet manufacturing
any medical products, this should be explained to the investigator.

This FDA representative may still want to go through the factory to make sure it is not in operation—firms should have a policy covering this situation. It is advisable, in this situation, to allow the investigator to walk through the factory to verify later that it was not in operation. If the factory is not in operation, advise the investigator when operations will begin. The investigator will consider the request and circumstances, then determine whether to proceed with the inspection.

Inspection Preliminaries

Before an inspection begins, an investigator will display credentials. The credentials have a picture of the investigator and identify him or her as a representative of the FDA.

After presenting credentials, the investigator will issue form FDA 482, Notice of Inspection. This form is issued to the owner, operator, or agent in charge of the factory or to the designated FDA contact. The bottom portion of the Notice of Inspection contains excerpts from section 704 of the FD&C Act. The investigator will complete the top portion of the form by filling in the firm name, address, name of the individual given the signed form, date, and time of inspection. The investigator then signs the form.

The FDA contact person should always be prompt. An investigator may become suspicious if kept waiting and may wonder if the firm is busily correcting GMP deficiencies. After suspicions are aroused, a firm may receive a more comprehensive inspection because the investigator may be looking for areas that have been corrected or temporarily corrected.

Conduct During the Inspection

Awareness of what is going on at all times by the contact person of the firm during the inspection is important. Therefore, once started, the inspection should be given priority. If the contact person is distracted by other business, the inspection may be prolonged and the investigator's questions concerning suspected deficiencies may go unanswered. Familiarity with the circumstances surrounding any deficiencies listed on form FDA 483 (the list of deviations presented at the close of the inspection) is vital in discussion of these with the investigator.

During inspections, the FDA contact person must deal with many issues such as viewing of records, copying, photos, tape recordings, differences of opinion, immediate corrections, promises, samples, notes, etc. All of these issues would be addressed by a company procedure.

There should be a procedure for responding to requests for production records, change control records, complaint files, and shipping records. All records required by the GMP regulations must be made available to the investigator for review and copying. Therefore, device master records, production records, and complaint files must be readily accessible. However, shipping records are not required by the device GMP regulation for noncritical devices; therefore, firms have the option of allowing access to these records unless these records are the only source that shows compliance with the requirements in 820.184 for quantity released to distribution, control numbers, etc. The procedures covering review of records by the investigator should identify who will retrieve records, the investigator or one of your employees; how many records can be reviewed at one time; and who should be present to answer questions raised by the investigator.

Because all records required by the GMP regulations must be available for copying, management should decide on a policy concerning record copying during inspections. The following questions need to be answered in this policy and the answers recorded in the inspection procedure.

Will company employees photocopy the records? If so, will the FDA be billed for copying charged? The FDA is authorized to pay for any photocopies made on the company machine when the company pays for a commercial photocopier.

If the company does not have a photocopying machine or does not want the investigator to use it, will the investigator be permitted to make copies outside the plant? If so, a plant employee should accompany the investigator.

In all situations, the company contact person should make duplicate copies and keep these together as a record of the documents that the investigator copied.

If any records copied by an investigator contain confidential information, it should be identified, i.e., by a "confidential" stamp. This identification does not automatically prevent release of these records under the Freedom of Information (FOI) act; however, the FOI officer filling a request is then made aware that the firm considers the information confidential. Confidential information is not released under the FOI.

Caution: Do not make every page of a document as confidential. Be specific and mark only those items that are genuinely confidential. Marking everything confidential forces the FOI officer to review each page and independently make the determination of what is confidential.

As with photocopying of records, management should decide on a policy regarding picture taking by the investigator during an inspection. Include this policy in the inspection procedure.

If your firm disagrees with any observation made by the investigator, be sure to discuss with the investigator the reason for the observation. You may find that there was a misunderstanding that can easily be corrected. When explaining a situation or answering questions, be honest. Don't make up answers, as this could lead to additional problems. If you don't know the answer, say so. There is no FDA penalty for not knowing an answer, and there is no requirement that a firm answer hypothetical or "what if" questions. If questions arise about photocopying, photography, records, or any other topic, it is best not to force a confrontation. Arguments about an investigator's observations may lead to loss of dialogue.

If there are questions for which you don't have an immediate answer, promise to research the question. A list of these unanswered questions is a reminder to get the answers and give them to the investigator. The investigator usually records the questions, and resolving unanswered questions may avoid negative items on form FDA 483 and in the establishment inspection report prepared by the investigator at the end of the inspection.

If possible, any GMP deficiencies that the investigator notes and with which you agree should be corrected immediately. The investigator should be made aware of these corrections, as this will show intent to comply with the regulations and commitment to quality assurance.

If correction cannot be made during the inspection, management may want to consider providing an estimated timetable for correction. However, the firm should not present or commit to a timetable that may be difficult or impossible to meet. If a timetable cannot be developed immediately, try to get one to the FDA as soon as possible.

As with any production change, it is a good idea to discuss possible corrective actions with affected company personnel before promising correction to the FDA. This concept was discussed in Section 5, and may prevent promises that have adverse effects on other areas of production. Hastily conceived corrections can cause greater problems in the long run.

Any commitments made to the FDA should have top management concurrence. It can be detrimental to the firm to be committed to a course of action that cannot be completed or that management refuses to pursue. Therefore, only persons with the authority to do so should make commitments.

Occasionally during an inspection, investigators collect samples. These may be used to:

Verify conditions in the factory
Establish interstate movement of finished devices and their components
Fulfill a request from the FDA's Center for Devices and Radiological Health (CDRH)

The FDA may request samples for a number of reasons, such as surveys of device manufacturers and investigation of user complaints. Whenever an investigator collects samples, duplicate samples should be collected and stored by your firm. If problems are uncovered by the FDA, testing of these duplicate samples by your firm may confirm FDA results or form a basis for discussion of FDA findings.

Before leaving your premises with a sample, the investigator will issue a form FDA 484, Receipt for Samples. This serves as a record of the samples that were taken. Where indicated, interstate movement of the shipments from which these samples were taken will be documented by the investigator with copies of shipping records. The investigator will then prepare an affidavit (form FDA 463a, 463, 1664a, or 1664b) referencing these documents. A responsible firm individual will be asked to verify, by signature, that the documents referenced in the affidavit pertain to the shipment(s) in question. Therefore, your firm should include in its inspection procedure the company policy on the signing of affidavits.

Having accurate and complete knowledge of what an investigator has done in an important part of handling an FDA inspection. Use good notes to record this information. Comments and suggestions made by the investigator, unanswered questions, and promises should all be recorded. General information on the areas of the plant the investigator visited, to whom he or she spoke, etc., can help when commenting on form FDA 483 items, making corrections to the facilities or QA system, or advising top management of the results of an inspection.

Notes will also be useful in fulfilling promises or obtaining answers to previously unanswered questions. When the items on the FDA 483 are presented, accurate notes help to prevent surprises. Good notes can also help to prepare well thought out and adequate answers to FDA 483 items even before these items are presented at the close-out meeting.

Close-out Meeting

At the end of an FDA GMP inspection, the investigator conducts a close-out meeting. This meeting is usually held immediately after the inspection, but it may take place a day or so later, especially if the completed form FDA 483 is long. During this meeting, the investigator discusses with company management the observations recorded on form FDA 483.

Representatives of the firm will be given a copy of the completed form FDA 483, which should be checked for accuracy and completeness against notes. Misunderstandings may have occurred during the inspection that gave the investigator the false impression that deficiencies existed. Close-out meetings present an opportunity to correct such misunderstandings.

Top management should be present at the close-out meeting to answer questions about any corrective actions to be taken and schedules for these actions.

The investigator should be reminded of any corrections that have been made. Mention your plans to make corrections, and provide a timetable for these future actions. Answers given at this meeting will be recorded by the investigator. Again, it is important that the individual promising corrections and setting up timetables have the authority to do so. Future inspections will cover those areas where correction was promised.

After the Inspection

Completion of the inspection by the FDA should signal the start of certain activities by the firm, such as discussion of deficiencies with appropriate departments and employees to advise them of corrections to be made and time frames involved.

Unresolved form FDA 483 items should be reviewed by company technical and legal personnel. If a decision is made that corrective action is not needed and there is disagreement with the investigator's opinion regarding the deficiency, state this, along with the rationale, in a letter to the FDA District Office responsible for inspection of your firm. Even if a firm agrees with all the items on the FDA 483, it is a good idea to respond to each item in a letter to the District Office. This reply shows a commitment to quality assurance and "officially" presents the company's case to the FDA. This reply should help resolve any doubts that the inspection report might raise about a firm.

The final step for a firm is to determine what can be learned from the inspection, so that the business can operate in a better state-of-control, improve quality assurance, and assure future GMP compliance.

The following is a concise summary of the major points made in this section. This summary should help your firm formulate an inspection plan.

Basic Points for an Inspection Plan

1. Be prepared for the eventual inspection by trying diligently to comply with applicable medical product regulations and preparing an inspection plan. If needed, assistance is available from the Division of Small Manufacturers Assistance, Center for Devices and Radiological Health, (800) 638-2041; and other FDA offices.

2. Receptionists should know who to call when an FDA investigator visits.

3. Determine that an FDA investigator is calling by examining his or her credentials.

4. Receptionists or initial contact persons should inform all key employees that an FDA investigator is present.
5. Someone, but not a large number of individuals, should accompany the investigator and be with the investigator at all times.
6. If the investigator is not familiar with the firm, describe the product line and operations before entering the manufacturing area.
7. At the beginning, review with the investigator all company policies and programs. Employees should accentuate positive aspects of these programs.
8. Employees should be cooperative, avoid conflict, and know when to terminate discussions with the investigator.
9. Don't start an argument with, get uptight with, or lie to the FDA investigator.
10. Understand the investigator's questions before answering. If needed, ask for an explanation. Refer each question to the most suitable employee.
11. Don't state that a particular event is impossible with your product—the investigator may have a report that covers the impossible event.
12. Don't try to compromise the compliance role of the FDA investigator or threaten to call his or her supervisor.
13. Correct deviations as soon as possible.
14. Keep duplicate copies or samples of material given to the FDA investigator.
15. During the close-out meeting, make sure that all deviations are adequately discussed. If there is disagreement, present all of the company information and any regulations and official interpretations that support your viewpoint.
16. Immediately submit to the local FDA District office a written reply to the FDA 483. Make sure you address all of the observations. State how and when you expect to make corrections. If you disagree with an observation, give reasons and references for your position.
17. Be reasonable in setting schedules for corrective actions—don't state impossible deadlines or drag out completion schedules.
18. A follow-up report should be distributed to appropriate company employees.

C. Regulatory Sanctions

Responsible officials who are in positions of authority in regulated firms have a primary legal duty to implement whatever measures are necessary to ensure that their products, facilities, and operations are in compliance with the law. The law presumes that these individuals are fully aware of their responsibilities.

Whenever the FDA determines, as a result of an inspection, investigation, complaint or other source, that a product is or may become adulterated or misbranded, several actions may be taken. These actions may be in the form of a warning letter to the firm, such as a Notice of Adverse Findings (NAF) letter or a Regulatory Letter; or result in the seizure or detention of a product or an injunction; or result in prosecution of the firm. The actions vary depending on the degree of danger to the public, or willingness of the manufacturer to correct violations. Following are several sections of the Food, Drug and Cosmetic (FD&C) Act that are commonly used in misbranding or adulteration charges. In this reprint, some key words are italicized for emphasis. Added notes are in brackets.

Adulteration

Section 501(351). A drug or device shall be deemed to be *adulterated*—

(a)(1) If it consists in whole or in part of any filthy, putrid, or decomposed substance; or

(2)(A) If it has been prepared, packed, or held under insanitary conditions whereby it may have been *contaminated* with filth, or whereby it may have been rendered injurious to health;

(c) If it is not subject to the provisions of paragraph 9(b) of this section [Paragraph 9(b) refers to drugs] and its strength differs from, or its purity or *quality falls below*, that which it purports or is represented to possess.

(h) If it is a device and the methods [refers to Good Manufacturing Practices] used in, or the facilities or controls used for its manufacture, packing, storage, or installation are not in conformity with applicable requirements under Section 520(f)(1) or an applicable condition prescribed by an order under section 520(f)(2).

Misbranding

Section 502(352). A drug or device shall be deemed to be *misbranded*—

(a) If its labeling is *false* or *misleading* in any particular.

(b) If in a package form unless it bears a label containing (1) the name and place of business of the manufacturer, packer, or distributor; and (2) an accurate statement of the quantity of the contents in terms of weight, measure, or numerical count . . . .

(f) Unless its labeling bears (1) adequate *direction* for use; (2) such adequate *warnings* against use in those pathological conditions or by children where its use may be dangerous to health, or against unsafe dosage or methods of duration of administration or application, in such manner and form, as are necessary for the protection of users . . . .

(j)   If it is *dangerous* to health when used in the dosage or manner, or with the frequency or duration prescribed, recommended, or suggested in the labeling thereof.

A device may be considered misbranded for other administrative reasons, such as failure to register the firm, formally list the product, or failure to submit a premarket notification (21 CFR Part 807).

When it is consistent with the public interest, it is the FDA's policy to advise regulated firms to potentially violative products, practices, or conditions; advise firms of violations requiring correction; and give firms any opportunity to make corrections voluntarily before initiating legal or administrative action.

The Notice of Adverse Findings (NAF) and Regulatory Letters are used primarily to draw a company's attention to violations and, thereby, obtain prompt correction. Also, these letters are a prior warning and notification to responsible company officials of possible civil or criminal action to be taken by the FDA.

Responsible individuals should not assume that they will receive a Notice of Adverse Findings or Regulatory Letter before the FDA initiates administrative action or recommends an injunction, seizure, civil penalty, and/or criminal proceeding. The FDA is under no legal obligation to warn firms or individuals that they or their products are in violation of the law before initiating formal regulatory action. For example, the agency ordinarily will not issue a letter but will take other action such as seizure and injunction when:

The violation reflects a recent history of repeated or continuous conduct of a similar or substantially similar nature during which time the firm and/or individual(s) have been notified of a similar or substantially similar violation.

The violation is intentional or flagrant.

The violation represents a reasonable possibility of injury or death.

The regulatory actions the FDA can pursue for violations of the FD&C Act such as NAF letters were briefly mentioned above; more detailed descriptions follow.

Notice of Adverse Findings Letter

A NAF letter may be issued when an inspection reveals that:

A firm and/or individual(s) is(are) in violation of the law or regulations;

There is information that an existing condition or practice may lead to a violation if left uncorrected; and

The agency has concluded that the nature of the violation does not require immediate action.

The issuance of an NAF does not preclude the initiation of other concurrent action, such as seizure or administrative detention, as part of an overall enforcement strategy.

Regulatory Letter

A Regulatory Letter is intended to effect correction of deficiencies noted during an inspection, from an investigation of a product complaint, or from information received from other sources. A Regulatory Letter may be issued by the FDA instead of seizing a product or obtaining an injunction. It is a specifically worded and formated enforcement letter written to top management of a firm by top management of an FDA field or headquarters unit. It contains a formal warning to the firm that specific sections of the law have been violated and, unless corrective action is taken, the agency is prepared to impose legal and/or administrative sanctions. Sanctions include seizure, prosecution, injunction, and civil penalties. A formal response to this letter msut be made to FDA within 10 days of receipt.

Seizure

A seizure is a civil court action against a specific quantity of goods whereby the FDA seeks to remove these goods from commercial channels. After seizure, no one may tamper with the goods except by permission of the court. The owner or claimant of the seized merchandise is usually given approximately 30 days by the court to decide on a course of action. If no action is taken, the court will recommend disposal of the goods. If it is decided to contest the government's charges, the case will be scheduled for trial. A third option allows the owner of the goods to request permission of the court to bring the goods into compliance with the law. The owner of the goods is required to provide a bond (money deposit) to assure that the orders of the court will be performed; and the owner must pay for FDA supervision of any activities by the company to bring the goods into compliance.

Detention

An administrative detention prohibits the distribution or use of
adulterated or misbranded devices encountered during inspections.
The detention usually lasts up to 30 days, possibly longer, until
the FDA has considered what action it should take concerning the
devices, or has initiated legal action if appropriate. Devices that
are detained may *not* be used, moved, altered, or tampered with in
any manner by any person during the detention period.

Restraining Orders and Injunctions

A Temporary Restraining Order (TRO) is sought by the FDA before
an injunction and is designed to stop the alleged violative practice
until the court can hear evidence that may lead to an injunction. A
TRO imposes restraint upon a defendant for not more than 10 days,
but this period may be extended by the courts.

   An injunction is a court order that restrains a person or firm
from violating the law, e.g., to prevent interstate distribution of
violative products, and to correct conditions in the establishment in
which the violation occurred. It is not mandatory for the FDA to
demonstrate that the law has been violated to obtain an injunction,
but only to show that there is a good probability it may have been
violated. Injunctions are considered and sought by the FDA when
imminent health hazards have been identified. With regard to legal
actions, injunctions and temporary restraining orders have the
highest priority within the FDA because these are used to stop imminent health hazards.

Citations

A citation is a notice that the agency is instituting criminal pro-
ceedings—it is not a warning. A citation provides the person
against whom such proceeding is contemplated an opportunity to
present his or her views. Citations are used only when a prosecution recommendation is definitely being considered by the agency.

Recalls

The Food and Drug Administration prefers to promote compliance by
means other than through the courts. Recall by the manufacturer of
violative products from the market is generally the fastest and most
effective way to protect the public. A recall may be initiated by the
manufacturer or shipper of the product, or may be requested by the
FDA. The first step in a product recall is for the manufacturer or
distributor to contact the nearest FDA field office for guidance. The
FDA can provide technical assistance to small and large manufacturers
on how to conduct an effective recall.

An FDA Statement of Enforcement Policy, published in the *Federal Register* of June 16, 1978, contains guidelines on recall procedures and industry responsibilities. It is recommended that manufacturers develop plans that can be put into effect immediately if a recall emergency arises. Accurate and complete product and shipping records are vital to the success of a product recall. Products should be labeled (direct or by code) to show date and place of manufacture.

Recently, the FDA has observed that when a firm discovers a risk presented by a medical device, the firm often voluntarily notifies appropriate persons of this risk in order to reduce or eliminate it. In some cases these notifications meet the definition of recall in 21 CFR Part 7.3(g). Because of concern that a notification might be classified as a recall, firms have sometimes delayed issuing a notification while discussions are held with the FDA. To try to eliminate delays in situations where public health might be at risk, the FDA published "Medical Device Notification and Voluntary Safety Alert Guideline" in March 1984, which contains procedures that firms should use in notifying or alerting health professionals who prescribe or use a medical device. These procedures also describe the steps used by the FDA in the notification and safety alert process.

part two
SPECIFIC APPLICATIONS

Chapter 4

MICROENCAPSULATION: SCALE-UP CONSIDERATIONS AND PRODUCTION TECHNOLOGY

Victor A. Crainich, Jr.

CDS, Inc., Kettering, Ohio

I. INTRODUCTION

The general field of microencapsulation technology, representing a
multiplicity of associated chemical and physical processes, has been
practiced for over 50 years. Initially, only physical processes were
developed and introduced into commerce. Examples of these processes were spray-dried flavors and pan-coated medicaments. Then,
in the 1950s, chemical processes evolved at the National Cash Register
Co., where coacervation techniques were developed and commercialized for carbonless copy paper.

Today, a myriad of candidate physical and chemical processes
exist in commerce worldwide and often represent competitive routes
through the somewhat mystical paths of product development, process
development, engineering scale-up, facility design, and finally, manufacturing. The configuration of a final microencapsulated product
has, heretofore, nearly always been the result of, and limited to,
that fraction of the total worldwide delivery system technology to
which the product developer may have exposure or equipment availability. Thus, even from the embryonic stage of an applied research program, organizations will tend to proceed through product
development utilizing their "pet" processes or "available" equipment.
More often than not, this "close-minded" approach, in the absence
of assistance from a superior being, will lead the product development project along the road to disaster and failure. These obstinate
research approaches alone can often explain many of the numerous
product failures that have been experienced when attempts have been
made to integrate microencapsulation technology into product application and development plans. Case histories abound. Each company,
each research institute, or each university researcher walks a very

narrow path through development. Certainly, this is often dictated by project time limitations, by financial restraints, and even by "politics." However, I would suggest that a greater share might be caused by a limited knowledge of alternate microencapsulation technologies—not necessarily as practiced in the laboratory, but the multifaceted technical disciplines, experiences, and know-how required to convert a newly envisioned product application into a profitable manufacturing mode.

However, researchers and developers should not be offended by the accusation of knowledge gaps. For this present chapter is by no means intended to be a condemnation. On the contrary, this writer does fully recognize that such voids in the technology have been caused by an almost complete lack of publication of these critical downstream developmental phases of microencapsulation technology.

First, due to confinement and restriction to laboratory environs, microencapsulation academicians do not often obtain the experience, or even exposure, to the engineer's scale-up or manufacturing challenges associated with microencapsulation processes, even though they may even have participated in its early stage development. This is a pity, since such exposure could certainly assist them in their present and future process and product development perceptions. Second, academicians and company researchers need not feel offended by an accusation of downstream microencapsulation technology gaps; for the public domain is almost wholly deficient of definitive written publications or explicit verbal dissertations. All researchers, except the naive, know the basic reasons for this gap: "Industry does not talk."

For although an industrial microencapsulation developer and manufacturer may have his basic process skills, composition, or product application fully patented, he is highly reluctant, and often forbidden, to disclose the associated process paths, equipment requirements, scale-up data, and other mandatory "know-how" necessary to manufacture a microencapsulation product reproducibly and profitably. A wide chasm of public knowledge on the subject does exist. However, it is not likely to a change in any major way, since industry tends to guard such information as one would the family jewels. Unsurprisingly, some industrial firms seem to have a policy against even sending their technical personnel to seminars where microencapsulation is discussed, since jewels may have been lost in the past. Other industrial firms, out of the necessity to disclose their technology to outside engineering design and construction firms, may even have lost some of their jewels. Unfortunately, these jewels may even emerge at a competitor's facility with whom the engineering firm may also consult. These types of technology "leaks" are not necessarily intended. But the engineering firm, probably being a novice to the field of microencapsulation technology, does not clearly distinguish "the jewels" from its own proprietary data. As a result, when discovered, industry retracts even further into its shroud of secrecy. No one can truly blame these reactionary measures, since their company's profitability, and perhaps even their survival, may depend on retention of specific proprietary information and know-how.

Therefore, on one hand, the applied researchers may operate in a vacuum, since published data is unavailable. And on the other hand, industrial firms encourage an ever-increasing cloak of secrecy, and thus hinder the researchers' true perspective and understanding of many real problems in microencapsulation product and process development. Industry will often absorb a high internal development cost, i.e., the "trial-and-error" research approach, rather than disclose their shortfalls and difficulties to outside organizations.

During the past 32 years, this writer has had extensive exposure to all functional aspects of microencapsulation technology from research to final full-scale manufacturing. Thus, the opportunity to associate and apply research concepts to the potential manufacturing effects has been large, real, and continuing. During that lengthy period, a voluminous number of engineering experiences, both good and bad, have been acquired. In the past, the suppression of these experiences has contributed to the industrial cloak. In the present capacity, this direction is not likely to change in any major way.

Nevertheless, the writer does firmly believe that there is certain pertinent information and experiences that can be disclosed and presented in a cursory manner without too severely infringing upon the company's microencapsulation and delivery system technologies base. That is the objective of this chapter. It is sincerely hoped that its presentation will contribute to offering microencapsulation researchers a broadened perspective of the microencapsulation challenge that must be addressed and resolved before a microencapsulated product and its associated process can be scaled up and manufactured in a cost-effective manner.

As stated above, a broad range of appropriate subjects will be presented, but in a cursory manner only, so as to fulfill the basic scope and intent of this chapter and publication. It is hoped that individual subjects of interest can be critiqued in future publications in a more detailed manner.

II. COST DEVELOPMENT

A. Manufacturing Costs

It is by intent that we first discuss the cost development to manufacture a microencapsulated compound when, in fact, it is almost the very last cost entity to be definitively known. It is the ultimate

objective. For only after the process development, product development, engineering scale-up, facility construction, equipment acquisition, manufacturing start-up, product quality, and marketing tests
are all successful can anyone truly define manufacturing costs. Any
earlier calculations are based merely on a myriad of engineering
assumptions and estimates, as expressed by the experiences and
technical insight of the cost engineer. The product manufacturing
costs may be the last engineering data known. Yet for a new
product concept involving microencapsulation, they are usually the
initial "acid test" for whether a product development will even progress forward.

In CDS' initial product development discussions with new customers, we are invariably asked, "How much will it cost to microencapsulate my compound?" We know that the potential customer's
inquiry is sincere. So we try to give them a sincere answer: "Any-
where from $0.20 per pound to $1000.00 per pound." After a predictable moment of astonishment and silence, we explain that our response is genuine, but was truly based on the nonspecific nature of
the question asked. For the cost to microencapsulate can vary quite
vastly. However, products currently manufactured fully support
the cost range given.

Obviously, the customer's inquiry requires clarity and additional
specifications before one can more definitively answer the question
of manufacturing costs. For although cost parameters such as production volume, process definition, and process yield are important—
as they are in all manufacturing systems—microencapsulation technology necessitates the elucidation of a number of additional unique
technical properties and features. These include the polymer ratio,
polymer composition, the microencapsulation process selected, particle
size, and particle size distribution. Some of these critical parameters
will be commented upon in this chapter.

It is, however, fully recognized that the prospective product
marketer cannot wait until all development activities have actually
been performed, and manufacturing has been initiated, before a
manufacturing cost and product marketing price is established.
Fortunately, it is not necessary to wait until the manufacturing stage,
if highly experienced engineering functions are utilized. In this
case, experience in the scale-up of multifaceted microencapsulation
processes and pilot scale-manufacturing equipment performances is
mandatory. Then, on this basis, it is often possible to begin "order-
of-magnitude" cost projections as soon as initial laboratory samples
are prepared and definitized. CDS has generated such costs on a
number of occasions, thereby offering the potential marketer an
early indication of expected manufacturing costs and, therefore,
product pricing and marketing considerations.

B. Engineering

As a requisite to the success of any applied research program, a point in time arises when it is beneficial to expose and integrate the engineering disciplines into the product development project. For if it is important to obtain an early understanding of "order-of-magnitude" manufacturing costs, early exposure is mandatory. However, cost engineering need not be directly involved with applied research projects until at least the initial phase of developmental microencapsulated samples have been demonstrated by the marketer and a significant number of the desired or predetermined product objectives have been achieved. For example, it would be unrealistic to generate an engineering cost for a microencapsulated product where it is desired to have a particle size of 100 μm when the laboratory samples to date have been produced with a 500-μm mean particle size. The experienced process engineer will know that the laboratory experiments still require modifications, which, in turn, could ultimately affect the accuracy of the estimated cost. The process must be modified, product yields may vary, and most certainly the ultimate process may dictate different equipment requirements.

So it is desirable to involve the process engineering staff as soon as the requirement for product costing projections is indicated. But what accuracy can be expected from an engineering cost at this early stage? As might be expected, the answer is: "It depends." The answer depends primarily on:

1. The experience of the engineer and his or her prior familiarity with the expected scale-up design and manufacturing equipment performance
2. The relative cost of polymer materials and materials to be microencapsulated
3. The engineer's process yield estimates, which will contribute further sensitivity to the product cost estimate

For example, if we were to microencapsulate a very expensive compound, i.e., gold or diamonds, using a high-cost polymer, then we must seriously assess process yields and be less concerned about materials and labor costs. To the contrary, if an inexpensive material is to be microencapsulated, labor, materials costs, and production volume will normally be the major contributors to the cost estimate.

Obviously, there are many additional parameters that will ultimately contribute to the final manufacturing cost of microcapsules, but they are not significant for first cost projections.

"Order-of-magnitude" costs generated from preliminary laboratory samples will, by definition, carry a large cost variance. At this earliest stage, a cost projection of ±50% would not be unrealistic.

C. Scale-up

Engineers involved in microencapsulation systems perform scale-up or pilot plant operations for two primary reasons:

1. To produce larger quantities of microencapsulated materials than are reasonably available from laboratory-scale facilities.
2. To develop engineered manufacturing costs

Larger quantities of microencapsulated materials are often required to initiate:

    a. Product performance tests
    b. Field efficacy tests
    c. Marketing assessments
    d. Manufacturing equipment performance

Engineered cost represents a comprehensive evaluation of all direct labor, materials, process yields, process equipment components, utilities, and facilities that are expected to contribute to total manufacturing costs.

If a particular microencapsulation process is being scaled up for the first time, costs development is particularly challenging to the project engineer.   Some of the considerations that must be addressed for the first time may include the following:

1. Direct Labor
    a. The number of labor hours required
    b. Personnel qualifications
    c. Projected future labor rates
2. Materials
    a. Sole/multiple sources
    b. Future materials costs
    c. Inventory requirements
    d. Supply capabilities
    e. Quality variability
    f. Source of shipping points
    g. Procurement frequency
    h. Packaging requirements
    i. Procurement volume/materials cost effects
    j. Freight costs
3. Process yields
    a. The translation of laboratory scale-up to manufacturing yields
    b. Expected batch-to-batch process yield variability
    c. Operation error and/or equipment malfunctions

4. Process equipment
   a. Projected future equipment cost
   b. Source and availability
   c. Customization requirements
   d. Process adaptability
   e. Performance history
5. Utilities
   a. The projection facility geographic location
   b. Projecting future utility operational cost
   c. Projecting, estimating, and calculating utilities consumption
   d. Predetermination of equipment and utility configurations
   e. Infrastructure status
6. Facility
   a. Land availability
   b. Engineering costs
   c. Facility construction costs
   d. Equipment installation costs
   e. Personnel acquisition and training
   f. Manufacturing start-up period

There is considerable concern, by this writer, that when process engineers review the above outline, they may conclude that the scale-up parameters and cost considerations given are not new, since they seem to be identical, or at least similar, to other chemical scale-up activities. Certainly that initial conclusion would be true, except for the fact that all of the listed parameters must be defined, analyzed, and estimated in the context of addressing a microencapsulation process. Why does that make the engineering cost estimating activity unique? This chapter will try to contribute to answering the question.

D. Equipment Evaluation

Assuming that a new process is being scaled up, it is extremely important during the engineering scale-up phase to adequately identify the specific equipment that will ultimately be required in the manufacturing facility. For equipment design and performance specifications will have a significant impact on the acquisition cost of the equipment.

If a defined microencapsulation process has unique performance requirements, it is highly likely that the perceived process equipment will require unique features and design modifications. It is possible that the microencapsulation process may even dictate a requirement for completely new, customized equipment design.

These unique equipment design demands are not particularly unusual when microencapsulation processes are being engineered. How, then, should engineers address this problem during the equipment

evaluation phase? First, it is desirable to possess or have access
to highly flexible and adaptable pilot-scale equipment. If the
equipment is not available in-house, then it may be necessary to
rent the equipment or test in a vendor's facility. For example, a
pilot-scale reactor should have the designed capability to accomodate
a variety of mixing conditions, including agitation designs, speed
ranges, and mixing configurations. For even with an expertly pre-
planned pilot-scale facility, it seems to be almost always necessary
to evaluate certain equipment or design configurations that are not
available in-house. Thus, testing in the manufacturer's testing facilities often becomes necessary.

Unavailability of in-house pilot equipment in itself often generates
a unique problem related to many microencapsulation systems. With
such systems it is often difficult, if not impossible, to preestablish
a material's identical physical conditions in a vendor's facility as
would be experienced in one's own pilot plant. For example, if it is
desired to evaluate drying equipment that requires a filter cake of a
microencapsulation compound as process feedstock, how do we ensure
that the characteristics of the feedstock are identical to what would
actually be generated in a manufacture mode?

Immediately a problem exists: Even the predictable static conditions caused by the need to package and ship the filter cake material
to a vendor's destination can cause abnormal drying test conditions
and results that may not adequately simulate the sequential process
operations of an actual manufacturing mode. Fusion of microcapsules,
wet-state permeability, bulk handling of a shear-sensitive microcapsule, diffusion, and premature drying are just examples of some of
the raw material deviations caused by attempting to ship an "in-
process" test material. It is easy to reflect upon the disastrous experimental results of a number of equipment trials where these parameters were not adequately considered.

As a result, it is possible that a novice engineer might wrongly
conclude that certain drying equipment design configurations are inadequate, when, in fact, the real problem might be a poorly simulated feedstock. How, then, are equipment test results to be interpreted? It almost always demands comprehensive engineering experience to offer proper and adequate test planning and test results
assessment. This microencapsulation engineering experience is almost
never communicated in the public domain.

Aside from projecting the cost of manufacturing equipment, it may
also be important to project the cost of the equipment evaluation
function itself. This function comprises:

1. The cost of producing "test" quantities of microencapsulation
    materials, which, more than likely, will not be recyclable nor
    salable.
2. Packaging and freight costs

3. Vendor testing facility costs
4. Analytical costs

These "one-time" costs are often overlooked by the process engineer when estimating the project development cost requirements.

E. Facility

Facility cost development and estimation is dependent on a number of parameters:

1. Land cost or availability
2. Geographic location
3. Manufacturing capacity
4. Facility expansion capability

Upon first analysis, one might not conclude that land acquisition cost would be affected by the microencapsulation processes. However, unless individual end-use microcapsule markets justify (for instance, carbonless paper or perhaps a herbicide), the construction of an individual large-volume facility, it may be most desirable to acquire land that would allow the construction of a multifacility complex which, in total, would be capable of producing and servicing a variety of processing requirements.

Is the facility dedicated to a specific microencapsulation process? A specific microencapsulated product? A specific customer? The latter two may even affect geographic location. Corporate management may have an inherent desire to locate a new microencapsulation facility proximal to existing facilities. Precedent has shown this decision to be erroneous: "Force-fitting" a microencapsulation facility into the infrastructure of an existing facility may require too many design and layout compromises to be made of the new facility.

This writer believes that, because of the many unique operating features demanded by a microencapsulation facility, a geographic location should be selected independent of an organization's current geographic location. Then, when unbiased alternate locations are listed, and one location also happens to coincide with an existing location, this selection will offer an additional economic or logistic advantage. As mentioned earlier, the only rational exception to this selection approach would be when the new microencapsulation facility will be a large-volume, through-put facility and directly aligned to a coordinating, fully integrated manufacturing process. One example of such an exception would be carbonless paper microcapsules, a paper manufacturing installation, and a paper coating facility. Another example would be the subsequent microencapsulation of herbicides following their manufacture, wherein freight costs could be prohibitive.

Manufacturing design capacity has always been a difficult decision for the design engineer. The classical and academic approach to establish facility capacity suggests that the capacity be calculated from historical market data and forecasts. However, historically, with respect to microencapsulated products, such data sources have hardly ever proven fruitful or correct. This is due primarily to the fact that the microencapsulated product may be a new, untested product such that realistic or insufficient marketing data existed.

Yet establishing a facility's design/operating capacity is undoubtedly one of the key parameters to establishing the total capital cost of a new facility. It will determine building area and volume requirements, and it will also determine service and process equipment sizing. Historically, in several cases, new manufacturing facilities have been cost estimated, project approved, authorized, and designs begun, and only then does new marketing data indicate higher capacity requirements. Even worse, there have been incidences where such marketing data became available only after the plant had been constructed and major process equipment either committed, fabricated, or already installed. At this point, facility capacity cannot be effectively modified without disproportionately affecting facility capital construction cost as well as targeted completed schedules.

Therefore, a facility's expansion capability and the additional cost to integrate this design parameter into the original cost development can be extremely important. Thus, in developing capital cost estimates, three options exist: (a) Design the facility to a capacity that is discernibly greater than current marketing data indicates; (b) design the facility for nominal 100% capacity, based on available marketing data; or (c) design the facility with expansion capability. If engineering design experience related to microencapsulation facilities is available, the latter approach, can be integrated into a facility design at relatively low capital investment cost. Historically, this design capacity "hedge" can more than justify its incremental additional capital investment.

F. Capital Equipment

The development of costs projected for facility capital equipment should be divided into service equipment and process equipment.

Service equipment is represented by steam generation and condensation recovery, compressed air, electrical distribution, general water, fire protection and related nonprocess safety systems, general facility heating, ventilating and air conditioning (HVAC), and security systems. Certain HVAC systems, if required for process requirements rather than personal comfort, would be considered process equipment. The same analogy would apply to inert gas and treated water if they are required for process utilization. "Treated water" could include deionized water, distilled water, or any other facility-related, process-dictated treatment, including waste treatment.

Therefore, it should be evident that the majority of equipment required for a microencapsulation facility is process equipment and may comprise up to 90% of the capital equipment costs required.

As with any chemical process, service equipment can be acquired from a multiplicity of potential competitive vendors as "off-the-shelf" commodities. When service capacities are defined, the cost for service capital equipment can be readily generated to a relatively high degree of accuracy.

Process equipment costs should not be generated until engineering has completed process flow diagrams (PFDs) and piping and installation diagrams (P&IDs). These engineering drawings will illustrate all process equipment requirements, their interrelationships, controls, and process flow rates.

Process capital equipment costs will comprise all equipment illustrated on PFDs. Such costs should include equipment acquisition, field pretesting if necessary, freight, equipment installation, and consumable spare parts. Maintenance, spare parts, and maintenance contracts would not normally be included in initial facility capitalization, but would instead be included in normal operating costs.

As mentioned earlier, to achieve a properly designed microencapsulation facility a considerable amount of process equipment must be custom-designed for maximum performance. Thus, early product cost development must be estimated based almost solely on the engineers' experience with the microencapsulation process, equipment performance, and the specific manufacturing facility. Final cost estimates cannot be generated accurately until process equipment field evaluation and testing is completed, because testing data and results can often indicate the need for equipment modifications.

III. SCALE-UP PLAN

To scale up a batch microencapsulation process from laboratory quantities, where perhaps a few grams of microencapsulation are processed, to a full-scale manufacturing facility, where up to 100 kg of microcapsules are produced, normally requires a number of scale-up stages or phases. It is highly recommended that scale-up be evaluated in a multiplicity of scale-up capacities, with each state increasing by a multiple factor of 5—7. Thus, if an initial laboratory research scale batch yields ca. 200 g of product, three stages of scale-up plus the full manufacturing scale must be evaluated. These would be represented, for example, by process scale-up batch sizes of 1.5, 10, and 70 kg, prior to a full manufacturing scale. Pilot-scale reactors are shown in Figs. 1 through 4.

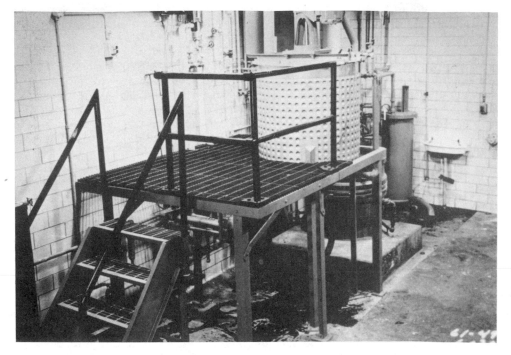

Fig. 1 Pilot plant aqueous reactor (200 gal).

During each stage of scale-up, complete process and product data should be collected and analyzed so as to define the process equipment requirements and product quality achieved. The process engineer must assess a number of scale-up considerations, such as:

1. Raw material variability
2. Process control latitude
3. Product quality variations
4. Product yield projection
5. Process equipment limitations

A. Raw Materials

During the early product development stages, it is important to evaluate the lot-to-lot quality variability of raw materials that will be expected from candidate vendors. For example, the vendors can expect to offer raw materials whose specifications satisfy a range of physical and chemical properties. However, it would be a severe mistake to assume that the microencapsulation process can be

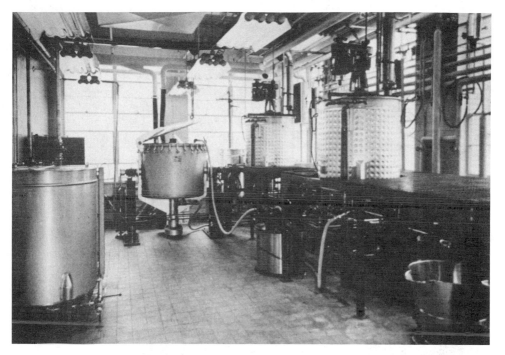

Fig. 2 Pilot plant solvent reactors (200 gal) and support equipment.

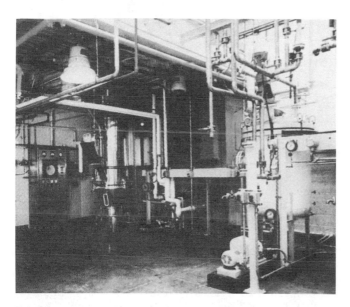

Fig. 3 Pilot plant pharmaceutical reactor. (Courtesy of Eurand America.)

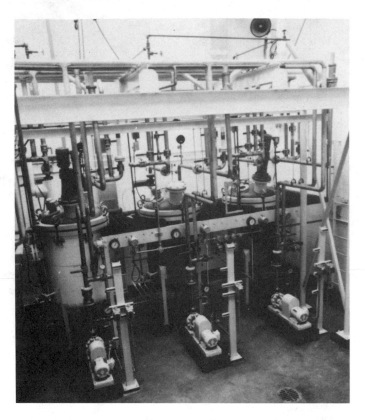

Fig. 4 Pilot plant aqueous reactor. (Courtesy of Eurand America.)

satisfactorily utilized within the complete range of raw materials
specifications offered. Experience has clearly illustrated that such
an assumption, when translated to the manufacturing scale, can be
financially disastrous. What may appear to be subtle changes in a
raw material's physical or chemical properties may cause manufactured products to yield microencapsulated products outside their
own specification range and thus cause severely reduced yields. In
some cases, when not discovered early, raw material changes have
even yielded malfunctioning converted end products. Converted
products are defined as the final form and application of the microcapsules, as they are utilized and/or consumed by the end-user.
    During the scale-up process, it can often be advantageous to
assess alternative supply sources for raw materials. This latitude
not only allows an increased assurance of supply, but may generate
more competitive pricing from vendors. However, experience has

shown that when identifying raw materials for microencapsulation systems, developing multiple or even dual sources of raw materials is almost never a straightforward task. This is particualrly true of the monomers, prepolymers, and polymers that are used in microencapsulation processes as the encapsulant or carrier. Unfortunately, the differences in the processibility and effectiveness of raw materials from different vendors are not always easily delineated from the chemical/physical properties normally specified by them. Therefore, it is often only after trial and error, tedious analysis of lot-to-lot variations, and the resultant microencapsulation product quality that raw material differences are all taken into account.

Thus, individuals who have never experienced all of the processing problems associated with changing or expanding raw material sources for microencapsulated processes might conclude that insufficient scientific definition of these processes must exist; and perhaps, the whole technology may be more of an art that a science. Those individuals who have had extensive microencapsulation experience, and in particular scale-up experience, would tend to agree. But why aren't these processes clearly definable in order for raw materials quality to be correctly specified to the vendors? Several of these processes, such as various coacervation techniques, have been utilized in commercial products for over 30 years! The answer is both simple and complicated. First, the microencapsulation processes utilized in manufacturing most commercial products during the 30-year period have not remained constant. For example, microcapsules for carbonless paper have undergone four major changes, all of which required different monomer/polymer systems. Second, total predetermination of raw materials requirements based solely on written specifications for acceptance-rejection criteria have always proven fruitless, even though major R&D efforts have been expended by highly experienced microencapsulation research chemists and highly skilled polymer chemists of the vendors. As a result, a more direct, "results-oriented" approach to raw materials acceptance has been taken by at least three microencapsulation firms. In these firms, in addition to the more classical detailed specifications, each new lot of raw material is also committed to a laboratory-scale microencapsulation prior to the materials being fully accepted for production. This may seem to be a very archaic and nonscientific approach to resolving an ongoing technical problem. But it satisfies the objective and it does save considerable money, for this technical approach to the problem has markedly reduced manufacturing losses. Following is one case history: Although the specific organization cannot be disclosed, one firm scrapped over $400,000 in final product before a raw material deviation (not specification) was identified by preparing lab-scale microencapsulation batches.

How does the process for raw materials selection relate to scale-up studies? It relates very clearly, for it further emphasizes the need to completely correlate and project detailed laboratory and pilot plant processing data to the anticipated manufacturing process. In addition, the data generated can offer the candidate vendor(s) an early signal or warning that raw material controllable variables (physical/chemical properties) must be kept to an absolute minimum—and often to a considerably narrower specification range than vendors might normally guarantee. Frequently, new raw material grades may evolve from the vendors to accommodate the higher quality requirements which, more often than not, creates a premium price for these "special" raw materials. From a process cost savings viewpoint, the price differential is usually justified.

B. Process Control Latitude

When new microencapsulation processes are scaled up and project responsibilities are shifted from the R&D laboratories, it is a valuable tool and guideline for the R&D chemist to prepare and transfer a written procedure of the new microencapsulation process to the process engineer. In this regard, microencapsulation projects are treated similarly to any other chemical process development project. However, during the scale-up phase it is exceptionally critical to analyze the "process parameter flexibility" of the microencapsulation process. Process procedure flexibility analyses, depending on the type of microencapsulation process being addressed, include a number of operating parameters such as temperature, presssure, rate of addition, order of addition, emulsification criteria, reaction time, heating rate, cooling rate, washing time period and number of cycles, filtration conditions, drying conditions, classification, and blending conditions. Any and all of these operating parameters can be critical. Production-scale process control panel boards are illustrated in Figs. 5 and 6.

It has been concluded from extensive experience that a vast number of operating parameters relating to a microencapsulation process will have an ultimate effect on the microencapsulated product quality and the manufacturing yield. Therefore, process control instrumentation can and does play a critical role in assuring maximized product quality and yield. When designing and constructing new facilities for our firm or our licensees, process control considerations are among the most critical analyses. As cited elsewhere, microcapsule product quality and reproducibility in a manufacturing mode is not only difficult without adequate process control, it is often a technical and financial disaster!

How does process control design and operation differ from other types of chemical reactions? In most cases, it differs dramatically,

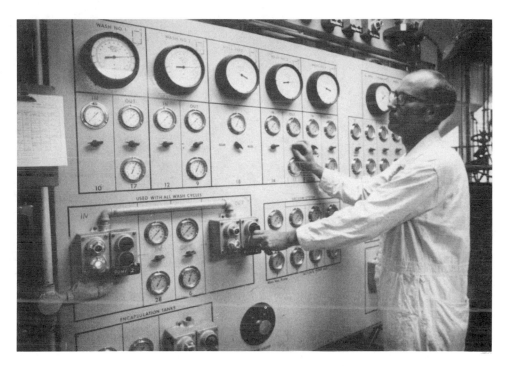

Fig. 5 Production-scale process control panel board.

since microencapsulation processes are often nonreversible reactions (in situ polymerization, interfacial polymerization), or if reversible, will follow a phase-diagram hysteresis loop. Even those microencapsulation systems in which desired operating conditions may have been disrupted or become "out of control," and then the conditions are ultimately reversed, will yield a microencapsulated product of altered quality. Complex coacervation systems are examples of processes that will exhibit hysteresis.

On the other hand, certain solvent-based phase-separation microencapsulation processes are frequently reversible. The resultant resolubilization and redeposition of polymers can greatly affect the quality of final polymer film formation, and therefore the quality of the microencapsulated product itself.

During engineering scale-up studies, critical operating parameters will be intentionally altered to ascertain the resultant effect on product quality and yield. Results from these studies will then aid in the definition and sophistication of process control equipment ultimately required in the manufacturing facility.

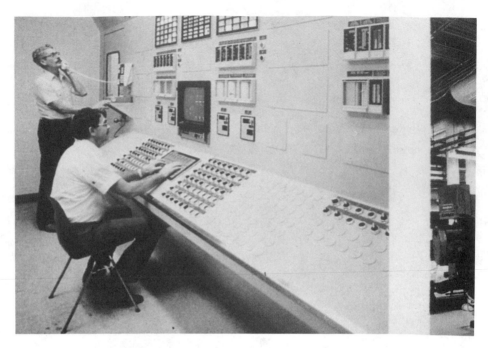

Fig. 6 Production-scale process control panel board. (Courtesy of
Eurand America.)

C. Product Quality Variations

One dangerous practice that has often occurred in microencapsulation
product development projects is the premature establishment of product specifications. After many shocking prior operational experiences, it has finally been more broadly accepted that product specifications cannot and should not be established based solely on laboratory-scale experimentation. It has been shown time and time again
(and for many of the technical reasons being discussed in this chapter) that, because of the multiple scale-up stages, mass effects,
equipment design variations, as well as process control limitations,
resulting product quality may vary significantly during scale-up experimentation. Thus, microencapsulated product specifications should
evolve from the actual scale-up test data generated and not from
laboratory experimentation.

It is easy to recall product specifications being prematurely established by the applications research program management at the
time new products were being developed for new potential markets.
The same "new product specification" was simultaneously transmitted
to the marketing group, who, unfortunately, often transmit the antic-

ipated new product specifications to potential customers. More critically, if the product is a pharmaceutical and the specifications have been prematurely transmitted to the Food and Drug Administration (FDA), it is quite possible to become committed to a product specification that is very difficult and expensive to fulfill in a manufacturing mode. Unfortunately, there have been a few commercial microencapsulated products that have suffered this ill fate, for it was only after considerable additional scale-up and manufacturing costs were expended in vain that realistic product specifications finally evolved.

D. Product Yield Projections

One of the key aspects of any microencapsulation scale-up study is to adjudge the product yield projections that can be anticipated from a new process being scaled up to a full manufacturing facility.

During preliminary scale-up, detailed analytical analyses and mass balances for each processing step and each material transfer are undertaken. It may be readily obvious to identify those microencapsulation processing stages where critical losses may be occurring. Since yields will have a significant and direct impact upon the economics of the final product, it is always important to ensure that yields are optimized. Optimization normally occurs as a culmination of scale-up studies that access and correlate the process, process modifications, and associated equipment performance. Although there are exceptions, in most scale-up scenarios the parameters related to optimized microencapsulation processes indicate a definitive requirement for nonstandard process equipment, or at least significant modifications in "off-the-shelf" items. Depending on the process and the product form, this equipment may include emulsifiers, the primary reactor, washing vessels, filters, dryers, blenders, and classifiers.

It is beyond the scope of this chapter to detail the myriad of microencapsulation processing aspects necessary to optimize any specific process or product being produced. However, it may be of interest to cite several actual product yields that have been experienced by various commercial processes. Microencapsulation yields for carbonless paper are approximately 98%; microencapsulated aspirin has a processing yield of about 94% on certain grades. Microencapsulated fragances normally have lower yields of 80—90%, depending on fragrance volatility and equipment design.

E. Laboratory Transition

It is anticipated that the very first stages of scale-up, perhaps up to a 1- to 2-kg batch, can and should be performed within the laboratory environment. This stage offers the engineer an opportun-

ity to work directly with the applications research chemist in evaluating the initial stages of the process, as well as the equipment that
may be utilized. At this first stage of scale-up, the process variables are most readily and easily evaluated to assess deviations from
a norm. In many cases, depending on the equipment required, it is
often possible to make, simultaneously, a multiplicity of laboratory-
scale batches having various process parameters and then access
the end product caused by these process variables. Evaluating process parameters at this stage allows for minimal materials loss during
the scale-up development. During this first stage, process parameters such as those referenced previously are most critically assessed
so that they may be firmly established during the future stages of
scale-up. Additionally, during the first stage of scale-up, evaluation of various equipment variations is desirable to ensure compliance
with the specifications that may have been determined. Thus, the
second and third stages of scale-up are devoted primarily to equipment evaluation rather than to process variables. This is to ensure
that the equipment will operate within the range where the process
variables have been established and where the final product from
those scale-ups will still fulfill the product specifications. As mentioned earlier, the first stage of scale-up can normally be accomplished within the laboratory environment. However, the laboratory
equipment may not necessarily be analogous to equipment that may
be required for scale-up in the second and third stages, and in the
manufacturing stage. A key activity during the first stage is for
the engineer to extrapolate and perceive future manufacturing equipment requirements.

F. Pilot Plant Transition

When process development is transferred from a laboratory scale into
the pilot plant (1—2 kg), it is often advantageous to allow the research chemist to transfer with the project. This practice provides
improved communications and a greater efficiency in interpreting experimental results. In most cases, there is a greater technology gap
in the process equipment capabilities between the laboratory scale
and the pilot plant scale than exists between the pilot plant scale
and the ultimate manufacturing. This is due primarily to the fact
that process equipment design at the pilot plant and the manufacturing scale tend to be similar in design configuration, whereas laboratory equipment is related more to research-oriented projects. As
mentioned earlier, unless a very flexible pilot plant is designed and
maintained, the second and third stage of pilot plant efforts may be
accomplished, at least partially, in the vendor's facility. Since the
vendor's equipment is likely to be very customized, this adds
credibility to the scale-up project. In the past, it has often been

necessary to perform a myriad of equipment evaluations at the vendor's facility. Equipment evaluations are performed throughout the free world.

Field equipment evaluations, in themselves, have created additional problems during the scale-up phase. For example, if you are interested in filtration equipment, then you must ship to a vendor a feedstock for that filter. For obvious reasons, you will want to simulate the filtration process as closely as possible. To accomplish this, it is necessary to carry the microencapsulation process through the entire system up to the stage required for the filtration and then ship the filter feedstock (slurry) material to the vendor. Although this task may sound fairly straightforward, it is, in fact, very difficult to simulate an ongoing process internally by actually interrupting the process and evaluating the equipment externally. For example, the stability of the microcapsule slurry materials may differ due to time and environmental exposure than if they were being processed wholly internally and sequentially with other stages of the process. Thus, an evaluation of a filter outside the pilot plant facility can create new problems, which are not to be associated or confused with the actual process itself. For example, during the winter months it may be difficult to ensure that an aqueous slurry does not freeze during transit. It may also be necessary to be concerned about the volatility of the materials that have been encapsulated.

Evaluating drying equipment in a vendor's facility creates perhaps even greater problems. In this case, it is necessary to ship a filter cake in a nondried state to the vendor for use a feedstock for the drying evaluation. At the very least, very tight scheduling is required to ensure that the minimum exposure time of filter cake is maintained. If filter cake materials are allowed to dry during transit or before being processed in the drying equipment, the test is not valid. More often than not, when materials are shipped they are stored in a static state and have an opportunity to aggregate. Thus, the feedstock becomes completely useless for test purposes. To ensure that the lag time required to ship material to a vendor has, in fact, not altered the properties of the product, it is necessary to simultaneously retain material within the pilot plant in a static condition and then process the material simultaneously with the vendor's experimentation. Then, when the field test is evaluated, it can be compared to retained samples. These few examples should enlighten the readers of several difficulties that are unique to progressing microencapsulation products during an engineering scale-up program. For there are many aspects to consider that would not be experienced in a normal chemical processing scale-up operation. It may be a trite statement, but it is certainly true that there is no substitution for experience when engineering microencapsulation processes through the pilot plant stages.

IV. EQUIPMENT CONSIDERATIONS

If the process to be scaled up is represented by coacervation, interfacial polymerization, in situ polymerization, phase separation, or
gelation chemical processes, then there are a number of process
equipment operations to evaluate and consider during a scale-up program. If a mechanical process is being engineered, such as pan
coating, spray coating, or fluid bed coating, then the equipment com-
plications are much less. In this section we will discuss the candidate equipment necessary for various chemical processes.

A. Emulsification

It is usually desirous to microencapsulate materials to yield a very
specific and reproducible particle size distribution range. If the material to be microencapsulated is a liquid, then it is necessary to
emulsify to a specific particle size prior to its encapsulation (reservoir systems). If the material to be microencapsulated is a solid,
then it is also necessary to precondition the particles to the desired
size. If available raw materials are too large, the particles must be
premilled.
    There are commercial product requirements for microcapsules rang-
ing from 20 nm up to 5000 μm. Liquid-core microcapsules having a
particle size greater than 300 μm can usually be emulsified in the
same reaction vessel where microencapsulation takes place. Liquid
droplets 2 to 300 μm in size require preemulsification prior to microencapsulation. Emulsification should be performed in a different
vessel than the reactor itself. A number of designs and styles of
emulsifiers are available from vendors that can be utilized to develop
droplets for microcapsules. The emulsifiers have the ability to emulsify droplets from 300 μm down to perhaps 1 or 2 μm in diameter.
To produce droplets below 2 μm usually requires a different approach
to emulsification. There are several mechanical approaches. One of
these approaches is ultrasonic equipment. Another approach utilizes
high-pressure fluid streams. The latter equipment is produced by
Microfluidics. A production model of the equipment is shown in Fig.
7. Microfluidics equipment will emulsify oil droplets down to particle
size of 400 nm. This equipment is often used for producing liposomes, i.e., microcapsules containing lipid walls.
    It is normally an objective during the emulsification operation to
produce a narrow particle size distribution. One question that is
often asked is: "How narrow a particle size distribution can be produced?" The reply to this inquiry is very dependent on the type
of equipment used, but it is also dependent on the operating conditions in which emulsification occurs.
    In a typical emulsification step, it would normally be expected
that the particle size distribution would comprise a size range where-

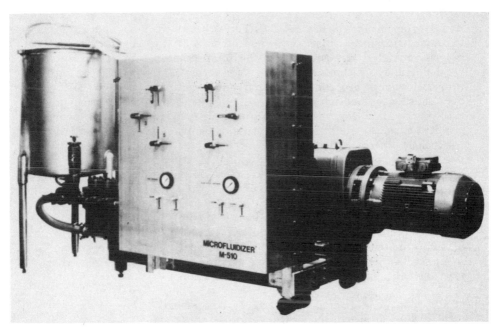

Fig. 7 High-pressure emulsifier. (Courtesy of Microfluidics.)

in 90% of the particles are ±50% of the mean particle size. That is, microcapsules having a mean size of 200 μm would comprise a distribution where 90% of the particles were in a size range of 100 to 300 μm. If larger particles are desired, say, 2000 μm, then particles having a 90% distribution of 1000 to 3000 μm can be expected. Microcapsules having a much tighter distribution are required, in some cases, and can be produced. However, the key word is patience. That is, considerable emulsification time is required. A good commercial example of this approach is carbonless paper, as produced under the NCR brand name. It is produced by a coacervation process. These capsules have a cluster or aggregation configuration. Individual droplets are approximately 2 μm and are clustered to approximately 8 μm. To achieve a narrow size distribution of particles of 2 μm requires prolonged batch-scale emulsification. During the process oil droplets are actually emulsified through a continuous recirculation system for over 6 hr prior to the actual encapsulation step.

B. Reactors

Batch-type encapsulation systems require custom-designed reactors in which microencapsulation is performed. In the reactor, the polymeric wall is deposited onto the oil droplet reservoir or onto a solid particle. Without a doubt the reactor itself and its configuration components are the most important portion of the process design of a microencapsulation system. It has been illustrated time and time again that poor reactor design results in low yields or poor-quality microcapsules. As with most aspects of microencapsulation technology, reactor design configurations for microencapsulation vessels are not published in the open literature. The obvious purpose for this omission is that each firm fiercely attempts to retain its own experiences rather than divulge this know-how to the public—including its competitors.

Through the years, several reactor designs have been directed specifically for microencapsulation systems. It is beyond the scope of this chapter to discuss all of the engineering details required to design a functional encapsulation reactor. Suffice it to say that the following aspects are worth consideration:

1. The geometric design ratio of the vessel
2. The bottom head configuration
3. The number of baffles and the baffle design, that is, the cross-sectional area and location in the vessel
4. The heat exchange mechanism
5. The agitator, the number of mixing blades, and their configuration

All of these design parameters, and more, must be taken into consideration in relation to the microencapsulation process to be utilized. In the past there have been horrible experiences when it had been falsely concluded that the reactor design requirements for two systems were not in themselves different. For instance, one very serious case occurred where a facility was being used for encapsulating a pharmaceutical, and was converted to run a second pharmaceutical product. Both processes required the same basic encapsulation system, as well as the same solvents. However, when the attempted conversion was made, disaster resulted. What had not been initially considered was the density difference of the two products. This change, in itself, created a significant difference in the mixing configuration. A completely different type of reactor and agitator system were indicated. This is perhaps the best example of where each individual process and the material encapsulated supports and justifies its own customized design. Examples of production-scale reactors are shown in Figs. 8 through 11.

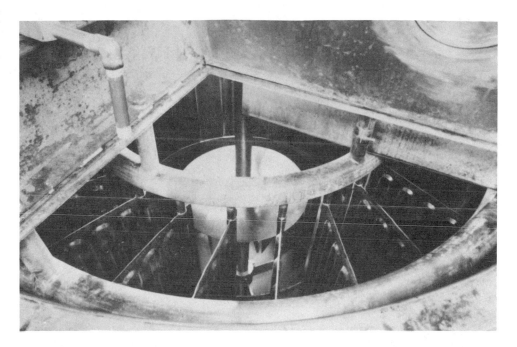

Fig. 8 Aqueous reactor (2000 gal) with cooling system.

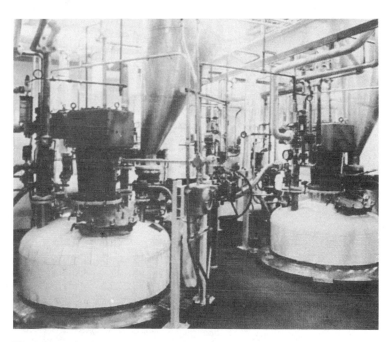

Fig. 9 Dual aqueous reactors (500 gal). (Courtesy of Eurand America.)

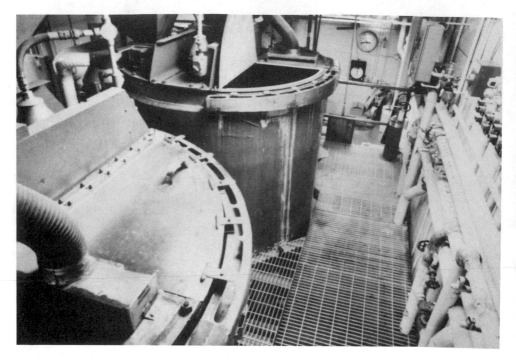

Fig. 10 Dual solvent reactors (1000 gal).

C. Treatment Equipment

In some processes, after the microcapsules are produced in a reactor, it is necessary to wash the microcapsules to elute the continuous phase, i.e., solvent or water. When certain microcapsules are produced down to as low as 1 to 2 μm, it is easy to note that the microcapsules are not readily separated from the continuous phase in a simple settling tank. Therefore, clarification and purification of the microcapsules might be accomplished through clarifiers or centrifugal separators. A production-scale wash and settling tank is shown in Fig. 12.

The next step in the microencapsulation process might be filtration. If one is interested in removing the bulk of the continuous phase from the microcapsules, a drying operation is necessary after filtration or centrifugation. In the laboratory, capsule concentration can be accomplished very readily with a Büchner filter or centrifuge. However, in the pilot plant or in the manufacturing plant, Büchner-design filters are very large, cumbersome, and very labor-intensive. In some microcapsule processes containing large (greater than 1000

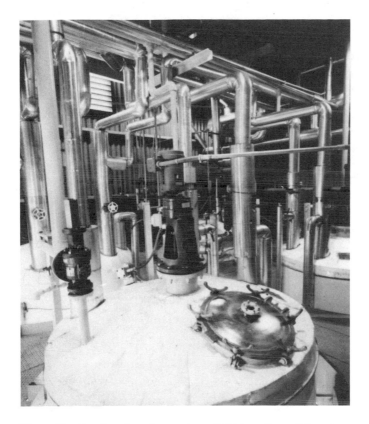

Γig. 11   Dual solvent reactor (1000 gal). (Courtesy of Eurand America.)

μm), liquid-core microcapsules, a large-scale Büchner filter may be the only solution, due to microcapsule frangibility. However, batch filters have one major drawback: They possess a very high volume-to-filtration area ratio.   Other types of standardized filtration equipment designs are more practical and effective in filtering microcapsules on a manufacturing scale.   Two of these designs are rotary vacuum drum filters and plate-and-frame filters.   Whether one is seeking a continuous filtration system or a batch filtration system may dictate which filtration design will be most efficient.   However, in both cases, the filtrate is transported through a very thin filter cake media, which also allows efficient additional washing cycles and high-concentration filter cakes.   There are other operational differences as well.   During filtration, it is desirous to develop a relatively moderate pressure drop across the filter cake.   However, if

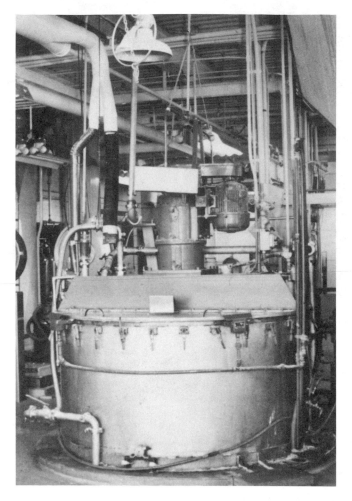

Fig. 12   Solvent wash tank (1000 gal).

the microcapsules are very large, it is obviously difficult to develop
a pressure difference across a rotary drum filter containing a very
thin filter cake.   Thus, since a pressure differential is required to
retain the microcapsules to the filter media while it is being filtered,
the filter cake will not form properly.   One solution to this problem
is a continuous belt filter.   A continuous belt filter might be considered as being nothing more than a rotary filter that is unwound
to a flat surface.   A continuous belt filter offers many advantages
that cannot be achieved with a rotary drum, including operating at

a significantly lower pressure drop. Since the filter cake can be formed in very thin layers, washing efficiency is also improved immensely.

As far as plate-and-frame filters are concerned, it is preferable to operate the filter press under a vacuum, as opposed to a pressure filter may be more efficient when removing higher quantities of the bed to no more than 1 atm, whereas a pressure filter will often develop or cause microcapsule aggregation. A pressure filter may be designed to operate up to 4 to 5 atm across the filter cake, thus resulting in excessive microcapsule filter cake compaction. A pressure filter may be more efficeint when removing higher quantitites of continuous phase, but with many microencapsulation systems it also causes downstream drying problems.

Over the past 30 years, in chemical microencapsulation processes, there have been a myriad of engineering approaches taken to isolate the capsules as dry, free-flowing powders. Both chemical and mechanical treatment techniques have been evaluated. Often, a combination of drying systems is necessary to obtain dry, free-flowing microcapsules. Chemical systems relate to treating the surface with chemicals such as surfactants or drying powders, such as silicates, talc, starches, etc. The sole objective of any such chemical additive is to inhibit aggregation during the drying operation.

Perhaps one of the more challenging process equipment development phases that this reader has experienced has been the drying of microcapsules. I believe that during the past 30 years every known technique for mechanically drying microcapsules has been attempted. Spray dryers, tower dryers, fluid-bed dryers, flash dryers, tray dryers, rotary trays, each in a batch or continuous configuration have been evaluated. Of all of these, batch fluid-bed dryers have demonstrated to be the most efficient. A production-scale continuous fluid-bed dryer is shown in Fig. 13.

While some mechanical microencapsulation techniques now utilize fluid beds for coating solid particles, fluid beds were used much earlier in drying microcapsules that had been produced by chemical systems. As early as 1965, we were experimenting with various fluid-bed dryer design configurations and, in fact, closely assisted the Fitzpatrick Company in designing and operating the very first pilot- /and production-scale agitated fluid-bed dryers. All of this was accomplished before mechanical microencapsulation via fluid-bed coaters was publicized or even practiced. One limitation of fluid-bed drying (or fluid-bed coating) is the particle size limitation. There have been some publications, as well as some company literature, which have claimed to produce dry, small microcapsules via fluid-bed techniques. This writer adamantly disagrees. In my opinion, microcapsules below 100 μm cannot be dried efficiently in batch-size fluid-bed configurations. There is scientific rationale for this posi-

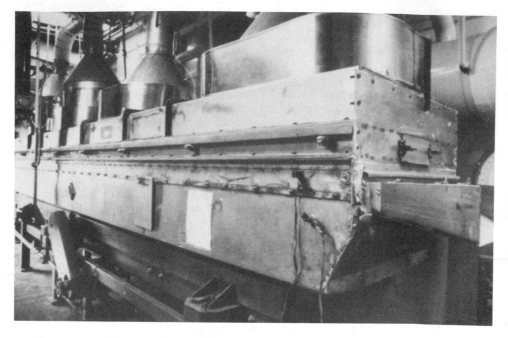

Fig. 13 Production-scale vibratory dryer.

tion: The velocity of microcapsules or particles moving in an airstream are influenced by Stokes' law. All spherical particles will
achieve a respective terminal velocity that is dependent on their
respective particle size. The terminal velocity of a particle is proportional to the square of the particle diameter, whereas the ability
to fluidize particles is closely proportional to the diameter of the particle. Thus it can be calculated, as well as demonstrated, that particles of 100 μm have a terminal velocity of 1 ft/sec. Any time the
airstream in a fluid bed reaches 1 ft/sec or greater, particles of
100 μm or less will be entrained in the airstream and will then be
exhausted from the expanded fluid bed and will be trapped on the
fluid-bed filter. Particles greater than 100 μm in a bed having an
air velocity of 1 ft/sec will expand into the open chamber and tend
to fall back to the bed plate and then recycle. However, particles
of, for example, 10 μm have a nominal terminal velocity of only 0.01
ft/sec. Pilot-/and production-scale fluid-bed dryers are shown in
Figs. 14 through 16.
     Spray-drying equipment can be used for particles less than 100
μm, as long as the potential problem of microcapsule frangibility is
addressed, for there is a very short time zone between the dispersal

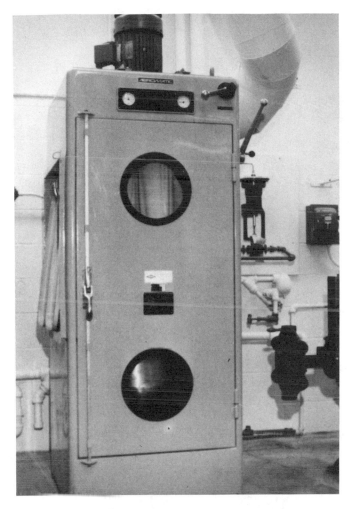

Fig. 14 Pilot-scale aqueous fluid-bed dryer.

of the microcapsule slurry on the atomizing disk until the capsules impinge against the wall of the spray dryer. Before impingement, the capsules must be completely dry or they will collect on the dryer wall. Therefore, high temperatures are usually required to dry capsules in spray-drying equipment. A modified approach to spray drying is tower drying. Tower dryers are tall, 40 to 100 ft in elevation, and have been utilized for drying small microcapsules. In this equipment it is also advantageous to have air passing through the dryer countercurrent to the direction of the microcapsules. This

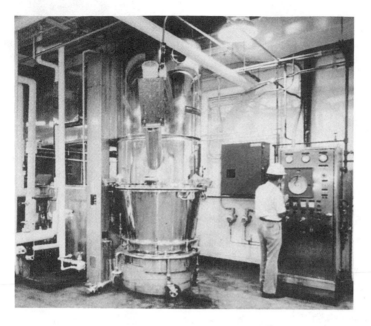

Fig. 15 Pilot-scale fluid-bed dryer.   (Courtesy of Eurand America.)

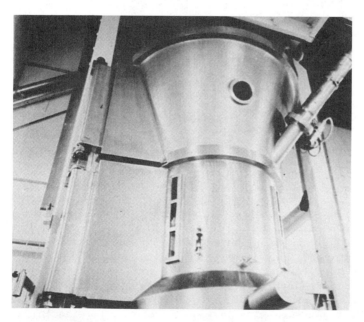

Fig. 16 Production-scale fluid-bed dryer.   (Courtesy of Eurand America.)

will increase the retention time in the dryer and also allow for lower operating temperatures. As indicated, to ensure that terminal velocities are not exceeded, the countercurrent flow rate must be less than the terminal velocity of the particles that are being dried.

V. MICROENCAPSULATION PROCESSING TECHNIQUES

There have been many open literature/references relating to the various processing techniques to produce microcapsules through mechanical or chemical processes. If one were to discuss all of these processes in any detail, it would justify a book. However, since many of these processes tend to compete with each other as alternatives for microencapsulation, I believe it is at least worthwhile to comment on several of the key processes from a manufacturing perspective.

A. Coacervation

Coacervation processes, both simple and complex, often require a multiplicity of processing equipment during scale up and in a manufacturing facility. The types of materials that are microencapsulated by these processes, as well as the polymers themselves, generate many parameters or variables that will complicate standardization of equipment. All of the coacervation techniques use water as the continuous phase. Therefore, water-soluble polymers are used for coacervation. Commercial products that utilize coacervation techniques include carbonless paper, fragrances, mineral oil for cosmetics, liquid crystals (used in temperature indicators), and various herbicides and pesticides. The largest capacity manufacturing demand that requires the coacervation system is unquestionably carbonless paper, for perhaps up to 20 to 30 million pounds per year, dry basis, microcapsules are produced.

B. Interfacial Polymerization

Interfacial polymerization is a specialized technique for microencapsulation that requires two monomers, one contained within the core material to be encapsulated (discontinuous phase), the second in the continuous phase. The two monomers react at the interface between the core and the continuous phase, causing polymerization. Although polymerization in itself is not instantaneous, it is a very rapid reaction when compared to coacervation techniques. Typical microencapsulating polymers that are developed via interfacial polymerization techniques are polyamides, polyesters, polyurethanes, and polyureas. Several commercial pesticides utilize this technique. One is

used for Knox-Out 2FM (microencapsulated Diazinon). A second is
Altosid SR-10, which is an insect growth regulator. A third com-
mercial product that utilizes interfacial polymerization is Monsanto's
Lasso ME.

C. Phase Separation

Phase-separation techniques are normally associated with microencapsulation systems solvents containing continuous phases. Although
by strict definition certain aqueous systems could be defined as
phase separation, in phase separation techniques, a polymer is generally phased out (desolvated) from the solvent continuous phase.
This polymer (discontinuous phase) will deposit around (reservoir)
a liquid droplet or a solid particle as a polymer wall. The polymer
can be deposited either by temperature differential, by the introduction of a second polymer, or by the evaporation of the solvent. Commercial products that utilize phase-separation techniques include
aspirin (Bayer Time Release), acetaminophen (Tylenol), and potassi-
um chloride (Micro-K).

D. Mechanical Microencapsulation Techniques

Mechanical techniques include pan coating, spray coating, and fluid-
bed coating. Pan coating has been commercially available and utilized for 50 years. One of the more common commercial products that
utilizes this microencapsulation technique is Contact. Spray coating
is utilized in the microencapsulation of many flavors commercially.
Fluid-bed coating, referred to as Wurster coating, is now being
heavily utilized for various pharmaceuticals.

When a microencapsulation product is defined or developed, there
are normally competitive processes that can alternately yield a similar product performance. Often the final determining factor in the
selection process is the availability of the particular process equipment and/or the manufacture's own process experience.

VI. PROCESS ALTERNATIVES

It is my understanding that even today all chemical microencapsulation processes are carried out as batch processes rather than in a
continuous mode. This should not suggest that continuous microencapsulation processes are not feasible. Techniques were designed,
installed, and favorably tested through the pilot plant scale over 15
years ago. The systems were proven to be technically feasible.

Converting any chemical process from a batch to a continuous
process requires economic justification, which in most cases also de-

mands large-volume capacity requirements. Thus, one might logically conclude that carbonless paper would be more economically produced on a continuous system than a batch system, since it is produced in large volumes. Thus, labor costs could be reduced. However, after very intensive pilot-scale engineering evaluation, this was concluded not to be the case. There were several significant opposing issues: (a) In converting to a continuous process, one objective is to reduce labor costs. This, in fact, did occur when considering carbonless paper, but the labor cost represents only a very small fraction of the total manufacturing cost. Thus, very little cost savings could be realized. (b) Raw materials costs for carbonless paper are very high. Therefore, continuous processes that require prolonged start-up and shut-down periods, and during which all in-process materials are lost, become cost-prohibitive. (c) Capital equipment costs for continuous processes are much greater. (d) In most continuous processes the control systems become extremely important. Thus, often critical process parameters cannot be satisfactorily controlled with available process control technology.

Chapter 5

LARGE-SCALE PRODUCTION PROBLEMS AND MANUFACTURING OF NANOPARTICLES

Jörg Kreuter

Institut für Pharmazeutische Technologie, J. W. Goethe-Universität Frankfurt, Frankfurt, Federal Republic of Germany

I. INTRODUCTION

An essential requirement of modern drug therapy is the controlled delivery of a drug or an active substance to the site of action in the body in an optimal concentration-versus-time profile. One attempt to achieve this goal was the development of colloidal drug carriers. Chiefly because of their small particle size, these systems offer advantages for many medical, veterinary, agricultural, and industrial applications. In medicine, colloidal preparations lend themselves to parenteral administration and may be useful as sustained-release injections or for the delivery of a drug to a specific organ or target site. Colloidal carrier systems that have been developed so far include liposomes and nanoparticles.

Nanoparticles are solid colloidal particles ranging in size from 10 to 1000 nm (1 μm). They consist of macromolecular materials in which the active principle (drug or biologically active material) is dissolved, entrapped, and/or to which the active principle is adsorbed or attached [1].

II. POLYACRYLIC NANOPARTICLES

A. General Aspects of Emulsion Polymerization

All the methods commonly used at present for the production of polyacrylic nanoparticles are modifications or special cases of emulsion polymerization [1]. A short review of the theory of this process, therefore, may be useful for understanding problems that may arise during scaling up.

Initially, it was believed that during the process of emulsion poly-merization, the localization of the polymerization would be at the sur-face of the monomer droplets [2]. However, the finding that the re-sulting polymer particles are smaller than the monomer droplets moved the hypothetical location of the polymerization initiation and chain growth into the emulsifier micelles [3, 4]: According to the classical theory of Harkins, Smith, and Ewart [5–7], the monomer is initially contained in the monomer droplets as well as in the emulsifier micelles. Radicals are then generated in the continuous phase (water) by the decay of water-soluble initiator molecules or by high-energy irradia-tion. Because of the much larger total surface area of the micelles in comparison to the total surface area of the monomer droplets, for statistical reasons practically all radicals hit and enter a micelle, thus initiating the polymerization [1].

The observation that the number of micelles present does not af-fect the number of particles formed and that the kinetics of poly-merization initiation is virtually the same if no surfactant is present led to a revision of the classical Harkins-Smith-Ewards theory [8–12]: Since the initiator is present only in the surrounding aqueous phase, the initial location of the polymerization is in this phase. The gen-erated oligomers grow as more monomer molecules are absorbed and enpolymerized. At a certain molecular weight or particle size, the oligomers become insoluble, thus forming the small separate particles of the polymer latex.

The particle formation is independent of the rate of polymerization [13], but dependent on the polymer concentration in the aqueous phase [10]. This indicates that the particle formation is thermody-namically controlled. In the case of methyl methacrylate, for in-stance, particle formation observed by Tyndall scattering occurs at a polymer concentration of 0.03 g/100 ml [13].

The particles are stabilized either by hydrophilic groups present in the polymer or by emulsifier present in the medium. They con-tinue to grow by absorbing more monomer, which is present in the surrounding aqueous phase, in the emulsifier micelles, and/or in the monomer droplets, and which diffuses to the growing latex particles. Termination of the polymerization occurs by reaction of the macro-radicals with a small radical or with another macroradical either in the aqueous phase or in the precipitated phase, i.e., the polymer particles [14]. Subsequently, if more and more radicals in the aque-ous phase become absorbed or terminated, no more new particles are formed and the polymer particles become the main location of poly-merization. By absorbing more monomer, the particles grow gradual-ly until the monomer is completely converted to polymer.

Consequently, the number of particles depends on the initiator concentration, the reaction temperature, and the surfactant concen-tration [5, 10, 15, 16]. Increasing initiator concentrations as well as increasing emulsifier concentrations lead to an increase in particle number. The molecular weight is inversely related to the particle number [15]. Flocculation of particles leads to deviations from these regularities [1, 12].

Initiation by high-energy radiation rests upon the same theories of emulsion polymerization [17] or emulsifier-free polymerization [1, 10, 14, 18].

B. Preparation of Nanoparticles Using an Aqueous Continuous Phase

Poly(alkyl Acrylates)

The monomers that have been used for the preparation of poly(alkyl acrylate) nanoparticles include methyl methacrylate, butyl methacrylate, 2-hydroxethyl methacrylate, methyl acrylate, acrylic acid, methacrylic acid, and also styrene. The monomers have to be purified from polymerization inhibitors using conventional methods [19]. The monomer is then dissolved or emulsified in water, a buffer solution such as phosphate-buffered saline, or the drug or bioactive substance solution (or suspension, in the case of antigens).

The polymerization may be initiated by γ-irradiation or by chemical initiation.

Gamma-irradiation has the advantage that it can be carried out at room temperature or below. Oxygen present in the aqueous phase does not have to be removed. The polymer yield is dose-dependent; in the case of methyl methacrylate, about 85% of the monomer is converted after 100 krads, about 98% after 500 krads, and almost total conversion is obtained after 2500 krads [20]. The polymer yield is inversely related to the dose rate. A dose rate of 2.2 krad/min leads to a polymer yield of 98% at a total dose of 500 krads. The particle size of poly(methyl methacrylate) nanoparticles thus produced is about 120 to 150 nm [21]. The molecular weights of these particles are between 20,000 and 80,000, depending on the initial monomer concentration and the electrolyte concentration in the surrounding medium [14].

Chemical initiation has the advantage that it does not require radioactive irradiation facilities. The disadvantage is that temperatures above 65°C have to be employed. For this reason, the polymerization cannot be carried out in the presence of heat-sensitive drugs or biological materials. The polymerization is initiated by the formation of radicals caused by the decay of the initiator at elevated temperatures. Since oxygen interacts with these radicals and inhibits or retards polymerization, it has to be reduced by gassing with nitrogen for 1 hr. After this, the monomer is added and the system stirred at about 100 to 500 rpm and heated at a rate of about

2 to 3°C/min [21, 22]. At about 45°C, the initiator (see Table 1) dissolved in water (4 vol% of the total reaction volume) has to be added, and the heating is continued until the desired polymerization temperature is reached. The medium is then kept at this temperature for 2 hr. After this, the medium is heated to 90°C in order to enpolymerize trace monomeric residuals.

High initiator concentrations (>5 mmol) lead to precipitation and flocculation. Lower initiator concentrations lead to the formation of a stable latex [21]. In the latter system, the particles are stabilized by electric repulsion generated by the persulfate groups, which are covalently linked to the polymer molecules and are not removable by dialysis [15].

The monomer concentration influences strongly both the molecular weight as well as the particle size. The temperature effect is less important for the molecular weight and much less significant for the particle size (Table 1). The initiator concentration even has a contrary effect: Increasing initiator concentrations decrease the molecular weight very significantly but increase the particle size slightly. For this reason, it has to be concluded that the mechanism of the growth of the polymer molecule itself and the mechanism of particle growth and stabilization are different. It can be further concluded that one particle consists of more than one polymer molecule: At a density of 1.06 g/ml and an approximate diameter of 150 nm [25], the molecular weight ought to be about 10^{11} if one particle consists of one molecule. However, the observed molecular weights (Table 1) demonstrate that one particle consists of about 2×10^5 to 10^7 polymer molecules. The particle formation is, as discussed in Section II.A, thermodynamically controlled [13]: Whereas an increase in initiator molecules leads to a decrease in molecular weight at a given monomer concentration, the particle size will increase because more stabilizing sulfate groups can be formed on the polymer surface.

If the drug or bioactive material was not added before polymerization, it is usually added after the nanoparticle is brought to the optimal temperature for drug or bioactive material sorption. The nanoparticles can be stored in suspension or may be freeze-dried, depending on the stability of the sorbed material.

Poly(alkyl Cyanoacrylate)

Poly(alkyl cyanoacrylate) nanoparticles are formed by an anionic polymerization mechanism due to OH⁻ ions present in water. Although the mechanism of particle formation is similar to that for the polyacrylate nanoparticles in the previous section, the fact that the solvent/surrounding medium creates the initiator leads to a smaller molecular weight (∿3000) for the resulting polymer [26]. As a consequence, the formed particles are initially more flexible and sticky and therefore may coagulate irreversibly. In addition, since the

Table 1 Influence of Monomer Concentration, Initiator Concentration, and Temperature on Particle Size and Molecular Weights of Poly(methyl Methacrylate) Nanoparticles

Potassium peroxodisulfate concentration (mmol)	Particle size (nm)								Molecular Weight ($\overline{M}_w$)			
	Methyl methacrylate concentration (mmol) at two temperatures								at two temperatures			
	10		33.75		80		156.25		80		156	
	65°C	85°C	65°C	85°C	65°C	85°C	65°C	85°C	65°C	85°C	65°C	85°C
0.3	85	72	129	128	181	170	256	262	—	434,000	—	—
1.65	98	88	151	169	212	193	248	248	—	—	—	—
3.0	92	72	135	149	223	177	250	258	289,500	220,500		400,000

Source: Ref. 23; see also Refs. 21 and 24.

monomers are less soluble in water, at monomer concentrations optimal for nanoparticle production (1.0 to 2.0%), the monomer does
not dissolve totally and monomer droplets are formed. These monomer droplets normally do not polymerize during classical emulsion
polymerization [4]. However, because of the formation of the initiating ions by solvent dissociation, the probability that the monomer
droplets will be hit by a polymerization-initiating ion is increased.
Therefore, polymerization also may occur within the monomer droplets.

As a result of these problems, the addition of stabilizers such as
surfactants or protecting macromolecules is required. These stabilizers may be added in amounts of between 0.1% and 5%. They have
to be selected carefully because they can influence the body distribution [27, 28] as well as the sorption behavior of drugs onto the
particles [29, 30].

C. Preparation of Nanoparticles Using an Organic Continuous Phase

Until now, two methods of preparation of nanoparticles using emulsion polymerization with a continuous organic phase have been developed, the method of Birrenbach and Speiser [31] and the method
of Sjöholm and co-workers [32, 33]. Both processes use organic
solvents as the continuous phase. The polymerization mechanism is
similar to the classical emulsion polymerization with a continuous
aqueous phase. Because of the large amounts of organic solvents
and emulsifiers required and the toxicity and nonbiodegradability of
the polymer, these processes have not been further developed.
For more details see Ref. 1.

D. Scaling-Up Problems

As discussed in the previous sections, the process of emulsion polymerization is thermodynamically controlled. For this reason, the
scaling up of nanoparticle production using this process should be
easy if a homogeneous temperature distribution can be achieved in
the reaction vessel. This corresponds to our experiences: The initial monomer concentration is the major parameter governing particle
size and molecular weight. The conditions for this parameter are
the same in small and large batches: But since, in chemically induced polymerization, the number of initiating radicals generated depends on the initial initiator concentration as well as on the temperature (see Sections II.A and II.B.1), a homogeneous temperature distribution throughout the reactor as well as a constant heating rate
is required. Therefore, the stirring speed, which is normally not a
critical factor, may have to be increased in larger reactors. Never-

theless, with batches up to 5 liters, the largest size we have worked with so far, we had no problems in maintaining the same conditions as with 100-ml batch sizes.

In γ-irradiation-induced emulsion polymerization, the situation is different. Water has a large shielding effect toward γ-irradiation. For this reason, in reaction flasks with a diameter greater than 5 to 7 cm, the system has to be stirred (100 to 400 rpm). This stirring has no direct influence on the polymerization kinetics but will enable the supply of the polymerization medium with a homogeneous radiation field. However, since the residence time of the polymerization medium in high-dose irradiation areas is limited in large vessels even upon stirring, the reactor size has to be limited. In addition, an extensive irradiation dosimetry at several places in the reactor is required in larger vessels for calculating the dose density and the appropriate irradiation dose. In our experiences with γ-ray-induced emulsion polymerization, no significant differences in particle size, molecular weight, and polymer yield were obtained between unstirred reaction flasks of a diameter smaller than 5 cm and reaction flasks with a diameter of 12 cm stirred at 100 rpm (1-liter bottles). No experience exists with larger batch sizes.

Some formulations and production protocols for specific particle sizes and molecular weights are given in Refs. 21—23, 34, and 35.

As explained in Section II.B.2, the polymerization of poly(alkyl cyanoacrylates) is also thermodynamically controlled, leading to a homogeneous particle size distribution of the polymer latex formed [36]. Because of this thermodynamic control, the stirring rate also has very little influence on the particle size [36]. However, as also mentioned briefly in Section II.B.2, the molecular weight of the resulting polymer is very small in comparison to classical emulsion polymerization with poly(alkyl acrylates), due to the polymerization initiation by OH^- ions and partial termination by H^+ ions, both dissociation products of the continuous phase [37]. Therefore, the effect of pH during polymerization of poly(alkyl cyanoacrylates) is very complex. Its influence on the molecular weight is small [26, 39]; the smallest particle sizes and the most homogeneous particle size distributions are obtained around a pH of 2 to 3 [36].

The small molecular weights lead to a number of problems: The initial polymer particles are rather soft and sticky and therefore coagulate without addition of stabilizers [40]. For this reason stabilizers [39], but also the type of acid used to monitor the desired pH [36], have a significant influence on the particle size and a smaller influence on the molecular weight [38]. The stabilizers used most commonly include poloxomers, polysorbates, dextrans, and cyclodextrins [38, 39]. With cyclodextrins it is possible to obtain particle sizes slightly above 1 μm [39].

The particles grow by capture of further oligomers and adsorption of monomer, which subsequently polymerizes within the nanoparticles [38]. As a result, the particles become more rigid and stable and the danger of coagulation decreases with progressing polymerization.

Because of the low solubility of the monomeric cyanoacrylates, monomer droplets are formed before onset of the polymerization, which may coalesce at the reactor wall, the air/medium interface, and around the vortex created by the stirrer. For this reason, basic materials such as metals cannot be used as materials for the inner reactor or container wall. The creation of the polymerization-initiating ions by the solvent/dispersion medium also enables the initiation of polymerizaiton within the droplets or in the coalesced phase. For this reason, the pH must be maintained below 4 until the monomer droplets disappear. Stabilizers as used for the control of the particle size also facilitate the dispersion of the monomer droplets.

The dispersion of the monomer droplets is, of course, also improved by increasing stirrer speeds. However, if the stirring speed is too high, too much additional air/medium interphase is created and more polymer lumps are formed.

For these reasons, the scaling up of the production of poly(alkyl cyanoacrylate) nanoparticles is much more difficult than in classical emulsion polymerization of poly(alkyl acrylates). Nevertheless, in our experience with batches up to 5 liters, the nanoparticle yield improves and the problems decrease with larger-size batches. This is probably due to the fact that the surface-to-volume ratio decreases and that the hydrodynamics is often less homogeneous in small reaction flasks.

For this reason, we believe that larger batch sizes do not create additional problems in comparison to smaller batches. It has to be kept in mind, though, that the reactor wall surface must be made of a nonmetallic material.

In any case, the formation of larger polymer particles and lumps cannot be avoided totally. However, since these lumps are very large, they can easily be removed by filtration through filters with a pore size of 5 to 20 µm.

III. REFERENCES

1. J. Kreuter, *Pharm. Acta Helv.*, *58*:196 (1983).
2. H. Staudinger and W. Frost, *Ber. Dtsch. Chem. Ges.*, *68*:2351 (1935).
3. H. Fikentscher, *Angew. Chem.*, *51*:433 (1938).
4. H. Fikentscher, H. Gerrens, and H. Schuller, *Angew. Chem.*, *72*:856 (1960).
5. W. V. Smith and R. E. Ewart, *J. Chem. Phys.*, *16*:592 (1948).

6. W. D. Harkins, *J. Amer. Chem. Soc.*, *69*:1428 (1947).
7. W. D. Harkins, *J. Polym. Sci.*, *5*:217 (1950).
8. C. P. Roe, *Ind. Eng. Chem.*, *60*:20 (1968).
9. I. D. Robb, *J. Polym. Sci. A1*, *7*:417 (1969).
10. R. M. Fitch, M. B. Prenosil, and K. J. Sprick, *J. Polym. Sci. C*, *27*:95 (1969).
11. R. M. Fitch and C. Tsai, *J. Polym. Sci.*, *Polym. Lett.*, *8*:703 (1970).
12. R. M. Fitch, *Brit. Polym. J.*, 5L467 (1973).
13. R. M. Fitch, M. B. Prenosil, and K. J. Sprick, *Amer. Chem. Soc.*, *Polymer Preprints*, *7*:707 (1966).
14. J. Kreuter, *J. Polym. Sci.*, *Polym. Lett.*, *20*:543 (1982).
15. H. Ono and H. Saeki, *Brit. Polym. J.*, *7*:21 (1975).
16. G. S. Whitby, M. D. Gross, J. R. Miller, and A. J. Constanza, *J. Polym. Sci. A1*, 549 (1955).
17. G. J. K. Acres and F. L. Dalton, *J. Polym. Sci. A1*, 3009 (1963).
18. F. Fiquet-Fayard, *J. Chim. Phys.*, *56*:692 (1959).
19. K. Tessmar, in *Methoden der Organischen Chemie (Houben-Weyl)*, Vol. XIV/1 (E. Müller, ed.), G. Thieme, Stuttgart, 1961, pp. 1033–1072.
20. J. Kreuter and H. J. Zehnder, *Radiation Effects*, *35*:161 (1978).
21. U. E. Berg, J. Kreuter, P. P. Speiser, and M. Soliva, *Pharm. Ind.*, *48*:75 (1986).
22. J. Kreuter, U. Berg, E. Liehl, M. Soliva, and P. P. Speiser, *Vaccine*, *4*:125 (1986).
23. U. E. Berg, Immunstimulation durch hochdisperse Polymer-suspensionen. Diss. ETH Nr. 6481, 1979, pp. 35–69.
24. V. Bentele, U. E. Berg, and J. Kreuter, *Int. J. Pharm.*, *13*: 109 (1983).
25. J. Kreuter, *Int. J. Pharm.*, *14*:43 (1983).
26. M. A. El-Egakey, V. Bentele, and J. Kreuter, *Int. J. Pharm.*, *13*:349 (1983).
27. D. Leu, B. Manthey, J. Kreuter, P. Speiser, and P. P. DeLuca, *J. Pharm. Sci.*, *73*:1433 (1984).
28. L. Illum, S. S. Davis, R. M. Müller, and P. West, *Life Sci.*, *40*:367 (1987).
29. T. Harmia, P. Speiser, and J. Kreuter, *Int. J. Pharm.*, *33*:45 (1986).
30. T. Harmia, J. Kreuter, P. Speiser, T. Boye, R. Gurny, and A. Kubis, *Int. J. Pharm.*, *33*:187 (1986).
31. G. Birrenbach and P. P. Speiser, *J. Pharm. Sci.*, *65*:1763 (1976).
32. B. Ekman, C. Lofter, and I. Sjöholm, *Biochem.*, *15*:5115 (1976).
33. B. Ekman and I. Sjöholm, *J. Pharm. Sci.*, *67*:693 (1978).

34. J. Kreuter, in *Methods in Enzymology*, Vol. 112 (R. Green and
     K. J. Widder, eds.), Academic Press, Orlando, Fla., 1985,
     pp. 129–138.
35. J. Kreuter and I. Haenzel, *Infect. Immunity*, *19*:667 (1978).
36. S. J. Douglas, L. Illum, S. S. Davis, and J. Kreuter, *J.
     Colloid Interface Sci.*, *101*:149 (1984).
37. H. W. Coover, Jr., and J. M. McIntire, in *Handbook of Ad-
     hesives*, 2nd ed. (I. Skeist, ed.), Van Nostrand Reinhold, New
     York, 1977, p. 569.
38. S. J. Douglas, S. S. Davis, and S. R. Holding, *Brit. Polym.
     J.*, *17*:339 (1985).
39. S. J. Douglas, L. Illum, and S. S. Davis, *J. Colloid Interface
     Sci.*, *103*:154 (1985).

Chapter 6

PHARMACEUTICAL MANUFACTURING OF LIPOSOMES

Francis J. Martin

Liposome Technology, Inc., Menlo Park, California

I. INTRODUCTION

Liposomes are now recognized as a drug delivery system that can improve the therapeutic activity and safety of a wide range of compounds. A prerequisite to the successful development and commercialization of liposome products is the capability to scale production methods in compliance with currently accepted good manufacturing practices, at acceptable cost and using processes that provide the high degree of reproducibility required for finished pharmaceuticals. A number of reviews have described studies of liposome production methodology and properties, their use as carriers for drugs, and interactions with a variety of cell types [1–7]. Many of these highlight the fact that liposome behavior can vary substantially with certain formulation variables, most notably chemical composition, size, surface charge, and drug payload. Therefore, it is essential to form liposomes using processes that control these variables.

In this chapter the key pharmaceutical issues that must be addressed in the manufacture of liposome-based products are discussed, including sterility assurance, pyrogen control, stability, and solvent handling and residues. Descriptions of the more useful processing methods disclosed in the scientific and patent literature are provided, including an assessment of the scale-up potential of each.*

---

*Many of the recent advances in liposome production technology have yet to be published in peer-reviewed scientific journals, and some may never be. In the interest of being current, information obtained from *issued* U.S. Patents will be cited in this chapter.

Finally, one highly efficient liposome production method is discussed in greater detail to exemplify a process that appears to be
well suited to industrial-scale pharmaceutical operations. Several
variations are examined that provide liposomes of uniform size (which
are "sterilizable" by filtration) and encapsulate up to 70% of the
aqueous medium in which they are formed. Free (unencapsulated)
drug is removable by standard ultrafiltration techniques and, if required for adequate shelf-life stability, selected formualtions can be
successfully lyophilized in the presence of certain cryoprotectants.

A. Utility of Liposomes

Liposomes provide a range of advantages in drug delivery. When
administered parenterally, either by the intravenous, subcutaneous,
or intramuscular route, liposomes can protect an encapsulated drug
from degradation and provide controlled "depot" release over an extended period of time [8–10]. This feature can reduce the side
effects of the drug by controlling the rate at which free drug becomes available in the bloodstream. Liposomes can also alter the
tissue distribution of an uptake of certain drugs, in a therapeutically
favorable way (such as targeting to elements of the reticuloendothe-
lial system), and can increase the convenience of therapy by allowing
less frequency drug adminsitration.

The utility of liposomes for drug delivery by inhalation has also
been demonstrated. Liposomes used for inhalation can be tailored,
according to lipid composition, to release an entrapped drug following administration to the lung at a selected release rate, which may
vary in half-life from a few minutes to many hours [11]. Further,
to the extent that the drug is sequestered in the liposomes, side
effects related to rapid uptake from the respiratory tract into the
bloodstream are reduced [12].

The compatibility of liposomes with both lipophilic and hydrophilic
drugs, and the ability to vary lipid composition to achieve a selected
release pattern, are also advantageous when administering a drug
topically or to mucosal tissues [13]. An added advantage for drug
delivery to mucosal tissue is that liposome surfaces can be modified
to provide a degree of bio-adhesion, enhancing the residence time of
the liposomes at target sites such as the eye [14].

B. Comparison with Other Hetergeneous Systems

The pharmaceutical industry has successfully produced other heterogeneous systems, such as emulsions and suspensions, on a large
scale. The most successful example is represented by the phospholipid-stabilized triglyceride emulsions used for hyperalimentation.
Products such as Intralipid are produced in large quantities and,

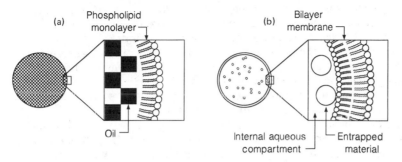

Fig. 1 Diagrammatic representations of (a) a phospholipid-stabilized triglyceride emulsion droplet and (b) a phospholipid bilayer vesicle or liposome. In the case of the emulsion droplet, phospholipid molecules form a monolayer at the oil-water interface—the headgroups in contact with water molecules and the acyl chains dissolved in the oil core. Although drugs may be loaded (dissolved) in the oil phase of emulsions, there is no real barrier to keep them from moving (partitioning) into the water phase. Liposomes, in contrast, consist of a phospholipid bilayer membrane that wraps around an aqueous compartment—sealing it from the external medium much like a cell. Water-soluble drugs can be encapsulated in this aqueous core and held there, or, alternatively, released at a rate regulated by the composition of the membrane. Lipid-soluble drugs can be incorporated into the bilayer membrane itself.

since they are administered in fairly large doses by intravenous (IV) infusion, require tight control over pharmaceutical quality. Some of the raw materials and much of the apparatus, solvents, quality and process control systems, and process validation approaches developed for parenteral emulsions will almost certainly apply to the production of liposomes as well.

However, this is where the similarities between liposomes and emulsions end. Perhaps the greatest contrast between the two systems is rooted in thermodynamics and is a direct consequence of their very different structures. In emulsions the oil phase is dispersed into small droplets in excess water by high-energy processing methods such as homogenization or high-shear mixing. To prevent coalescence of the oil droplets, an amphipathic emulsifier is included that orients as a monolayer at oil/water interfaces, significantly reducing interfacial tension (Fig. 1a). The headgroups of the emulsifier molecules are in contact with water (up to 15 water molecules are bound to each headgroup) and the acyl chains dissolved in the triglyceride core. The inclusion of charged species in the emulsifier system leads to the establishment of a surface potential that may also stabilize the suspension.

Although the emulsifier in these formulations acts to stave off the inevitable, coalescence of the oil phase will eventually take place. This is evident from the tendency of such emulsions to "oil out" with time or under stress conditions such as freezing, centrifugation, filtration, or temperature cycling. In a thermodynamic sense, then, emulsion systems are not at an energetic minimum—a fraction of the energy used to create the emulsion is stored in the system and there is a pressure to relieve this energy over time.

Liposomes, in contrast, are at true energy minimum. The basic structural element of a liposome resides in its thin but durable membrane, a similar structure to biological membranes. As illustrated in Fig. 1b, liposomes consist of a lipid bilayer matrix that wraps around an aqueous volume—sealing it from the external medium, much like a cell. The central aqueous core can range in diameter from 20 nm to several micrometers, and liposomes can contain from one to hundreds of concentric bilayers, each creating its own aqueous compartment (much like the layers of an onion).

As shown in Fig. 2, these bilayer membranes form spontaneously when certain amplipathic molecules (such as phospholipids) are exposed to excess water. The phospholipid molecules align next to one another, forming biomolecular sheets with the polar "headgroups" in close contact with water on either side of the structure and the

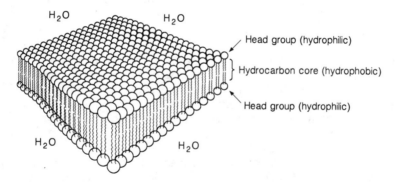

Fig. 2 Schematic representation of the lipid bilayer matrix that serves as the basic structural element of liposomes (and cells). When exposed to water, phospholipids spontaneously assemble into these bimolecular sheets, a segment of which is illustrated here. The polar "headgroups" of the individual phospholipids are in contact with water molecules on either side of the structure, while the apolar acyl "tails" form a thin oil phase sandwiched in between. Covalent bonds are not formed during bilayer assembly, but the summation of the hydrophobic interactions among the many methylene groups present in the core of the membrane leads to remarkable stability.

apolar "tail" groups mixing to form a very thin oil phase sandwiched in between. The bilayer configuraiton satisfies the dual chemical nature of the lipids, the headgroups fully hydrated and the hydrocarbon tails content to mingle with one another within the core of the membrane. Although covalent bonds are usually not formed during bilayer assembly, the summation of the apolar forces among the many methylene groups, what Tanford refers to as the "hydrophobic effect" [15], explains the remarkable stability of the structure.

Liposomes are at a thermodynamic minimum free energy so long as the packing density of the phospholipids present in each monolayer of the bilayer structure is roughly the same. In the case of very small liposomes, produced by high-energy processing such as homogenization or sonication, packing differentials may develop due to the extreme curvature of the membrane. This can lead to physical instability such as coalescence and fusion [16]. But this situation is the exception rather than the rule.

Just as in the case of emulsion systems and other aqueous colloids, the introduction of a surface charge into the liposome can be used to prevent close approach of the particles and thus reduce the changes for aggregation. Acidic phospholipids and ionic surfactants have been used extensively for this purpose.

II. KEY PHARMACEUTICAL ISSUES   *(Classification)*

A. Lipid Solvents

With few exceptions, liposome products will contain more than one bilayer-forming component. In the simplest case, a neutral phospholipid such as phosphatidyl choline (PC) is mixed with a lipid-soluble antioxidant such as alpha-tocopherol or butylated hydroxytoluene (BHT). In more complex systems charged species, sterols, and a drug may be included in the bilayer. Traditionally, to ensure a true moelcular mixture, the bilayer-forming elements selected for a particular formulation are dissolved in a suitable organic solvent. Chloroform, ether, methylene chloride, methanol, and combinations of these have been used for this purpose in the past, but upon reflection these may not be the best choices with respect to safety. From the point of view of the patient, residues of such processing solvents in the drug product must be kept well below toxic levels. From the perspective of the manufacturer, highly volatile, flammable, explosive, or toxic solvents should be avoided if possible to protect operators. For these reasons a solvent such as ethanol may be preferred.

Differential solubilities of bilayer components in organic solvents are often encountered and must be taken into consideration in order to avoid crystallization of a single component during solvent-stripping operations. This is an important point, which has been overlooked quite often in the past. Lipids such as cholesterol, and PCs of differing degrees of saturation and drugs (in the case where a hydrophobic compound is being encapsulated) may have very different solubilities in single solvents or solvent mixtures. This is particularly true for solvent systems consisting of a mixture of a nonpolar solvent such as chloroform and a more polar one such as an alcohol. The more volatile, water-immiscible solvent is likely to evaporate at a faster rate than the alcohol, leading to changes in solvent power as solvent removal progresses. This effect may lead to crystallization of one component, cholesterol for example, before drying is complete. Problems associated with phase separations are easily avoided by selecting proper solvents and solvent removal conditions. Data from preformulation workups, including measurements of the solubilities of individual components of the mixture in candidate solvents, are useful in this regard.

In choosing a processing solvent, considerations other than safety and solubility must be taken into account. Since solvent removal tends to concentrate contaminants, the purity and reproducibility of the solvents as well as the quality control measures used to assess purity are also viewed as critically important. With respect to the economics of a process, solvent recovery and disposal can add significant expense, so recycling of solvents is an attractive option, particularly in cases where difficult-to-separate solvent mixtures can be avoided.

Residual solvents such as ethanol and hydrocarbons may lead to physical destabilization of liposomes by interfering with the cooperative hydrophobic interactions among the phospholipid methylene groups that hold the structure together. So care must be taken to remove solvents to well below such destabilizing levels.

Setting processing solvent residue limits for key in-process intermediates or for a final dosage form depends critically on the intended use of the product. Solvent residue specifications for topicals will generally be less rigid than those for inhalation dosage forms. Specifications for injectables will tend to be the most stringent. Regulatory authorities are not likely to set such limits themselves— but will certainly require proof that whatever specifications are set by the manufacturer are safe, verifiable, and that residue vales that meet the specifications do not affect the quality or stability of the product.

Given the choice, it would be preferred to avoid solvents that are known to be carcinogenic or teratogenic, even though they may be substantially removed during processing. Quantitation of volatile solvent residues by headspace sampling followed by gas chromatography (GC) or high-performance liquid chromatography (HPLC) analysis is usually satisfactory. Reliable chemical and enzymatic assays for various alcohols are also available.

B. Pyrogen Control

By far the best approach to ensuring that parenteral liposome products meet the pyrogen limit requirements is to begin with raw materials with low pyrogen levels, design processes that are as sanitary as possible (i.e., microbiologically contained), and conduct all operations using depyrogenated apparatus. In this way, the process will not be expected to add significantly to the original pyrogen burden.

The lipid industry has for many years successfully produced phospholipids from natural and synthetic sources with low pyroburben for use in nutritional emulsions. Pyrogen levels in lipids can be reduced even further by passage of solutiosn of the lipids made in certain organic solvents through ultrafiltration membranes. The basic subunit size of lipopolysaccharide-type pyrogens (LPS) is about 10,000 to 20,000 daltons. In aqueous solutions and certain organic solvents, LPS molecules tend to aggregate into even larger structures (30,000 to 1 million daltons). LPS can, therefore, be removed quite effectively by passage of solutions through ultrafilters with molecular-weight cutoffs of about 10,000 daltons [17].

Considerable care must be taken in validating the assays used to detect and quantify pyrogen levels in lipid raw materials. Since LPS molecules are lipophilic and exhibit similar solubility behavior as phospholipids, they may incorporate into internal bilayers in MLV, interfering with assays (such as the *Limulus* amebocyte lysate test, LAL [18]) that have been designed to detect the more usual of the micellar or vesicular assemblies that are formed by LPS in aqueous systems [19].

Apparatus used to produce liposomes is depyrogenated in the usual ways, including chemical treatment (dilute acids or bases, oxidizing agents such as hydrogen peroxide, or alkylating agents such as acetic anhydride) or exposure to heat (dry or moist). Food and Drug Administration (FDA) draft guidelines on aseptic filling operations recommend that "a pyrogen challenge, where necessary, should be an integral part of the validation program, e.g., by inoculating one or more articles to be treated with 1000 or more USP units of bacterial endotoxin" and that the "*Limulus* lysate could be used to demonstrate that the endotoxic substance had been inactivated to not more than 1/1000 of the original amount." In line with this current thinking, when steps are taken to lower pyrogen levels in raw materials, it may be desirable to include endotoxin challenge testing to confirm that the ultrafiltration process used reduces the endotoxin burden sufficiently and reproducibily. The adequacy of depyrogenation procedures used for apparatus should also be confirmed by challenge testing. Validation of depyrogenation has been simplified with the development of reliable and quantitative LAL assays and the availability of endotoxin standards [20].

C. Sterility

Many of the liposome dosage forms under development must be produced in a manner that assures their sterility (parenteral and oph-
thalmic, for example). In the best possible situation the production
process would not only be designed to "build in" sterility, but the
product would be terminally treated after filling into the final vial to
guarantee it. Unfortunately, for most liposome-based systems under
development, terminal sterilization by heat or ionizing irradiation is
not an option. In many cases terminal sterilizaiton is ruled out because the active ingredient is heat- or irradiation-sensitive. Lipids
themselves are likely to hydrolyze rapidly at the high temperatures
required for sterilization. Gamma-irradiation not only aggravates
hydrolysis but also appears to accelerate peroxidation of unsaturated
lipids [21].

Two options exist for assuring sterility of liposome formualtions.
First, presterilize all raw materials and apparatus and conduct the
process—from beginning through the fill—aseptically. Although
this option may apply to very simple formulations (i.e., ones that
can be made in a few steps in apparatus that can be sterilized and
microbiologically contained), the approach may be expensive and
difficult to validate for the more typical liposome production processes, which take place in different reactors, have multiple transfer
steps, and cycle through pump heads and diafiltration cartridges
several times. The opportunity for contamination and batch failure
will certainly increase with the complexity of the process.

So, how can sterility be assured for liposome products? The same
way biological products are—by a combination of aseptic process design and filtration through sterilizing-grade filters immediately before
an aseptic fill operation. Although sterility assurance quidelines are
stringent and validation rather labor-intensive, this type of approach
is working well and becoming standard throughout the biotechnology
industry.

The only complication with liposomes is that they can be too large
to pass through the usual 0.45- or 0.22-μm-rated filters used for
sterilization. In this situation liposomes can be "down-sized" to an
average diameter and size distribution so that they pass through appropriately sized filters at acceptable rates.

As described in greater detail below, down-sizing by extrusion of
liposomes through selected capillary pore membranes or asymmetric
ceramic filters leads to a population of liposomes with an average
size in the range of 0.15 to 0.25 μm, with a tight distribution on
the high end. Although such liposomes are close in size to the
rates pore diameters of the sterilizing-grade filters, if properly
done, throughput is acceptable without producing untoward back-
pressures or blinding of the membranes. Of course, smaller liposomes, produced by homogenization or sonication, pass freely through
most sterilizing filters.

Validation of sterility assurance measures for liposome production processes is likely to follow the standards set by the industry, including media fills and challenge tests with selected microorganisms (including environmental isolates). Sterilizing-grade filters must be capable of removing the bioburden normally present in a product, and a function test of the selected sterilizing filter must be conducted as part of any validation program. A common bioburden may be on the order of 10^4 to 10^5 colony-forming units per liter, and a considerable body of evidence exists indicating that such a burden can be effectively removed by a single passage through sterilizing-grade filters with a rated pore diameter of 0.45 µm (a depth-type prefilter is often used upstream of the sterilizing filter in this case). Since organisms are known that can pass through a 0.45 µm rated filter, for sterilizing small-volume parenterals most plant operators would likely prefer an even smaller pore diameter filter (such as one rated at 0.22 µm) or serial passage through two 0.45-µm filters. It is also prudent to establish a correlation between microbial retention and a nondestructive test of filter integrity (such as the diffusion or bubble-point test) that can be conducted as a routine in-process control prior to all sterilization operations [22].

D. Stability During Processing

This chapter is concerned primarily with manufacturing of liposomes, so the focus of the following discussion is stability *during* processing. However, it must be recognized that, as with any other pharmaceutical, stability issues must be dealt with throughout the development of a liposome dosage form, starting with the selection of raw materials and formulation and proceeding all the way through to process design and packaging. In the case of liposome formulations, stability of both the active ingredient (drug) and the excipients, including lipids, must be considered. Since the active ingredient is formulation-dependent, stability issues related directly to it must be handled on a case-by-case basis. More often than not, the drug is less stable than the lipids, and conditions designed to preserve drug integrity will also ensure lipid stability.

Phospholipids derived from natural sources are subject to two major degradative reactions: peroxidation of double bonds, which may be present in acyl chains; and hydrolysis of the ester bonds linking the fatty acids to the glycerol moiety.

Hydrolysis of the sn-2 fatty acid of phospholipids usually occurs first and follows first-order kinetics as shown in the Arrhenius plot presented in Fig. 3 (inset). Also shown in Fig. 3, hydrolysis rates are negligible at low temperatures but can become significant at elevated temperatures (>40°C). Hydrolysis during processing should not present a problem, since the actual time of exposure to such

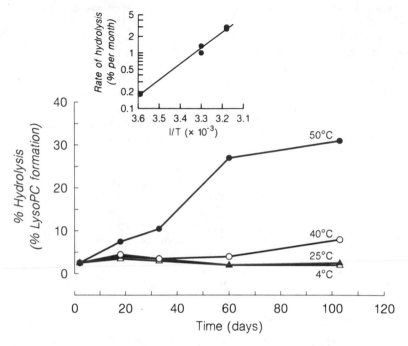

Fig. 3 Hydrolysis of phosphatidyl choline in aqueous liposome dis-
persons at various temperatures with pH being held constant at 6.5.
As illustrated in this graph, rates of hydrolysis are negligible at
low temperatures (4—25°C) but become significant at higher temperatures (>40°C).   As shown in the Arrhenius plot (inset), the
kinetics of hydrolysis appear to be first-order.

high temperatures in a production setting would be expected to be
short (a few hours at most). Hydrolysis rates are also strongly pH-
dependent, exhibiting a minimum at about 6.5 as shown in Fig. 4.
By careful selection of temperature, bulk pH, and processing time,
hydrolysis during processing can usually be kept to a minimum.
    Peroxidation can be controlled in a number of ways. Clearly, the
selection of the lipids is the place to begin. Natural egg and soy
phospholipids are abundant and inexpensive, but they contain a fair
number of double bonds. In the case of soy PC, the predominant
fatty acid is linoleic (18:2), representing about 70% of the total.
Egg PC is less unsaturated overall, but the presence of about 10%
long-chain, highly unsaturated fatty acids such as docosahexanoic
(22:6) and arachidonic (20:4) can introduce oxidative stability problems. As shown in Fig. 5, in the case of egg PC, peroxidation be-

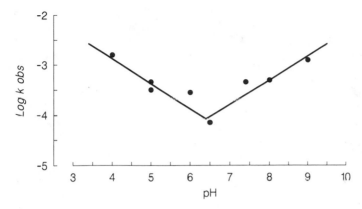

Fig. 4 Relationship between rates of hydrolysis of phosphatidyl choline in liposomes and pH. Rates of hydrolysis were measured at various temperatures at pHs ranging from 4 to 9 and observed rate constants (k_{obs}) calculated. As shown, hydrolysis rates are strongly pH-dependent—exhibiting a minimum at about 6.5 and increasing dramatically at both higher and lower pH.

gins with the most unsaturated species and, typical for such free-radical chain reactions, cascades through other susceptible fatty acids; the first to degrade is 22:6, followed in order by 20:4 and 18:2.

One attractive and cost-effective approach to improve the resistance of naturally derived phospholipids to oxidation is hydrogenation, either complete or partial. As shown in Table 1, in the case of egg PC the most offensive fatty acids, i.e., those that were shown to "kick off" oxidation above, can be selectively converted to saturated species by partial hydrogenation. Partially hydrogenated egg PCs with iodine values in the range of 30 to 40 appear to be ideal. Liposomes composed of these materials are not only highly resistant to oxidation, but also do not undergo thermal phase transitions at temperatures likely to be encountered during processing, shipment, or storage [23].

Of course, fully saturated phospholipids (either synthetic or fully hydrogenated natural lipids) are not subject to peroxidation at all, and these may be used in selected liposome formulations. When developing a formulation composed of saturated lipids, caution must be exercised to exclude the possibility that physical instability of the liposomes does not result during cycling through bilayer thermal phase transitions—particularly if they should occur at temperatures the product may encounter during production or distribution [24].

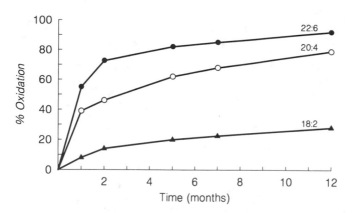

Fig. 5 Oxidation kinetics of three of the polyunsaturated fatty acids present in egg phosphatidyl choline liposomes, docosahexaenoic (22:6), arachidonic (20:4), and linoleic (18:2). Fatty acid analysis was conducted at the indicated time points for a sterilized liposome preparation stored at 38°C for one year. The vials were vented through a sterile filter so that air was free to diffuse into and out of the vials. The extent of oxidation is expressed as percent of the total initial value of each fatty acid remaining at each time point. As shown, the more unsaturated species oxidize first (22:6 and 20:4), followed by the less unsaturated linoleic acid (18:2). These data strongly suggest that the long-chain polyunsaturated fatty acids present in natural egg phospholipids initiate peroxidation, which, once started, cascades through other susceptible fatty acids. It must be emphasized that these results are "worst-case" conditions, since incubation temperature was relatively high, no antioxidants were included, and no attempt was made to exclude oxygen.

Rates of peroxidation may also be reduced by inclusion of lipid or water-soluble antioxidants, avoiding exposure to light, and by conducting operations and packaging of the product under an inert-gas atmosphere.

III. CONVENTIONAL LIPOSOME PREPARATION METHODS

Traditionally, the series of sequential unit processes shown in the flowchart in Fig. 6 is followed to produce liposomes. First, the bilayer-forming elements are mixed in a volatile organic solvent or solvent mixture (such as chloroform, ether, ethanol, or a combination of these). The predominant bilayer-forming element is usually a neutral phospholipid such as phosphatidyl choline. Cholesterol,

Table 1 Fatty Acid Compositions of Native and Partially Hydrogenated Egg Phosphatidyl Cholines[a]

Fatty acid	Native PC	Iodine value				
		40	30	20	10	1
16:0	30.1	29.1	30.3	29.7	29.1	29.5
18:0	11.9	14.8	20.1	30.3	42.9	56.7
18:1 trans	0.3	8.5	16.9	18.2	11.1	0.2
18:1 cis	30.8	32.4	22.0	9.9	4.3	0.1
18:2	15.6	3.6	0.4	0.0	0.0	0.0
20:0	0.0	0.4	1.1	2.2	3.4	5.3
20:1 trans	0.0	2.8	2.1	1.6	0.9	0.0
20:1 cis	0.0	1.0	0.0	0.0	0.0	0.0
22:0	0.0	0.5	1.4	2.9	4.4	7.1
22:1 trans	0.0	2.5	3.9	3.8	2.3	0.0
22:1 cis	0.0	2.0	0.0	0.0	0.0	0.0
22:2	0.0	1.0	0.0	0.0	0.0	0.0
20:4	3.8	0.0	0.0	0.0	0.0	0.0
22:6	5.4	0.0	0.0	0.0	0.0	0.0

[a]Fatty acid compositions of native and partially hydrogenated egg yolk phosphatidyl choline (>95%) are shown. Degrees of hydrogenation are indicated by iodine value. For reference, native egg yolk PC has an iodine value of about 65. Notice the levels of disaturated (18:2) and polyunsaturated (20:4 and 22:6) fatty acids in the native material, and how they decline as the degree of hydrogenation increases.

up to 40—50m% is often included to provide greater stability in biological fluids. As mentioned earlier, a charged species may be added (normally 5—20m%) to prevent aggregation. Common natural acidic lipids include phosphatidyl serine (PS), phosphatidyl glycerol (PG), phosphatidyl inositol (PI), phospatidic acid (PA), and cardiolipin. Positively charged surfactants have also been used (such as stearylamine), but these are not generally considered as safe as phospholipids for most therapeutic applications. Small amounts of antioxidants such as alpha-tocopherol or BHT are also included when polyunsatu-

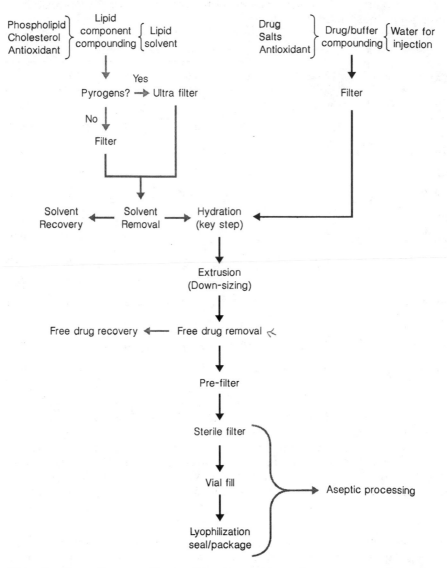

Fig. 6 Flow diagram illustrating the series of steps normally used to produce conventional liposomes. See text for details.

rated natural lipids are used. Once a suitable solution of the lipid components is made, the mixture may be filtered to remove minor insoluble components or ultrafiltered to lower pyroburdens. The solvent is subsequently removed under conditions (pressure, temperature) that ensure that no phase separations of the components of the mixture take place.

Following solvent removal, the "dry" lipid mixture is usually hydrated by exposure to an aqueous medium containing dissolved solutes, including buffers, salts, cheating agents, and, in the case of hydrophilic compounds, the drug to be entrapped. Hydration, more than any other step, influences the type of liposome formed (number of layers, size, and entrapped volume). The nature of the dry lipid, its surface area, and its porosity (thin to thick film, flaky to fine powder, granular pellets, etc.) is of particular importance. Rates of aqueous phase addition, temperature, agitation, and ionic conditions also influence the rate of liposome formation and their morphology. Other methods of drying the lipid mixture have been reported, including spray drying and lyophilization; as pointed out below, these may be more useful than thin-film methods for manufacturing. Depending on the solvent used, it may be desirable to condense, recover, and perhaps even recycle it.

Liposomes produced during hydration are generally heterogeneous in size but can be "down-sized" by extrusion or mechanical fragmentation. If desirable, unencapsulated drug can be removed by a variety of techniques such as centrifugation, dialysis, or diafiltration and recovered. Parenteral formulations are usually passed through sterile 0.22-μm depth filters to ensure the removal of any bacteria that might be present. In this case downstream operations, including vial filling, lyophilization, and vial sealing, are conducted under aseptic conditions.

A. Thin-Film Hydration

Multilamellar vesicles (MLV) are by far the most widely studied type of liposome and, as pointed out by Alec Bangham in 1974, easy to make [25]. In the laboratory, a mixture of vesicle-forming lipids in a volatile organic solvent is deposited on the surfaces of a round-bottomed flask as the solvent is removed by rotary evaporation under reduced pressure. MLVs ranging in size from tens of micrometers to several tenths of a micrometer form spontaneously when an excess volume of aqueous buffer is added to the dry lipid and the flask is agitated (the so-called hand-shaken dispersion). The drug to be entrapped may be included either in the lipid film (in the case of a lipophilic drug) or in the aqueous hydration medium (in the case of a hydrophilic drug).

Importance of Hydration Conditions

The time allowed for hydration and conditions of agitation are critical
in determining the amount of the aqueous buffer (or drug solution)
entrapped within the internal compartments of the MLV. For example,
as reproted by Szoka and Papahadjopoulos, the same amount of total
lipid can encapsulate 50% more of the aqueous buffer per mole of
lipid when hydrated for 20 hr with gentle shaking, compared to a
hydration period of 2 hr with vigorous shaking, despite the fact that
the two preparations end up with roughly the same particle size distribution [26]. If hydration time is reduced to a few minutes with
vortexing, a suspension will exhibit a still lower capture volume and
a smaller mean diameter.

As pointed out by Bangham [27], the hydration and entrapping
process is most efficeint when the film of dry lipid is kept thin.
This means that different sized round-bottomed flasks should be
used for different quantities of lipid. Glass beads and other inert,
insoluble particle have been used to increase the surface area available for film deposition. Hydration time, the method of suspension
of the lipids, temperature, and the thickness of the film can result
in markedly different preparations of MLVs, in spite of identical
lipid concentrations and compositions and volume of the suspending
aqueous phase. The unmistakable message from the literature is that
conditions under which the dry lipid first encounters the aqueous
phase are critical and must be carefully controlled.

Effect of Charged Lipids

The inclusion of negatively charged lipids such as PS, PA, PI, or
PG or positively charged surfactants such as stearylamine will tend
to increase the interlamellar repeat distances between successive bilayers in the MLV, swelling the structure with a greater proportion
of the aqueous phase. This effect leads to a greater overall entrapped volume. As illustrated in Fig. 7, the entrapment improvement is particualrly striking in low-ionic-strength buffers or nonelectrolytes because the electrostatic repulsive forces that give rise
to the effect are even greater under these conditions. Generally,
5–20 mol% of a charged species is used, although it is possible to
form respectable MLVs (albeit just a few layers) from purely charged
lipid such as PS. The presence of charged lipids also reduces the
likelihood of aggregation following the formation of MLVs.

Alternatives to Thin Film

Although thin-film hydration is readily carried out in the laboratory ,
and perhaps at a pilot plant scale, problems relating to limitations of
surface area are likely to be encountered at a manufacturing level.

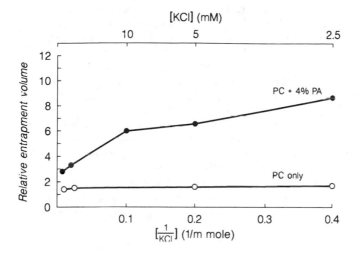

Fig. 7 Importance of surface charge on entrapment volume of liposomes. Liposomes were composed of phosphatidyl choline alone or
phosphatidyl choline plus 4 mol% phosphatidic acid (PA). Liposomes
were prepared by thin-film hydration in KCl solutions of increasing
ionic strength. Relative entrapment is greatest for the PA-containing
liposomes at low KCl concentrations. As expected, at higher salt
concentrations the beneficial effect of the PA is lost due to screen-
ing of the acidic groups by K^+ ions. In line with this explanation,
ionic strength had no effect on encapsulation values of the uncharged
liposomes.

One possible alternative, which was mentioned briefly above, uses
inert insoluble materials such as sorbitol and sodium chloride to increase the surface area available for film deposition [28]. Another
remedy that appears well suited to industrial-scale production uses
conventional spray-drying technology to remove the organic solvent
used to compound the liposomal lipids. The process is reported to
yield an extremely fine, flowable powder mixture, which can be
stored as such or hydrated to form MLV. Hydration is as simple
as introducing the powder slowly into the aqueous phase held in a
suitable processing vessel while mixing [29].

B. Hydration in the Presence of Solvent

One of the drawbacks of thin-film and powder hydration methods is
relatively poor encapsulation efficiency of water-soluble drugs.
Typically, when the vesicles are prepared by addition of an aqueous
drug solution to dry films or powders, only about 5—15% of the total

drug is encapsulated. Liposome down-sizing, if needed, further
reduces the percentage of free drug, since reducing the diameter
of liposomes generally results in the loss of encapsulated material
(see Fig. 19).

   MLVs with relatively high entrapment efficeincies can be produced by hydrating the lipid in the presence of an organic solvent.
A method pioneered by Paphadjopoulos and Watkins [30] begins with
a two-phase system consisting of equal volumes of petroleum ether
containing a mixture of bilayer-forming lipids and an aqueous phase.
The phases are emulsified by vigorous vortexing and the ether
phase removed by passing a stream of nitrogen gas over the emulsion. As the solvent is removed in the carrier gas, MLVs form in
the aqueous phase. A similar method was reported by Gruner et al.
[31], except that diethyl ether was used as the solvent, sonication
was used in palce of vortexing, and the aqueous phase was reduced
to a relatively small proportion in relation to the organic phase.
Typically the method calls for the lipids to be dissolved in about
5 ml of ether, and about 0.3 ml of the aqueous phase to be entrapped
is added. The two phases are emulsified by sonication while a gentle stream of nitrogen gas is passed over the mixture. The resulting MLV preparation encapsulates up to 40% of the aqueous phase,
and the concentration of solute molecules is in equilibrium across all
the bilayers, a feature that is claimed to translate into greater stability to leakage [32].

   A similar approach for producing liposomes by hydration in the
presence of an organic solvent system has been described that begins
with the preparation of a solution of the selected bilayer-forming
elements in a narrowly defined, two-component solvent system. Subsequent mixing of this lipid-in-solvent system with the aqueous phase,
followed by stripping of at least a portion of the solvent system,
leads to the formation of liposomes [33].

C. Small Unilamellar Vesicles (SUV)

The classical methods of dispersing phospholipids in water to form
optically clear suspensions use high-energy sonic fragmentation processes introduced in the early 1960s [34]. These were soon followed
by refinements that employed a high-pressure homogenization device
(a French pressure cell) to produce the same effect in somewhat
larger volumes. These types of SUV dispersions have been rigorously characterized by Huang [35] and others and shown to consist of
rather uniform closed bilayer vesicles of about 25 to 50 nm in diameter. Solvent injection methods have also been devised to produce
SUVs. These typically involve the slow infusion of a lipid solution
in ethanol into water containing a drug or other marker to be entrapped. All of these methods are discussed in greater detail below.

Sonicated SUVs

Methods for the preparation of sonicated SUVs have been reviewed in detail by Bangham [36] and others. Briefly, usual MLV, oligo-lamellar vesicles (OLV), or LUV preparations are sonicated following preparation, either with a bath-type sonicator or a probe sonicator, under an inert atmosphere (usually nitrogen or argon). Although probe sonication leads to more rapid size reduction, heat production, degradation of lipids, metal particle shedding from the probe tip, and aerosol generation may present problems. Although temperature can be accurately regulated in bath-type sonicators and the tube contain-ing the specimen is sealed (allowing for aseptic operations with little likelihood of personnel exposure to aerosols), these instruments are difficult to tune (i.e., regulate power output in a reproducible way) and are available only in small sizes. Flow-through sonic devices are available that are capable of processing larger volumes, but they have yet to be proven in liposome manufacturing, and it is likely that the same disadvantages will apply, including particle shedding, difficulty with energy regulation, and heat-exchange problems.

High-Shear Fragmentation

Dispersions of MLVs can be converted to SUVs by passage through a small orifice under high pressure. A French pressure cell was used by Hamilton and Guo for this purpose [37]. As shown in Fig. 8, an MLV dispersion is placed in the French press and extruded at about 20,000 psi at 4°C. One pass through the cell produces a heterogeneous population of vesicles ranging from several micrometers in diameter to SUV size. Multiple extrusions results in a progressive decrease in the mean particle diameter. Following about four or five passes, about 95% of the vesicles have converted to SUVs, as judged by size-exclusion chromatography. The resulting vesicles are some-what larger than sonicated SUVs, ranging in size from 30 to 50 nm. The method is simple, reproducible, and nondestructive. However, temperature control is difficult (the body of the pressure cell must be allowed to cool between extrusions or the temperature rise may lead to damage to the lipids or drug) and the working volumes are relatively small (about 50 ml maximum). Higher-throughput methods using various types of reciprocating-piston homogenizers (which lend themselves well to continuous-flow operations) have also been used to produce SUVs. These methods are discussed in greater detail below (Section IV.B).

D. Freeze-Drying SUV Dispersions

A simple method for preparing MLVs with high entrapment efficiency was developed by Ohsawa et al. [38] and Kirby and Gregoriadis [39]. The aqueous phase containing the molecules to be encapsulated is

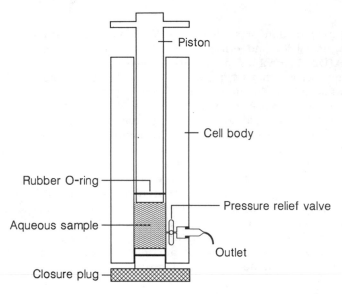

Fig. 8 Diagram illustrating a cross-sectional view of a typical French pressure cell. As the piston advances (by the action of the mechanical press, not shown), an aqueous suspension of large liposomes is forced at extremely high pressures (up to 20,000 psi) through a small orifice. The resulting shear forces mechanically fragment the liposomes, which spontaneously re-form into smaller vesicles.

mixed with a preformed suspension of SUVs and the mixture is freeze-dried by conventional means. Large MLVs are formed when the dry lipid is rehydrated, usually with a small volume of distilled water. Encapsulation efficeincies up to 40% have been reported for this method.

E. Injection of Water-Immiscible Solvents

Alternative "two-phase" methods for preparing liposomes with higher encapsulation efficiencies have been reported. One variation is based on the injection of water-immiscible solvents containing a mixture of bilayer-forming lipids into an aqueous medium. These methods produce relatively uniform unilamellar and oligolamellar vesicles with encapsulation efficiencies (trapping volumes) of between about 20% and 45%. The higher trapping volumes are presumably related to formation of relatively large unilamellar structures.

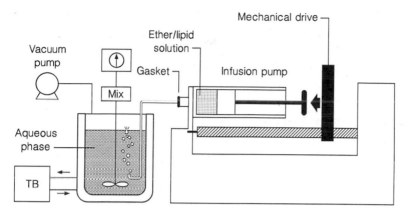

Fig. 9 Diagram illustrating the ether infusion method of forming liposomes introduced by Deamer and Bangham [40]. A mixture of bilayer-forming lipids is made in ether and the solution is placed in a syringe-type infusion pump. The aqueous phase is held in a jacketed vacuum vessel and temperature controlled by circulating fluid through the jacket from a temperature-controlled bath (TB). Pressure is regulated by a vacuum pump. The aqueous phase is agitated with a variable-speed mixer. As the lipid-ether solution is introduced, the ether flash-evaporates—leaving the lipid behind in the aqueous phase to form into small to intermediate-sized liposomes.

Ether Infusion

First introduced by Deamer and Bangham in 1976 [40], the ether infusion method provides a means of making liposomes by slowly introducing a solution of lipids dissolved in diethyl ether (or ether/ methanol mixtures) into warm water. Typically the lipid mixture is injected into an aqueous solution of the material to be encapsulated (using a syringe-type infusion pump) at 55–65°C or under reduced pressure. Vaporization of the ether leads to the formation of single-layer vesicles (Fig. 9). Depending on the conditions used, the diameters of the resulting vesicles ranges from 50 to 200 nm.

Fluorocarbon Injection

To overcome the hazards presented by diethyl ether, Cafiso et al. [41] identified a fluorocarbon solvent useful for injection. They found that Freon 21 ($CHFCl_2$) is an excellent solvent for phospholipids, is immiscible in water, and boils at about 9°C (at atmospheric pressure). Large unilamellar and oligolamellar liposomes form as a Freon 21-lipid mixture is injected into an aqueous medium at 37°C. The fluorocarbon boils off at practically the same rate as it is intro-

duced—leaving the lipid behind to hydrate and form liposomes.
Handjani et al. describe a similar approach and suggest an improvement that may preserve heat-labile molecules. Rather than injecting
into warm water, the solvent is infused into cool water under low
pressure—conditions that accomplish solvent stripping at a lower
temperature [42].

F. Injection of Water-Miscible Solvents

An alternative solvent-injection approach makes use of fairly safe
water-miscible solvents such as ethanol, glycerin, and polyglycols.
The principle is somewhat different form liposome formation during
water-immiscible solvent injection. In this case, during infusion the
solvent containing the lipid is diluted by an excess amount of the
aqueous phase rather than being vaporized as above. As solvent
power is reduced, liposomes form. The major drawback of the approach is the persistence of the solvent. However, such solvents
can be removed by diafiltration and, to the extent that "safe" solvents are used, residues are sometimes acceptable.

Ethanol Injection

An alternative method for producing small liposomes that avoids both
sonication and exposure to high pressure is the ethanol injection
technique first described by Batzri and Korn [43]. Lipids dissolved
in ethanol are rapidly injected into an excess of buffer solution.
SUVs form spontaneously. The procedure is simple, rapid, and
gentle to both lipids and the material to be entrapped. Unfortunately, the method is restricted to the production of relatively dilute
SUV suspensions. The final concentration of ethanol cannot exceed
about 10—20% by volume or the SUVs either will not form or they will
grow in size soon after formation. Removal of residual ethanol by
vacuum distillation can also present a problem, since its partial
vapor pressure at low residual concentrations is small compared to
that of water. Ultrafiltration represents a promising means of both
removing ethanol and concentrating the suspension if desirable. Still
another disadvantage is that some biologically active macromolecules
tend to inactivate in the presence of even low amounts of ethanol.

Alternative Water-Miscible Solvents

Solvents other than ethanol ahve been used to disperse lipids in an
aqueous medium and form liposomes. Polyhydric alcohols such as
glycerol, polyglycerol, propyleneglycol, and ethyleneglycol, as well
as glycerolesters such as monocetin, are claimed to adequately sol-
ubilize lipids and form reproducible suspensions of liposomes when
mixed with an excess aqueous volume [44]. Since these organic

solvents are relatively safe, they can be left in some formulations. The presence of such solvents may also protect the product during freezing (acting as a cryoprotectant), may reduce the sedimentation of some liposome suspensions, and may also serve as an isotonizing agent.

G. Large and Intermediate–Sized Unilamellar Vesicles

Large unilamellar vesicles (LUV) provide a number of important advantages as compared to MLVs, including high encapsulation of water-soluble drugs, economy of lipid, and reproducible drug release rates. However, LUVs are perhaps the most difficult type of liposome to produce. "Large" in the context of liposomes usually means any structure larger than 100 nm; thus large unilamellar vescicles refers to vesicles bounded by a single bilayer membrane that are above 100 nm in diameter. Some authors have referred to liposomes between the sizes of 50 and 100 nm as "large" [4], but these would be more appropriately referred to as intermediate-sized. Two primary methods are used to produce LUVs, one involving detergent dialysis, the other the formation of a water-in-oil emulsion. Intermediate-sized, single-layered vesicles can be generated from MLV dispersions by sequential extrusion through small-pore-size polycarbonate membranes under high pressure. A number of other techniques for producing LUVs have been reported, including freeze-thaw cycling [45], slow swelling in nonelectrolytes [46], dehydration followed by rehydration [47], and dilution or dialysis of lipids in the presence of chaotropic ions [48], but these may be less suitable for large-scale pharmaceutical operations.

LUVs Formed by Detergent Removal

Removal of detergent molecules from aqueous dispersions of phospholipid/detergent mixed micelles represents a radically different approach for producing liposomes. As the detergent is removed, the micelles become progressively richer in phospholipid and finally coalesce to form closed, single-bilayer vesicles. Shortcomings of the approach include leakage and dilution of the drug during liposome formation, high cost, and quality control, and the difficulty of removing the last traces of the detergent once liposomes have formed. Three methods of detergent removal appropriate for this purpose have been described in the literature and are treated separately below.

Dialysis. Kagawa and Racker [49] were the first to introduce detergent dialysis as a method for liposome preparation. Although these authors were interested primarily in reconstituting solubilized biological membranes, their method was immediately recognized as being applicable to the formation of liposomes as well. Detergents

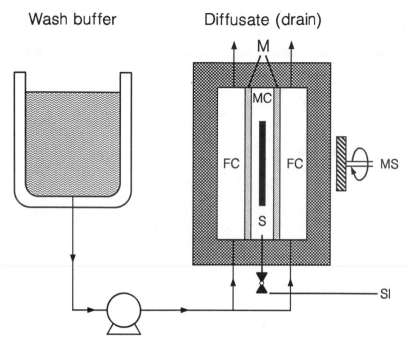

Fig. 10 Diagram showing a cross-sectional view of a flow-through dialysis cell of the type used by Milsmann et al. [50] to from liposomes by detergent removal. The membrane compartment (MC) contains a magnetic stir bar (S) and is filled with a suspension of phospholipid-detergent mixed micelles. A rotating magnet (MS) is used to drive the stir bar during dialysis. The dialysis membranes (M) separating the sample compartment from the two flow-cell (FC) compartments have a molecular-weight cutoff that allows detergent monomers to pass but not larger aggregates. Wash buffer is continuously pumped through the flow-cell compartments to accelerate detergent removal. The diffusate is diverted to a drain, or recycled after removing the detergent with an in-line affinity column or other absorbent material (not shown). The same principle can be adapted to continuously remove detergent (i.e., continuously produce liposomes), by pumping the detergent-mixed micelle suspension through the sample compartment at a rate that is properly balanced with the rate of detergent removal.

commonly used for this purpose exhibit a relatively high critical micelle concentration (on the order of 10 to 20 mM). This property facilitates their removal. Representative detergents used for this purpose include the bile salts and octylglucoside. During dialysis, liposomes in the 100-nm-diameter range form within a few hours. Milsmann et al. [50] were able to control conditions by removing the detergent with a flow-through dialysis cell of the type illustrated in Fig. 10. Their procedure results in a homogeneous population of single-layered vesicles with mean diameters of 50 to 100 nm.

Column Chromatography. The formation of 100-nm, single-layered phospholipid vesicles during removal of deoxycholate by column chromatography has been reported by Enoch and Strittmatter [51]. The method calls for mixing phospholipid, in the form of either small sonicated vesicles or a dry lipid film, with deoxycholate at a molar ratio of 1:2, respectively. Subsequent removal of the detergent during passage of the dispersion over a Sephadex G-25 column results in the formation of uniform 100-nm vesicles that are readily separable form small sonicated vesicles.

Bio-Beads. Another promising method for forming reconstituted membranes reported by Gerritsen et al. [52] may also be applicable to LUV preparation. The system involves the removal of a nonionic detergent, Triton X-100, from detergent/phospholipid micellar suspensions. This method is based on the ability of Bio-beads SM-2 to absorb Triton X-100 rapidly and selectively. Following absorption of the detergent, the beads are removed by filtration. The final particle size appears to depend on the conditions used, including lipid composition, buffer composition, temperature, and, most critically, the amount and detergent-binding activity of the beads themselves.

Reverse-Phase Evaporation (REV) Technique

LUVs can also be prepared by forming an water-in-oil emulsion of phospholipids and buffer in excess organic phse followed by removal of the organic phase under reduced pressure (the so called reverse-phase evaporation or REV method). The two phases are usually emulsified by sonication, but other mechanical means have also been successfully employed. Removal of the organic solvent under vacuum causes the phospholipid-coated droplets of water to coalesce and eventually form a viscous gel. Removal of the final traces of solvent under high vacuum or mechanical disruption (such as vortexing) results in the collapse of the gel into a smooth suspension of LUVs (this general sequence is shown in Fig. 11). With some lipid compositions the transition from emulsion to LUV suspension is so rapid that the intermediate gel phase appears not to form. The method, which was pioneered by Szoka and Papahadjopoulos in 1978, has gained wide-

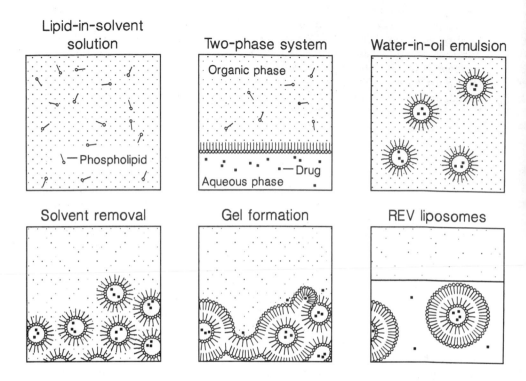

Fig. 11 Diagram showing the key steps in liposome formation by the REV (reverse-phase evaporation) technique. First bilayer-forming phospholipids are dissolved in ether (or another suitable water-immiscible organic solvent) to form a lipid-in-solvent solution. The aqueous phase containing the drug (squares) is added to form a two-phase system that is subsequently emulsified by mechanical means to form a water-in-oil emulsion. As the organic solvent is removed, the preparation becomes viscous and usually forms an intermediate gel. As the last traces of solvent are removed, the gel collapses into a smooth suspension of single-layered REV liposomes. See text for details.

spread use for applications that require high encapsulation of a water-soluble drug [53, 54]. Entrapment efficiencies up to 65% can be obtained with this method.

To prepare REV-type liposomes, the phospholipids are first dissolved in an organic solvent such as diethylether, isopropylether, or mixtures of two solvents such as isopropylether and chloroform (Fig. 11). Emulsification is most easily accomplished when the density of

the organic phase matches that of the buffer (i.e., about 1). For
this reason, ether (density of about 0.7) is often mixed with a solvent of higher density such as trichlorotrifluromethane (density of
1.4) to produce a solvent system with a density close to that of
water. The aqueous phase containing the material to be entrapped
is added directly to the phospholipid-solvent mixture, forming a two-
phase system (Fig. 11). The ratio of aqueous phase to organic
phase is usually about 1:3 for ether and 1:6 for isopropylether-
chloroform mixtures. Preparations using even greater proportions
of lipid and organic phase have been reported [53]. The two phases
are sonicated for a few minutes, forming a water-in-oil emulsion
(Fig. 11), and the organic phase is carefully removed under a partial vacuum produced by a water aspirator on a rotary evaporator at
20–30°C. The pressure is usually maintained at about 500 µm for
the removal of the bulk of the organic phase (using a nitrogen gas
bleed to regulate the vacuum) and then lowered cautiously to complete solvent stripping. Removal of the last traces of solvent trans-
forms the gel into large unilamellar liposomes (last panel in Fig. 11),
which have been used to encapsulate both small and large molecules.
Biologically active macromoelcules such as RNA and various enzymes
have been encapsulated without loss of activity. The principal disadvantage of the method is the exposure of the material to be encapsulated to organic solvents and mechanical agitation, conditions
that can lead to the denaturation of some proteins or introduce nicks
into nucleic acid strands. Although more involved than the thin-
film hydration approaches already mentioned, the high encapsulation
provided by the REV method is a real advantage, and with the development of safer solvent systems [65], there do not appear to be
any insurmountable obstacles to scale-up.

H. Unilamellar Vesicles by High-Pressure Extrusion

As mentioned earlier, MLV suspensions rich in acidic lipids such as
PS or PG tend to have large interbilayer distances due to electrostatic repulsive forces among the bilayers. They also have large internal aqueous cores for the same reason. Hope et al. [56], among
others, have shown that MLVs of this type, when repeatedly extruded
through very small pore-diameter polycarbonate membranes (80 to
100 nm), under high pressure (up to 800 psi), become progressively
smaller, the average diameter reaching a minimum of 60 to 80 nm
after about 5 to 10 passes. Moreover, as the average size is reduced, the vesicles become more and more single-layered. MLVs
prepared from pure PG convert to 60–70 nm single-layer vesicles
following about 10 passes through a 100-nm capillary pore membrane.
The mechanism at work during such high-pressure extrusion appears
to be much like peeling an onion. As the MLVs are forces through
the small pores, successive layers are "peeled" off until only one

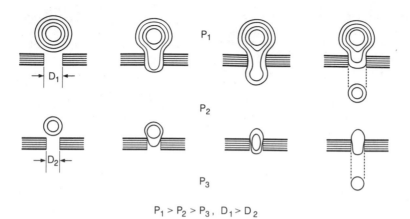

$P_1 > P_2 > P_3, \; D_1 > D_2$

Fig. 12 Cartoon illustrating the fate of a multilamellar liposome as it is passed under pressure through two polycarbonate membranes of different pore diameters. When pressure is applied, the MLV is forced through the first pore of diameter D_1 and emerges with fewer layers and a diameter that corresponds to the pore size. When the extrusion operation is repeated through a second capillary pore membrane of smaller diameter (D_2), single-layered liposomes appear which, once again, have a diameter that corresponds to the diameter of the final pore.

remains (Fig. 12). For this method to generate truly single-layered vesicles, however, the aqueous core of the starting MLV must be greater than about 70 nm in diameter. As said earlier, this appears to be the case for vesicles containing a significant proportion of acidic lipids. However, neutral vesicles or vesicles with only a few mole percent acidic lipids are not likely to convert to true single-lamellar vesicles using this technique because the diameter of the innermost bilayer is probably significantly less than 70 nm.

IV. METHODS FOR CONTROLLING LIPOSOME SIZE

Regrettably, for many of the academic studies that have used liposomes as drug carriers, particle size has not been rigorously controlled. Judging from the few studies that have controlled this parameter, it is clear that vesicle size can have dramatic effects on the in vivo behavior of liposomes [57]. Therefore, before liposome drug carriers systems can be taken seriously for pharmaceutical applications, their size will have to be controlled within reasonable and verifiable limits. An additional rather compelling reason for down-sizing heterogeneous preparations has already been mentioned: that is, to permit sterilization by filtration. Three possible approaches have been explored for achieving defined particle size distributions of liposomes: (a) fractionation of the desired size from a heterogeneous population; (b) homogenization of a polydisperse dispersion to yield a population of smaller vesicles with a narrower size distribution; and (c) extrusion of a heterogeneous preparation through various membranes of known pore diameter to yield liposomes with average sizes that bear some relationship to the rated pore diameter of the extruding membrane.

A. Fractionation

Two methods have become popular for fractionating defined-sized liposomes from a heterogeneous population: centrifugation and size-exclusion chromatography. Both can be used to enrich the product with the desired particle size, but are limited in terms of the volumes that can be easily handled.

Centrifugation

Liposomes sediment in a centrifugal field at a rate that is related to their size and density. Large liposomes composed of netural lipids such as PC can easily be pelleted at fairly low gravitational forces in a conventional centrifuge—much like separating blood cells from plasma. Under proper conditions the smaller liposomes will remain in the supernatant. This method is useful for making broad cuts between small and larger liposomes, but not for isolating narrow particle size distributions. Also, throughput is limited. Zonal rotors or continuous-flow centrifuges may be useful for pilot-scale operations, but probably not for manufacturing. Another disadvantage to centrifugation is that liposomes smaller than aobut 0.5 μm tend to require high gravitational forces and long spinning times in order to achieve effective separation from particles in the >0.2-micrometer range. Such centrifugal forces are achievable only by untracentrifugation, and the capacity of such instruments is limited.

Size-Exclusion Chromatography

Column chromatography has been used for many years as an analytical method to measure the particle size of liposomes. Preparative-scale chromatography has also been applied to isolate liposomes of fairly homogeneous sizes. This method is particularly useful for separating SUVs from larger structures. Typically, a column of Sepharose 4B is used [35]. As the column is washed with buffer, larger liposomes elute in the void volume while SUV appear with the included volume (Fig. 13). Larger pore-size chromatographic media

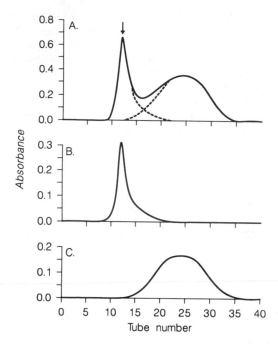

Fig. 13 Elution pattern of sonicated liposomes when chromatographed on a column of Sepahrose 4B. Absorbance was used to monitor the presence of liposomes in the eluting buffer. In panel A two peaks are apparent: The sharper one eluting with the void volume represents larger liposomes that were not converted to SUV during sonication; on the other peak, which is broader and occurs within the included volume of the column, represents SUV. As shown in panels B and C, when fractions containing these two peaks are isolated from the column, concentrated, and rechromatographed, the two populations are well resolved with excellent recovery. (Modified from Ref. 35.)

have been used in a similar fashion to fractionate populations of larger particles [58]. In general, however, such chromatographic separations are quite limited in terms of volumes and throughput, must be carried out in batches, result in significant dilution of the product, and require strict controls to ensure that no microbiological contamination of gel beds occurs.

B. Homogenization

When fairly small particles are desirable, such as the case with long-circulating liposomes or liposomes containing a lipid-soluble drug,

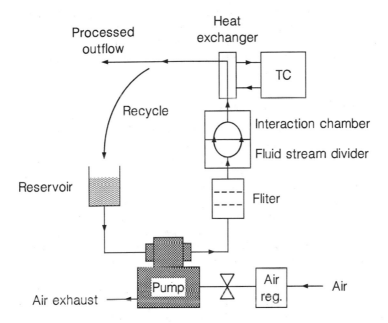

Fig. 14 Diagram illustrating the operation of a homogenizer used to down-size liposomes (Microfluidizer M110). The unsized liposome suspension is held in a reservoir and circulated (in this case with a pneumatic pump) under high pressure through a prefilter and into an interaction chamber where it is separated into two streams that subsequently impinge at extremely high velocities in dimensionally defined microchannels. Heat generated in the interaction chamber can be removed by a down-stream heat exchanger connected with a temperature-controlled bath (TC). The suspension is recycled until the desired particle size is achieved.

homogenization has proven to be a useful approach. In much the same way as milk or emulsions are homogenized, the average particle size and polydispersity of liposome dispersions can be reduced by passage under high pressure through a homogenizer. One such device marketed by the Biological Development Corporation under the trade name Microfluidizer (Fig. 14) has been shown by Mayhew and his colleagues [59] to generate vesicles in the 50–200 nm size range. Conventional homogenizers and high-shear mixers commonly employed in the dairy and pharmaceutical industries have also been reported to be useful for down-sizing liposomes [60, 61]. Such homogenizers are amenable to scale-up, and throughput rates are high. As with other high-pressure devices, however, heat regulation can sometimes present problems, and the shear forces developed within the reaction chamber can lead to local heat production and partial degradation of lipids. Another disadvantage relates to the empirical observation that conditions claimed to produce 200-nm liposomes actually yield polymodal distributions, including larger particles and a significant proportion of very small ones.

C. Capillary Pore Membrane Extrusion

A technique that has gained widespread acceptance for the production of liposomes of defined size and narrow size distribution, introduced by Olson et al. in 1979 [62, 62], is based on the extrusion of a heterogeneous population of fairly large liposomes through polycarbonate membranes under pressure (see Fig. 12). Polycarbonate membranes have uniform straight-through capillary pores of defined size and normally do not bind liposomes. This simple technique can reduce a heterogeneous population of MLVs or REVs to a much more homogeneous suspension of vesicles exhibiting a mean particle size that approaches the diameter of the pores through which they were extruded.

MLVs with a mean diameter of 260 nm can be obtained following a single extrusion through 200-nm pore size polycarbonate membranes; 75% of the encapsulated volume resides in vesicles between 170 and 370 nm (as measured by negative-stain electron microscopy). Upon additional extrusions through the same pore-size membrane, the average size is reduced further, finally approaching about 190 nm with greater than 85% of the particles in the 170—210 nm range. Compared to SUV preparations this still represents a rather broad distribution of vesicle sizes, but compared to the original MLV population, which ranges in size from about 500 nm to many micrometers, it represents a considerable reduction of both average particle size and polydisperisty.

In practice it is sometimes preferable to extrude sequentially through membranes of decreasing pore diameter. For example, a concentrated dispersion of MLVs may be difficult to extrude directly through a 100- or 200-nm pore size filter. In this case it may be advisable to begin the process by extrusion through a 1-μm filter followed by sequential extrusion through an 800-, 600-, 400-, and finally a 200-nm membrane. Alternatively, it is possible to use higher pressures and greater filtration area to extrude concentrated dispersions directly through the smaller pore size membranes.

D. Ceramic Extrusion

Although extrusion through polycarbonate membranes yields homogeneously sized liposome populations, the average diameters of which correspond closely to the diameter of the pores, the method is not without its drawbacks in large-scale processing. For one, the pores in the membrane tend to clog, particularly when processing concentrated suspensions and/or when the liposomes are rigid and of a size substantially greater than the membrane pore diameter. The clogged membranes cannot easily be cleared, because the filter housing configuration does not allow back-flushing, and replacing the filter may compromise the cleanliness of the extrusion operation.

One approach that overcomes the above-mentioned limitations makes use of ceramic membranes [64]. Extrusion of unsized liposomes through asymmetric ceramic filters yields sized liposomes having a selected average size of between about 0.1 and 0.4 µm, and a relatively narrow distribution of sizes. Such extrusion can be operated in a relatively problem-free manner, without heat buildup, at high throughput rates and volumes, in a large-scale operation, under sterile conditions with little risk of contamination.

In practicing the method a suspension of liposomes, containing a substantial portion of particles with sizes greater than about 1 µm, are passed through an asymmetric ceramic filter having an inner-side pore rating of about 1 µm (Fig. 15). As shown in Table 2, the resulting liposomes have an average particle size of between about 0.2 and 0.4 µm, depending on the number of times the liposomes are cycled through the membrane, and a standard size distribution of about 30–45%.

The suspension may be alternately passed through the membrane, in an outisde-to-inside direction, using the three-way divert valve system indicated in the process flow diagram in Fig. 15, to maintain the membrane in an unclogged condition, allowing high throughput, even when concentrated suspension of liposomes are processed.

The average size of the liposomes may be further reduced by passage through similar types of ceramic filters that have been rated at smaller inner-surface pore diameters.

V. PHARMACEUTICAL MANUFACTURING OF LIPOSOMES

Although it is likely that more than one of the processing approaches described above can be used to produce pharmaceutical-quality liposome products, several stand out with respect to ease of scale-up, reproducibility, and economics. Hydration of lipid mixtures in the form of flowable powders produced by spray-drying followed by homogenization or high-shear mixing is a good example of a process that may be useful for making topical liposome dosage forms, for example [29, 60]. Liposome production by hydration in the presence of solvents is another attractive approach [41, 43, 54]. In the following section three variations of a basic solvent-injection method are presented to highlight the key features that would be highly desirable when producing *injectable* liposome products. These include efficient, reproducible encapsulation, uniform size, and the option to

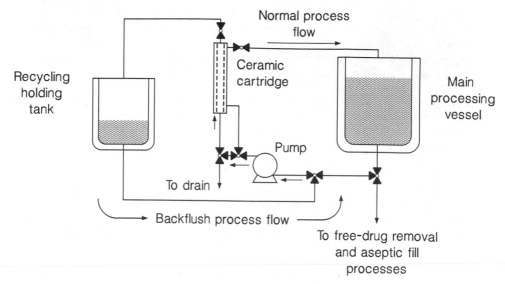

Fig. 15 Process flow diagram illustrating the key features of a system for down-sizing liposomes by passage through asymmetric ceramic membranes with pore diameters in the submicrometer range. The unsized liposome suspension in the main processing vessel is pumped through the valve system into the ceramic cartridge housing, where the fluid passes in an inside-to-outside direciton through the pores of the ceramic membrane and is returned to the main process vessel. The suspension is cycled through the filter until the desired particle size is reached. Should the membrane blind or unacceptable backpressure develop, the process flow can be reversed, to unclog the membrane, by switching the three-way divert valves so that the fluid flows from an outside-to-inside direction through the membrane. As shown, a recycling holding tank can be included to ensure that the pump does not run dry during back-flushing operations.

filter-sterilize the product immediately prior to filling. Untrafiltration as a means of removing unencapsulated drug and lyophilization as an option to preserve liposome dosage forms in an anhydrous state are also reviewed.

A. High-Encapsulation Processing

Accompanying the rapid growth of the liposome industry, breakthroughs have been made in the development of processing methods that provide high encapsulation efficiencies for water-soluble com-

Table 2 Size Reduction of Liposomes by Extrusion Through Asymmetric Ceramic Filters

Mean diameters (and standard deviations) of liposomes are shown following passage through an asymmetric ceramic filter with a rated inner-pore diameter of 0.45 µm. During the first passage, unsized liposomes (ranging in diameter from several tenths of a micrometer to 1–2 µm) are pumped in an inside-to-outside direction through the filter. The second passage is in the opposite direction (i.e., from an outdie-to-inside direction). Each subsequent odd-numbered pass is in an inside-to-outside direction, while each even-numbered pass is in the outside-to-inside direction. Notice that passage from the inside-to-outside direction results in down-sizing, while passage in the opposite direction does not.

No. of passes	Mean diam. (nm)	Std. dev. (%)
1	301.4	36.5
2	300.7	38.1
3	250.4	32.6
4	251.8	36.2
5	239.7	34.2
6	241.8	33.4
7	233.1	33.6
8	234.6	31.1
9	233.2	33.4
10	223.5	35.1

pounds (including peptides and proteins) and that are amenable to scale-up [65, 66]. One method, which is illustrated in the flowchart presented in Fig. 16 and the process diagram in Fig. 17, represents an improvement to earlier solvent-injection methods. Bilayer-forming elements are dissolved in a suitable chlorofluorcarbon solvent (S) and held in a jacketed tank at a temperature well below the boiling point of the solvent. The aqueous phase, including buffers, salts, antioxidants, and drug, is prepared in the main jacketed processing vessel, which is equipped with a mixer. Following compounding of both lipid and aqueous phases, the temperature and pressure in the main processing vessel are adjusted to be just above the boiling point of the lipid solvent.

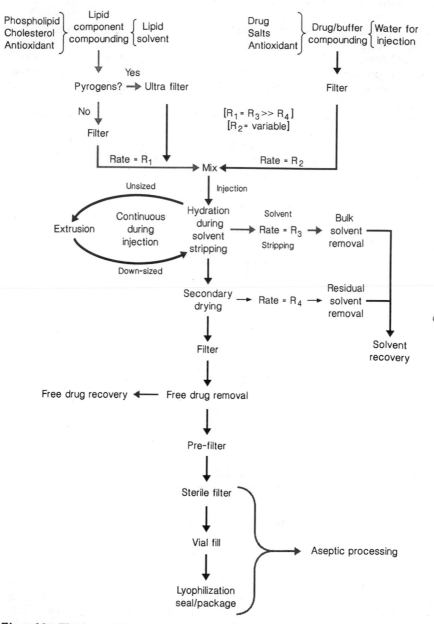

Fig. 16 Flowchart illustrating key steps in the high-encapsulation process, including the option of including an integrated down-sizing (extrusion) subsystem. When in operation, this subsystem produces liposomes of "sterile-filterable" size with the feature that volume (encapsulated drug) lost during down-sizing is recaptured by new liposomes forming as lipid-in-solvent injection continues. See text for details.

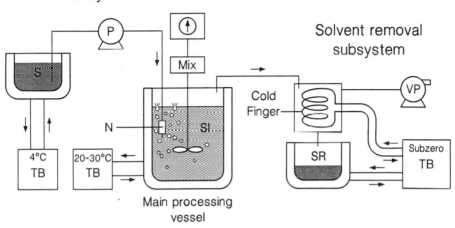

Fig. 17 Process diagram highlighting basic elements of a typical high-encapsulation solvent injection system [65, 65]. Temperature within the main processing vessel (SI) is regulated by circulating coolant fluid through the tank jacket form a temperature-controlled bath (TB). The main vessel is equipped with a variable-speed mixer. The lipid-in-solvent solution is held in a sealed reservoir (S), which is cooled by circulating coolant through the jacket. The lipid solution is usually maintained at a temperature below the boiling point of the lipid solvent (e.g., 4°C). The lipid-in-solvent solution is introduced into the main processing vessel by the pumping action of a fine metering pump (P) and injected through a nozzle (N) immersed in the aqueous phase. Once introduced into the main processing vessel, the lipid solvent vaporizes (bubbles). The lipid solvent vapor is removed by the solvent-removal subsystem consisting of a vacuum pump (VP), a cold finger condenser, and a solvent-recovery holding tank (SR). Pressure, temperature, and mixing rate are adjusted so that the lipid solvent is removed at the same rate as it is introduced.

Liposome formation occurs as the lipid-in-solvent mixture is injected into the aqueous phase. Mixing conditions, pressure, temperature, and injection rate are adjsuted to effectively strip the solvent as quickly as it is injected, without generating undue frothing. Lipid-solvent injection and solvent-stripping operations are continued concurrently until the desired encapsulation efficiency is achieved. Under proper processing conditions the liposomes formed are pre-

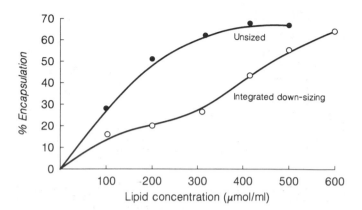

Fig. 18 Relationship between percent of the aqueous phase encapsulated and amount of lipid injected for unsized (0.1—2.0 µm) liposomes (filled circles) and liposomes that are being continuously down-sized to 0.2 µm as the injection operation proceeds (open circles). In both cases encapsulation appears to plateau at about 70%. For unsized liposomes this value is reached above 400 µmol/ml lipid. In the case of the 0.2-µm-sized liposomes, this same level of encapsulation is reached, but at lipid concentrations above 600 µmol/ml.

dominantly oligolamellar and range in size from several hundred nanometers to a few micrometers. An important feature of this approach is predictable entrapment of the aqueous phase as illustrated in Fig. 18. Continued infusion of lipids into the aqueous phase results in a steady increase in the fraciton of the aqueous phase entrapped, reaching a plateau value between 65% and 75%. The viscosity of the aqueous phase also increases as the lipid solids content increases.

Encapsulation efficiencies of about 70% probably represent the theoretical maximum. A this point the liposomes become packed as closely as possible for spherical structures. The approximately 30% that remains unencapsulated represents the volume left among the spheres due to their curvature (Fig. 19). Encapsulation values above 70% have been found with some preparations, but in these cases the liposomes are likely deforming from their usual spherical shape. Although additional lipid can be introduced after reaching this plateau encapsulation value, the newly introduced lipids probably will form internal bilayers (i.e., more multilamellar liposomes) rather than trapping additional aqueous volume.

In cases where the vesicle-forming lipids include charged components such as PG or PS, a gradual size reduction of the particles occurs with continued lipid-in-solvent injection until practically all the liposomes are below 1.5 µm in diameter.

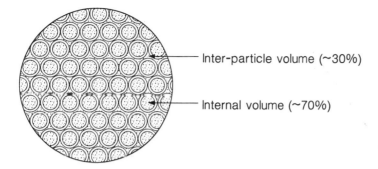

Fig. 19 Cartoon of a magnified cross-sectional view of "closed-packed" uniformly sized liposomes. The arrangement of the liposomes illustrates the maximal fraction of the total volume of water (or a water-soluble drug represented by the dots) expected to be encapsulated (about 70%) and that expected to remain within the inter-liposomal space due to the curvature of the vesicles (about 30%).

The suspension becomes quite viscous at a lipid concentration greater than about 350 to 500 μmol/ml, depending on the average diameter of the particles. The concentrated suspension has a paste-like consistency, and as mentioned below, is usable directly for some applications including topical dosage forms or alternatively as equilibrium storage forms for inhalation or injectable products.

The process may be carried out under sterile, microbiologically contained conditions by presterilizing the lipid and aqueous solutions (usually by filtration), presterilizing the chambers and connective tubing that are in contact with the liquid components (by heat or steam), and sealing the system to prevent contamination during operation.

B. High Encapsulation with Integrated Down-Sizing

Liposomes produced by the high-encapsulation injection process detailed above exhibit a broad size distribution, in the range of 0.2 to 1.5 μms. In order to be able to filter-sterilize such preparations the average particle size must be reduced to about 0.2 μm. This can be done with the extrusion methods detailed in Sections VI.C and VI.D. However, down-sizing such liposomes generally results in a loss of encapsulated materials. As shown in Fig. 20, the maximum entrapped volume provided by a given amount of lipid is reduced as the average diameter of a liposome decreases; a 200-nm-diameter liposome (which, in theory, is the largest possible size that would be sterilizable by filtration) holds 2.5 times the volume of a

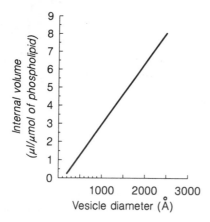

Fig. 20 Relationship between specific (internal) volume of a liposome
and its diameter for a given quantity of lipid. A steep drop in encapsulated volume is evident for very small liposomes. This explains
why SUVs are not ideal for applications where high aqueous drug
payload is desirable.

100-nm liposome and nearly 10 times the volume of a 50-nm vesicle
(a typical product of homogenization).

The high-concentration method is designed for producing a liposome suspension having a fairly high lipid concentration (up to 600–
700 µmol/ml), with average sizes in the range of 180–250 nm (which
are "sterizable" by filtration) and entrapment efficiencies of up to
60–70% for water-soluble molecules.

This system (Fig. 21) contains all of the components of the high-
encapsulation system (including the main processing vessel and the
temperature-regulating the vacuum systems shown in Fig. 17) with
the addition of a continuous liposome-extrusion subsystem. The down-
sizing subsystem is designed to continuously circulate the suspension
in the main processing vessel through the extrusion filter unit (FU)
as the lipid-in-solvent injection process proceeds. In this way volume lost form the liposomes during extrusion can be recaptured by
new liposomes forming during the injection of additional lipid. Although this subsystem may be placed in operation from the time of
initial solvent infusion, it is generally not necessary to begin extrusion until the lipid concentration reaches 50–100 µmol/ml. Below this
concentration the liposomes appear to self-size as noted above.

This approach offers several important advantages. First, continuous down-sizing during lipid-in-solvent infusion significantly reduces the viscosity of the suspension, at higher lipid concentrations,
allowing for infusion of additional lipid to levels that are substantial-

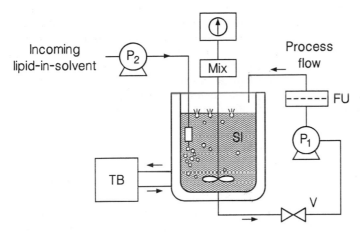

Fig. 21 Process diagram for a solvent-injection system equipped with an integrated "down-sizing" subsystem. All of the elements of the basic solvent-injection system illustrated in Fig. 17 are present, including the lipid-in-solvent infusion subsystem and the solvent-removal subsystem (not shown). The down-sizing subsystem consists of a valve (V), a positive displacement pump (P_1), and an in-line filter unit (FU). Down-sizing is achieved by continuously passing a portion of the volume present in the main processing vessel through the down-sizing filter while lipid-in-solvent injection and solvent-stripping operations are in progress. See text for more details.

ly higher than those achievable without integrated down-sizing. Second, as shown in Fig. 18, lipid infusion can be continued up to a final lipid concentration of 600 μmol/ml or higher, at which point encapsulation efficiencies are greater than 50% and as high as 70%. Without concurrent sizing, the liposome suspension would be too viscous to extrude above a lipid concentration of about 350 μmol/ml, even at high extrusion pressure. Third, the liposomes produced by this method are of a size that can freely pass through a sterilizing filter. This permits the product to be filter-sterilized immediately prior to an aseptic fill operation. Lastly, in the liposome concentrate form, solute molecules, including an aqueous-soluble drug, are in equilibrium throughout the system. No diffusion gradients exist that would tend to induce leakage of the drug from liposomes. Yet up to 70% of the aqueous volume in the concentrate form is encapsulated. Such a preparation may be used directly without free-drug removal for some applications where the 30% of unencapsulated drug might serve as an immediately avaialble "loading" dose, and the 70% of entrapped drug released at a selected rate from the liposomes with

time. Given its inherent leakage stability, the concentrate can be
used as a storage form for liposomes loaded with fairly permeable
drugs. In this case the concentrate would be diluted with isotonic
buffer solutions (such as 0.9% saline or D5W) by the end users and
administered before any significant leakage of the drug occurs.
Also, processing volumes (tankage capacity, etc.) can be kept to a
minimum by directly generating a concentrate that can subsequently
be diluted to provide the dose and volume desired for a particular
product.

C. Uniform-Size Processing

Although the integrated infusion/extrusion method described above
reduces larger particles to a defined diameter, it does not provide
for up-sizing of smaller particles that may be present. This may be
desirable for some applications where high aqueous payloads are required. Small liposomes (below 100 nm) have a limited internal
volume. The ideal size for some parenterally administered liposomes
would be about 200 nm, since these have maximal carrying capacity
while remaining sterilizable by 0.22-µm membrane filtration. A
modification to the integrated lipid infusion/extrusion system that
provides for removal and up-sizing of small particles is illustrated
in Fig. 22. Here a portion of the suspension is circulated by a
pump through a third subsystem containing a diafiltration cartridge
that has a rated pore diameter of about 0.1 µm. As the suspension
is circulated through the diafiltration cartridge, particles larger
than 0.1 µm are retained and returned to the main processing vessel,
while particles less than 0.1 µm appear in the filtrate. In order to
recover the lipid present in these small particles, the filtrate line
can be fed into an extraction chamber where it is mixed with fresh
lipid solvent. The conditions are adjusted so that the lipid is extracted by the solvent and re-formed into new liposomes as the lipid-in-
solvent aqueous phase mixture is infused into the main processing
vessel. The extrusion subsystem is also shown in Fig. 22 to exemplify a situation where lipid-in-solvent infusion, down-sizing, diafiltration, and up-sizing operations are conducted concurrently until
a uniform-sized product is obtained.

D. Free-Drug Removal

Once the uniform-sized liposomes are made and the desired encapsulation and viscosity reached, the concentrate can be diluted with
isotonic buffer and unentrapped drug removed by conventional
separation technology.

Even the smallest liposomes are enormous compared to most drugs.
The smallest possible SUV has an effective molecular weight of several million daltons, while most drugs are smaller than 1000 daltons.

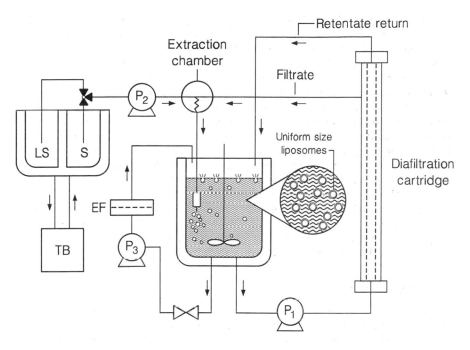

Fig. 22 Diagram illustrating equipment setup for producing uniform-sized liposomes with maximal aqueous-phase entrapment. All of the elements of the integrated down-sizing system shown in Fig. 21 would be in palce, including the lipid-in-solvent injection subsystem (P_2), the solvent-removal subsystem (not shown), and the integrated down-sizing subsystem (P_3 and the extrusion filter unit EF). In addition, a diafiltration loop consisting of a pump (P_1) and a diafiltration filter selected to retain vesicles above about 0.1 μm is included. As lipid-in-solvent injection, solvent removal, and integrated down-sizing operations are in progress, a portion of the volume present in the main processing vessel is circulated through this diafiltration loop. Liposomes with sizes above 0.1 μm are retained and returned to the main processing vessel, and ones below this diameter appear in the filtrate. To recover lipid present as small liposomes, the filtrate can be fed into an extraction chamber where it is mixed with incoming lipid-in-solvent solution (LS) or fresh lipid solvent (S). Conditions within the extraction chamber are adjusted so that lipid entering in the form of small liposomes is extracted (in a two-phase system) and re-forms into new liposomes as this lipid-solvent-water mixture is reinjected into the aqueous phase. The injection, solvent-removal, down-sizing, and up-sizing operations are continued until a uniform-sized product is obtained (as illustrated in the magnified view).

Moreover, drug-filled liposomes are hardy enough so that they do
not burst or leak their contents while being circulated through the
components of conventional ultrafiltration systems (including tubing,
pump head, and ultrafiltration cartridge). These properties make
the separation fo liposomes from enencapsulated drug a rather
straightforward job (Fig. 23). A wide range of equipment is available, from small to large scale, and ultrafiltration separations are
routinely carried out in the pharmaceutical industry. Various types
of membranes and equipment configurations can be used, including
hollow-fiber, spiral-wound, plate-and-frame, or other suitable systems. Since rather large pore diameter ultrafiltration membranes
manage very nicely to retain liposomes while washing out the drug
at high flow rates, diafiltration operations tend to be fairly rapid.
A typical ultrafiltration membrane used for this purpose may have
a molecular-weight cutoff of 20,000 to 100,000 daltons and even
larger. Subsequent processing steps such as sterile filtration (see
Section II.C) and aseptic fill are conducted in the usual manner.

E. Lyophilization

It is often the case that a drug (such as a biological or a drug that
is subject to nonenzymatic hydrolysis) is not stable in aqueous systems and therefore must be stored and distributed in dry form (as
a lyophilized cake, for example). Such a product would be accompanied with labeling that calls for reconstitution (with water for injection, saline, or D5W) immediately prior to administration. It goes
without saying that if a drug is not stable in the presence of water,
it is unlikely that a liposome-encapsulated form of the same drug will
be any more stable as a conventional aqueous suspension.

A number of reports have appeared over the last few years which
indicate that liposomes containing encapsulated drugs can be lyophilized and reconstituted with acceptable drug retention and without
significant changes in particle size. Nonreducing disaccharides such
as sucrose, lactose, and trehaolse are usually needed to act as cryoprotectants. It has been suggested that the presence of selected
concentrations of trehalose during the drying process preserves the
structure of drug-loaded liposomes in the anhydrous state by replacing water molecules normally bound to the lipid headgroups. Upon
rehydration water molecules quickly replace the sugars and the liposomes appear to reseal before significant leakage occurs [67, 68].

Since this pioneering work appeared, however, there have been
puzzling discrepancies in results obtained from different investigators,
both with respect to the relative effectiveness of the various sugars
and the degree to which liposomes can be preserved in the dry state
[69, 70]. As pointed out recently by Crowe and Crowe [71], who
looked into the problem systematically, these discrepancies appear to
be due in large part to differences in the methods used to produce

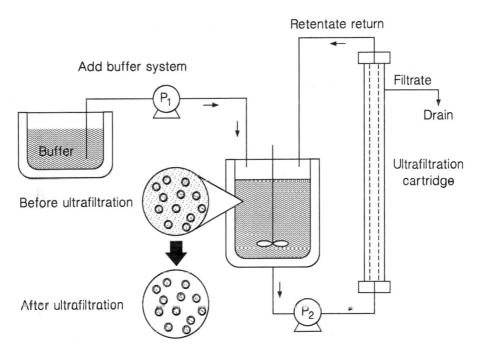

Fig. 23 Diagram illustrating a typical ultrafiltration system used to remove unencapsulated drug from a preparation of liposomes. Following formation, liposomes present in the main processing vessel are pumped through a standard ultrafiltration cartridge using pump P_2. Since liposomes are so large in comparison to most drugs, the ultrafiltration membranes can have rather high molecular-weight cutoffs— leading to rapid flow rates and washout of free drug. The volume is kept constant by balancing the addition of isotonic buffer held in a reservoir (using pump P_1) with the rate of permeate flow as ultrafiltration proceeds. The magnified views illustrate the distribution of drug before and after the ultrafiltration operation, before drug is distributed throughout the system, and after the drug is present only within the aqueous core of the liposomes.

liposomes, their chemical composition, and their physical properties. For example, there appears to be an optimal liposome size for the protective effect of trehalose. Small liposomes (<50 nm) and larger liposomes (>200 nm) appear to leak their contents more rapidly following reconstitution than particles in the 50- to 200-nm range. The relative concentrations of lipid and protective carbohydrate are critical. In the case of trehalose there is an optimal stoichiometry;

maximal retention of an internal marker dye occurs at a mass ratio of about 3:1, trehalose to lipid. There is also a suggestion that having the cryoprotectant present encapsulated within the liposome as well as in the suspension medium is an advantage. And, finally, the presence of charged species (such as PS) appears to improve retention compared with neutral liposomes.

Although freeze-drying is certainly an option for many liposome formulations, it is by no means universally applicable. Each drug may behave differently, and excipients and freeze-drying cycles must be optimized on a case-by-case basis. It is conceivable, for example, that the chemical nature of a drug or its loading requirements, possible interactions of the drug or its stabilizers with the liposome, osmolaity or ionic constraints, etc., may make it impossible to develop suitable freeze-drying conditions. It is just as easy to imagine formulations that would be straightforward to freeze-dry (a lipophilic drug, for example).

In practice there are many degrees of flexibility in formulating liposome-drug complexes (with respoect to excipient blends and composition). Although some compromises may be needed (such as long drying cycles or the presence of some free drug following reconstitution), in general, where dry storage is absolutely necessary to achieve an acceptable product shelf-life, development of freeze-dried liposome formulations, and the processes to make them, appears highly feasible.

VI. CONCLUDING REMARKS

Although the success or the failure of any liposome production technique will ultimately be judged on the basis of the economics of the process at a manufacturing scale, its suitability in a pharmaceutical setting (Good Manufacturing Practice compliance, etc.), and the therapeutic value provided by the delivery system itself, it is now clear that the key issues of stability, reproducibility, high encapsulation efficiency, particle size control, sterility assurance, and scale-up are being successfully addressed. Although the next step, to batch sizes needed to support an actual product launch, is not a trivial one, and unexpected problems will certainly be encountered, processing approaches now exist to produce pharmaceutically acceptable liposomes at a pilot scale (for preclinical and clinical supplies), and at least a few of these are amenable to linear scale-up. F. J. T. Fields was correct almost a decade ago in predicting that the pharmaceutical industry is resourceful enough that, given enough time and commitment, the obstacles confronting the development of efficient liposome produciton technology would eventually be overcome [72].

VII. REFERENCES

1. G. Gregoriadis (ed.), *Liposomes as Drug Carriers*, John Wiley, New York, 1988.
2. D. W. Deamer and P. S. Uster, in *Liposomes* (M. J. Ostro, ed.), Marcel Dekker, New York, 1983, p. 27.
3. G. Gregoriadis (ed.), *Liposome Technology*, Vols. 1, 2, and 3, CRC Press, Boca Ration, Fla., 1984.
4. P. R. Cullis, M. J. Hope, M. B. Bally, T. D. Madden, L. D. Mayer, and A. S. Janoff, in *Liposomes from Biophysics to Therapeutics* (M. J. Ostro, ed.), Marcel Dekker, New York, 1987, pp. 39.
5. D. Lichtenberg and Y. Barenholz, in *Methods of Biochemical Analysis*, Vol. 33 (D. Glick, ed.), John Wiley, New York, 1988.
6. J. H. Senior, *Crit. Rev. Ther. Drug Carrier Syst.*, 3:123 (1987).
7. P. Machy and L. Leserman (eds.), *Liposomes in Cell Biology and Pharmacology*, John Libbey Press, London, 1987, p. 6.
8. H. Schreier, M. Levey, and P. Mihalko, *J. Control. Rel.*, 5: 187 (1987).
9. E. Arakawa, Y. Imai, H. Kobayashi, K. Okumura, and H. Sezaki, *Chem. Pharm. Bull.*, 23:2218 (1975).
10. A. L. Weiner, S. S. Carpenter-Green, E. C. Sochngen, R. P. Lenk, and M. C. Popescu, *J. Pharm. Sci.*, 74:922 (1985).
11. P. J. Mihalko, H. Schreier, and R. M. Abra, in *Liposomes as Drug Carriers* (G. Gregoriadis, ed.), John Wiley, New York, 1988.
12. T. A. McCalden, R. M. Abra, and P. J. Mihalko, *J. Pharm. Exp. Ther.*, in press (1989).
13. P. S. Uster, in *Specialized Vehicles for Topical Delivery* (D. Osborne and T. Amman, eds.), Marcel Dekker, New York, 1989, in press.
14. L. S. S. Guo, C. T. Redemann, and R. Radhakrishnan, *Invest. Opthal. Vis Sci.*, 28:72 (1987).
15. C. Tanford (ed.), *The Hydrophobic Effect*, John Wiley, New York, 1980, p. 60.
16. J. N. Israelachvilli, D. J. Mitchell, and B. W. Ninham, *Biochim. Biophys. Acta*, 470:185 (1977).
17. W. Olsen, in *Aseptic Pharmaceutical Manufacturing* (W. P. Olsen and M. J. Groves, eds.), Interpharm Press, Prairie View, Ill., 1987, p. 101.
18. F. C. Pearson, *Pyrogens: Endotoxins, LAL Testing and Depyrogenation*, Marcel Dekker, New York, 1985, p. 119.
19. J. Dijkstra, J. W. Mellors, J. L. Ryan, and F. C. Szoka, *J. Immunol.*, 138:2663 (1987).

20. D. C. Morrison, in *Handbook of Endotoxin, Vol. 3: Cellular Biology of Endotoxin* (L. J. Berry, ed.), Elsevier, Amsterdam, 1985, p. 25.

21. C. Vigo-Pelfrey and N. Nguyn, personal communication.

22. W. P. Olson, *Process Biochem.*, *18*:29 (1983).

23. J. Lang, M. Man, C. Vigo-Pelfrey, and F. J. Martin, *Chem. Phys. Lipids*, in press (1989).

24. D. W. Deamer and J. Barmhall, *Chem. Phys. Lipids*, *40*:629 (1986).

25. A. D. Bangham, M. W. Hill, and N. G. A. Miller, in *Methods in Membrane Biology* (E. D. Korn, ed.), Plenun Press, New York, 1974, pp. 1–68.

26. F. C. Szoka and D. Papahadjopoulos, *Ann. Rev. Biophys. Bioeng.*, *9*:467 (1980).

27. A. D. Bangham, *Techniques in the Life Sciences*, B4/11, B420/ 1–25 (1982).

28. N. I. Payne, I. Browning, and C. A. Hynes, *J. Pharm. Sci.*, *75*:330 (1986).

29. G. Redziniak and A. Meybeck, U.S. Patent 4,508,703, April 2, 1985.

30. D. Papahadjopoulos and J. C. Watkins, *Biochim. Biophys. Acta*, *135*:639 (1967).

31. S. M. Gruner, R. P. Lenk, A. S. Janoff, and M. J. Ostro, *Biochemistry* *24*:2833 (1985).

32. R. P. Lenk, M. W. Fountain, A. S. Janoff, M. J. Ostro, and M. C. Popescu, U.S. Patent 4,522,803, June 11, 1985.

33. J. L. Taylor, U.S. Patent 4,394,372, August 19, 1983.

34. L. Saunders, J. Perrin, and D. B. Gammack, *J. Pharm. Pharmacol.* *14*:567 (1962).

35. C. H. Juang, *Biochemistry*, *8*:344 (1969).

36. A. D. Bangham, M. W. Hill, and N. G. A. MIller, in *Methods in Membrane Biology* (E. D. Korn, ed.), Plenum Press, New York, 1974, pp. 1–68.

37. R. L. Hamilton and L. S. S. Guo, in *Liposome Technology*, Vol. 1 (G. Gregoriadis, ed.), CRC Press, Boca Raton, Fla., 1984, pp. 37–49.

38. T. Ohsawa, H. Miura, and K. Harada, *Chem. Pharm. Bull.*, *32*: 2442 (1984).

39. C. J. Kirby and G. Gregoriadis, in *Liposome Technology*, Vol. 1 (G. Gregoriadis, ed.), CRC Press, Boca Raton, Fla., 1984, p. 19.

40. D. Deamer and A. D. Bangham, *Biochim. Biophys. Acta*, *443*: 629 (1976).

41. D. S. Cafiso, F. R. Petty, and H. M. McConnell, *Biochim. Biophys. Acta*, *649*:129 (1981).

42. R-M. Handjani, A. Ribier, and M. M. Maurelli, U.S. Patent 4,608,211, August 26, 1986.
43. S. Batzri and E. D. Korn, *Biochim. Biophys. Acta, 298*:1015 (1973).
44. H. Kikuchi and H. Yamauchi, U.S. Patent 4,687,661, August 18, 1987.
45. M. Kasahara and P. C. Hinkle, *J. Biol. Chem., 252*:7384 (1977).
46. J. P. Reeves and R. M. Dowben, *J. Cell Physiol., 73*:49 (1969).
47. R. L. Shew and D. Deamer, *Biochim. Biophys. Acta, 816*:1 (1985).
48. N. Oku and R. C. MacDonald, *Biochemistry, 22*:855 (1983).
49. Y. Kagawa and E. Racker, *J. Biol. Chem., 246*:5477 (1971).
50. M. H. W. Milsmann, R. A. Schwender, and H. Weber, *Biochim. Biophys. Acta, 512*:147 (1978).
51. H. G. Enoch and P. Strittmatter, *Biochemistry, 76*:145 (1979).
52. W. J Gerritsen, A. J. Verkleij, R. F. A. Zwall, and L. L. Van Deenan, *Eur. J. Biochem., 75*:4194 (1978).
53. F. Szoka and D. Papahadjopoulos, *Proc. Natl. Acad. Sci. USA, 75*:4194 (1978).
54. D. Paphadjopoulos and F. Szoka, U.S. Patent 4,235,871, November 25, 1980.
55. C. Pidgeon, S. McNeely, T. Schmidt, and J. E. Johnson, *Biochemistry, 26*:17 (1987).
56. M. J. Hope, M. B. Bally, G. Webb, and P. Cullis, *Biochim. Biophys. Acta, 812*:55 (1985).
57. K. J. Hwang, in *Liposomes from Biophysics to Therapeutics* (M. J. Ostro, ed.), Marcel Dekker, New York, 1987, p. 127.
58. Y. Nozaki, D. D. Lasic, C. Tanford, and J. A. Reynolds, *Science, 217*:366 (1982).
59. E. Meyhew, R. Lazo, W. J. Vail, J. King, and A. M. Green, *Biochim. Biophys. Acta, 775*:169 (1984).
60. G. Redziniak and A. Meybeck, U.S. Patent 4,621,023, November 4, 1986.
61. R. C. Gamble, U.S. Patent 4,753,788, Juen 28, 1988.
62. F. Olson, T. Hunt, F. Szoka, W. J. Vail, and D. Papahadjopoulos, *Biochim. Biophys. Acta, 557*:9 (1979).
63. C. A. Hunt and D. Paphadjopoulos, U.S. Patent 4,529,561, July 16, 1985.
64. F. J. Martin and J. K. Morano, U.S. Patent 4,737,323, April 12, 1988.
65. F. J. Martin and G. West, U.S. Patent 4,752,425, June 21, 1988.
66. G. West and F. J. Martin, U.S. Patent 4,781,871, November 1, 1988.
67. J. H. Crowe, L. M. Crowe, and D. Chapman, *Science, 223*:701 (1984).

68. J. F. Carpenter, L. M. Crowe, and J. H. Crowe, *Biochim. Biophys. Acta, 923*:109 (1987).

69. G. Strauss and H. Hauser, *Proc. Natl. Acad. Sci. USA, 83*: 2422 (1986).

70. T. D. Madden, M. B. Bally, M. J. Hope, P. R. Cullis, H. P. Schieren, and A. S. Janoff, *Biochim. Biophys. Acta, 817*:67 (1985).

71. J. H. Crowe and L. M. Crowe, *Biochim. Biophys. Acta, 939*: 327 (1988).

72. F. J. T. Fields, in *Research Monographs in Cell and Tissue Physiology; Liposomes: From Physical Structure to Therapeutic Applications*, Vol. 7 (G. C. Knight, ed.), Elsevier, New York, 1981.

Chapter 7

PRODUCTION OF DISPERSE DRUG DELIVERY SYSTEMS

S. Esmail Tabibi

MediControl Corporation, Newton, Massachusetts

I. INTRODUCTION

In general, a dispersion is defined as a heterogeneous mixture of two immiscible phases. The continuous phase is the medium in which no subdivided boundaries have been produced, while the dispersed phase consists of small particles/droplets with discrete boundaries separating the particles from one another.

There are varieties of dispersions within the context of the above defnition and, therefore, various descriptive terms define their characteristics, depending on their nature and composition. Some of these names are listed in Table 1.

Pharmaceutically important dispersion systems that are mostly used as drug delivery systems are dispersions of liquids and solids in gaseous media; gases, liquids, and solids in liquid media; and in some unusual cases, dispersions of gases, liquids, and solids in solid media.

It is beyond the scope of this chapter to discuss all of these delivery forms and their processes within the pharmaceutical industry. Therefore we will focus on emulsions (liquid/liquid dispersions), suspensions (solid/liquid dispersions), and liposomes (solid or liquid/liquid dispersions) from a processing viewpoint.

Generally a dispersed drug delivery system consists of the following ingredients:

A *dispersed phase*, which may be a solid active ingredient and/or solution of active ingredient in a suitable lipidic solvent

A *dispersant*, which aids the dispersion of the above phase in the continuous phase and acts in most cases as a physical stabilizer in the total system

317

Table 1   Some of the Known Names Used in Dispersion Systems

Continuous phase	Dispersed phase	
Solid	Solid	Alloys (14 K gold)
Solid	Liquid	Solid emulsions, gels
Solid	Gas	Solid foams (sponge)
Liquid	Solid	Suspensions, gel, sols, colloidal solutions
Liquid	Liquid	Emulsions
Liquid	Gas	Foams
Gas	Solid	Smoke, aerosols
Gas	Liquid	Aerosols, mists, fogs

A *continuous phase*, which is generally an aqueous solution of all other nontherapeutic but necessary ingredients.

A simplified flowsheet for a dispersion preparation is shown in Scheme 1. The indicated steps of milling and/or homogenization are crucial steps in obtaining a pharmaceutically elegant and stable dispersion, since the physical stability and shelf life of a dispersed drug delivery system is critically dependent on the particle size and size distribution of the dispersed phase in the continuous phase. That is to say, creaming, coalescence, sedimentaiton, and/or caking (whatever the instabilization phenomenon may be) is a function of particle size and its distribution. The rate of settling/floating (which is dependent on the density difference between phases) may be predicted by Stokes law, which indicates that the rate of settling/floating will decrease by reducing the particle size of the dispersed phase. Factors such as flocculation, random Brownian movement, viscosity change, etc., are also among the factors involved in the rate and fate of settling/floating that the formulator should consider when designing a dispersed drug delivery system.

II.   PROCESSING METHODS

Among the techniques introduced in the preparation of dispersed systems are the order of addition, rate of addition, temperature, and intensity of mixing or agitation. A glance at the flow diagram presented in Scheme 1 will indicate that the following conditions concerning the rate of addition may exist:

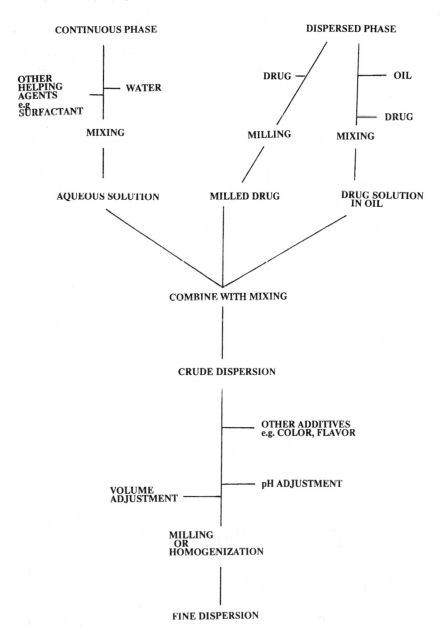

Scheme 1 Schematic representation of the processing of a disperse drug delivery system.

Slow addition of the continuous phase to the dispersed phase
Fast addition of the continuous phase to the dispersed phase
Slow addition of the dispersed phase to the continuous phase
Fast addition of the dispersed phase to the continuous phase

If we focus on the order of addition, the following conditions may exist:

Addition of dispersant to dispersed phase and then addition of
   that combination to the continuous phase
Addition of dispersant to dispersed phase and then addition of
   the continuous phase to the combination
Addition of dispersant to the continuous phase and then addition
   of the dispersed phase to the combination
Addition of dispersant to the continuous phase and then addition
   of the combination to the dispersed phase

Four other ways of addition also exist, in which the order of combining dispersant and the two phases in the above conditions are reversed.

It is obvious that if one would like to examine all the possible physical and chemical factors in this design, the number of probable ways of preparing a dispersion system will be prohibitively large. The existing data on this subject lead to the fact that rapid addition of the continuous phase to the dispersed phase with continuous agitation will produce the best results.

The "continuous agitation" mentioned above introduces the question of agitation techniques and their effects on the overall results. Milling or agitation generally can be achieved by five different processes: simple propeller or turbine mixing, colloid milling, ultrasound, homogenization, and Microfluidizer processing. Before discussing the mechanics of these processes in detail, we would like briefly to discuss the importance of agitation in dispersed systems.

A classical study was reported by Peck et al. [1] with respect to the effect of six different types of processing equipment. They studied emulsification of two dispersed phases, cod liver oil and liquid petrolatum, with three dispersants, gelatin, gum arabic, and a mixture of Tween 80 and Arlacel 80. The prepared emulsions were then evaluated. The rates of creaming were determined and reported. Particle size of the emulsions obtained was also measured initially, and after one and two months, by a photomicrographic method. The authors concluded, in general, that statistically significant differences existed among three dispersants, six pieces of equipment, and an interaction between dispersant and processing equipment. They also showed that the products produced by a Manton-Gaulin homogenizer operated at 8000 psi had the lowest creaming rates.

From this study one is able to deduce the importance of the agitation technique and its energy on the stabilization of a dispersed system.

III. PRODUCTION METHODS AND EQUIPMENT

Selecting a piece of equipment for the preparation of a dispersion drug delivery system will depend, in general, on the state of matter of the dispersed phase. Some processing techniques lend themselves to be used either with solid or liquid dispersed phases, but there are other processing techniques that may have little or no use in the size reduction of solid dispersed phases in the case of suspension systems. We will try to point out the difficulties involved in each case.

A. Simple Mixers

The mechanism by which simple mixers produce small particles is not well understood. Auerbach [2] and Kudryavstev [3] relate the mechanism as being cavitation, while Washington [4] explains the phenomenon by simple shear. Whichever the case may be, the simple mixer is usually used to produce coarse dispersions. These then may be utilized in the preparation of premixes to be used as feedstock for other, higher-energy processing equipment. Among the most frequently used simple mixers are propeller mixers, static mixers, turbine mixers, low-energy stator-rotor mixers, and anchor mixers. Since no orifice is involved in these processing techniques, they can be employed in various dispersion systems.

B. Colloid Mills

There are a variety of high-energy mixers that basically employ a revolving rotor, with 1,000- to 20,000-rpm rotation speeds, and a stator. The clearance between these two opposing faces may be as small as 1/1000 of an inch, into which a crude feedstock passes. These two pieces can be made of stainless steel or other suitable materials. The faces of these two pieces may be roughened by various grooves or may be smooth.

A typical cross-sectional view of a vertical colloid mill is illustrated in Fig. 1.

Shear energy is the dominant mechanism by which smaller particles are produced in this processing technique. As the feedstock passes the rotor, centrifugal force drives the mass away from the center toward the stator, causing the thinning of the film due to imparted turbulence and shear, which in effect reduces the particle size. This may increase the temperature and, therefore, result in

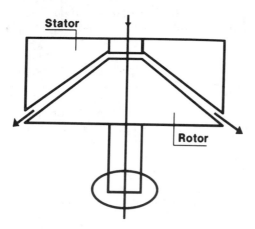

Fig. 1 A cross-sectional representation of liquid path in a vertical colloid mill.

possible physical or chemical instability. Among the disadvantages of this type of process equipment are the presence of a moving part (rotor) and the possible contamination of the product due to wear. Also, the presence of an uneven gap between the rotor and stator will cause a large polydispersity in the particle size of the product and, as a result, reduced stability. The need to change the moving parts very often adds an economic disadvantage to its use.

This technique can be used in suspension and emulsion production. Various configurations from different manufacturing companies are available. The power of the motors varies from 3 to 75 hp or even higher, with capacities from 80 to 14,000 liters per hour.

C. Ultrasonic Equipment

There are four different ways of producing ultrasonic energy [5].

1. Piezoelectric effects: Application of an alternating current with similar frequency as the vibrational frequency of crystal across the crystal will cause a powerful oscillation.
2. Electromagnetic effects, which is the same as the familiar moving-coil loudspeaker.
3. Magnetostriction effects: Due to the change in length of certain metals in a magnetic field, one may produce a large oscillation, for example, nickel in magnetic field.
4. Mechanical effects: The principle involved in this type of oscillation energy is similar to that of a whistle or organ pipe. The flow rate and pressure with which the fluid flows through

the pipe and causes resonancy in the blade of an organ pipe or whistle are conversely proportional to the fluid's viscosity.

Realizing the appropriate flow rate and pressure when the flowing fluid is not in the gaseous state is not a simple task. Before dealing with this subject, let us discuss the possibility of using any of the four modes of sonic energy formation in the manufacture of disperse systems.

Obviously, the first two methods are not useful for us, since the alternating current applied to either crystal or wire would pass through the dispersion system and therefore prohibit its general usefulness.

The third method may be applied in small-scale operations (as sonic baths or probes), but it suffers from an uneven distribution of energy.

The fourth one, which will be discussed here, has been made possible by means of the Pohlman whistle [6]. In this machine a jet of liquid is forced through an orifice that impinges on a blade, thus causing an oscillating vibration. This vibration then causes the stream of liquid to be forced up and down, producing powerful vibrations in the liquid (depending on the frequency of the blade and other parameters). This alternate up and down movement of the liquid causes the liquid to disrupt, forming actual cavities in the liquid. Collapse of these cavities (bubbles) then creates additional cavitation and shear forces [7].

The schematic presentation of a Pohlman whistle that has been constructed as commercial-scale equipment (Rapisonic) is illustrated in Fig. 2.

Among the disadvantages of ultrasonic systems are uneven energy distribution within the jet stream. This is because the energy of vibration is reduced by increasing the distance from the vibration center. Also, if the vibrating probe used inside the dispersion system is constructed of titanium, contamination of the sample may occur [4].

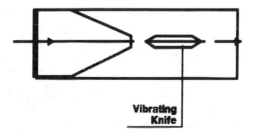

Vibrating Knife

Fig. 2 A diagramatic representation of a Pohlman whistle.

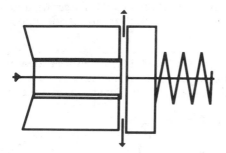

Fig. 3 A cross-sectional view of a homogenizing valve assembly.

D. Homogenizer

Soon after A. Gaulin presented his invention in Paris in 1900, the
processing machine was termed a "homogenizer." This equipment
basically consists of a homogenizing valve assembly through which a
liquid dispersion to be homogenized is pumped at high pressure by
a positive-displacement pump [8, 9].

The valve assembly is depicted in Fig. 3. A homogenizing valve,
which looks in general like a "plug," is forced against the valve
seat by an actuating spring. The gap between the valve and seat
can be adjusted. When a fluid, at low speed and high pressure, is
forced via a positive-displacement pump into the valve assembly, it
will generate pressure within the restricted area of the valve and
valve seat. This increased pressure then will cause the actuator
spring to compress, moving the valve away from the valve seat and
generating enough space for liquid to escape with increased velocity
in order to release the excess pressure. This high-velocity liquid
then impinges on the wear ring and causes the particles of the dispersed phase to be reduced, so that finally a "homogenized" product
discharges through the outlet. The time required for a fluid to pass
through the homogenizing valve is in the range of 0.0001 sec, but
it produces a large energy density in the liquid [9]. There are
various homogenizing valves for different applications. Some have
been presented in Fig. 4.

The standard flat-face valve, as in the original design, is useful
in a variety of dairy, food, and chemical applications, while a
grooved-face homogenizing valve and valve seat assembly is somewhat
more efficient [8]. A knife-edge valve design, on the other hand,
reduces the exerted pressure due to the enlargement of the restricted area, where the homogenization occurs. There are several different configurations, as shown in Fig. 4.

In all such spring-loaded valve and seat designs, the potential
for nonuniform homogenization exists due to the variety of mechan-

Conventional plug valve with seat　　**Knife-edge valve and seat**

Grooved valve and seat　　**Knife-edge valve design used for cell disruption**

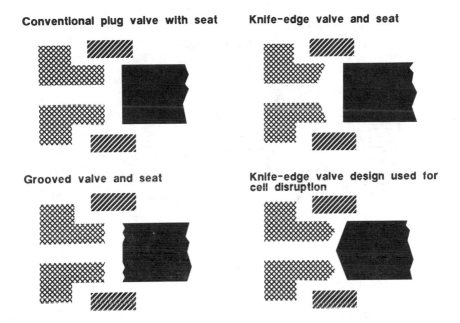

Fig. 4　Varieties of homogenizing valves.

isms, among them heat generated in the system, which may cause metal fatigue in actuating springs and uneven wear in the valve/seat area.

These homogenizers produce submicrometer-size droplets within the emulsion formulation. Mechanisms by which reduction in droplet size occurs is still not clear. Cavitation, turbulence, and shear are among the considerations [8, 9].

Gaulin Corporation has introduced a mixer/emulsifier called Hydro-Shear that has application in the pharmaceutics, cosmetics, and food industries [8]. This equipment differs in principal from a "homogenizer" in that the fluid undergoes a high-shear environment within a special chamber design. The chamber is constructed as two cones attached to each other from the wide sides with a tangential inlet in the center of the chamber. This tangential fluid flow causes a spiral motion toward the inner part of the chamber, and the fluid velocity increases progressively due to diameter decrease in the conical-shaped chamber. These progressive speed differences in the layers of flowing fluid generate a high-shear region and cause the reduction of the particle size of the dispersed phase, which finally discharges through the apex of the cones. This equipment produces a dispersed phase with particle sizes in the range of 2 to 8 µm. The company suggests this equipment for the preparation of premixes or crude

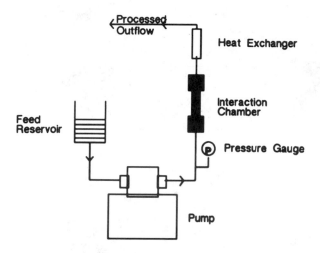

Fig. 5 A diagramatic representation of the Microfluidizer unit.

emulsions to be further processed. Also, this equipment will be useful in the processing of finished products that do not require fine
particles in the submicrometer range.

E. Microfluidizer

In 1985, a U.S. patent was issued to E. J. Cook and A. S. Lagace
[10] for new processing technology for the forming of emulsions in
the particle size range of 0.02-0.5 µm. This processing equipment
developed from this technology was later termed a Microfluidizer. A
premixed crude emulsion is pumped at high pressure into a unique
fixed architecture interaction chamber, forming liquid jets or sheets.
These jets or sheets then impinge upon each other in well-fixed and
precisely defined microchannels within the chamber, resulting in a
small zone of intense turbulence or cavitation, which causes the
dispersed phase to break into smaller droplets. Also, the uniform
application of this intense turbulence to each microunit of fluid passing through the chamber yields a vary narrow size distribution of
the dispersed phase, hence giving rise to more physically stable
emulsions.

The product may be processed in a batch or continuous mode.
The feedstock can be premixed, or the individual phases can be fed
separately by means of a coaxial feeding tube. In the latter case,
the interaction will occur upon the phases entering the processing
chamber [11].

Figure 5 schematically represents a prototype unit. The pump is
air-driven for laboratory (M-110) and pilot plant (M-210) Microfluid-

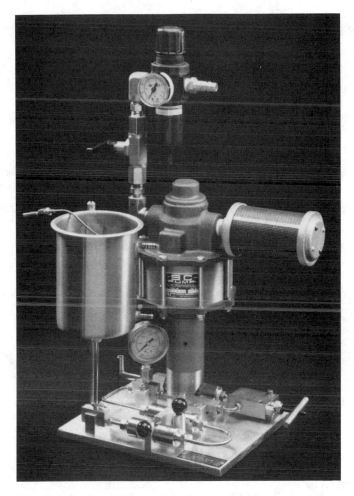

Fig. 6 Laboratory model Microfluidizer M 110T.

izer processors, while for larger manufacturing-scale equipment
(M-510), a triplex electric-powered pump is utilized.

Figure 6 and 7 show two models of Microfluidizer processing equipment.

The standard laboratory model can operate at pressures up to
15,000 psi, generated by a 100-psi air supply, which is available in
most laboratories. There are various laboratory models available for
different applications, some of which are capable of pressures up to
30,000 psi. The main part of a Microfluidizer unit is the "interaction
chamber." The flow path is presented schematically in Fig. 8.

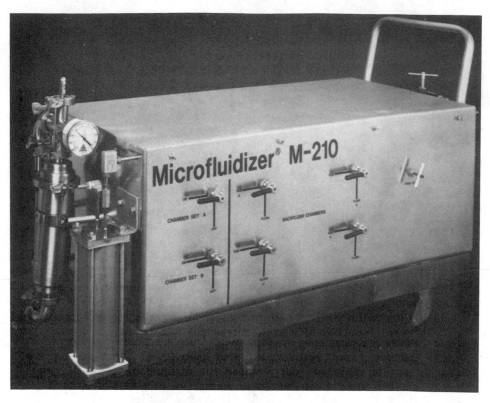

Fig. 7 Pilot plant Microfluidizer M-210.

    The fineness of the emulsion, its uniformity, and the intensity of
the liquid stream interactions can be controlled by operating factors
such as pressure, number of passes [11–14], and temperature at
which the operation takes place [13]. Also, there is another important factor that controls the above properties that in itself is
beyond the control of the operator. That is the configuration of
the inner parts of the interaction chamber [11]. Due to the importance of this parameter and the availability of various interaction
chambers for a variety of applications, it is advisable to consult
with the manufacturer (Microfluidics Corporation, Newton, MA) for
particular applications. Chamber designs are available, for example, for suspension processing cell rupture [15], liposome formation [16], emulsion processing, and microencapsulation [17]. These
chambers can be utilized with the same base model Microfluidizer
and, by analogy, is comparable to a variety of punches and die sets
in a tablet press.

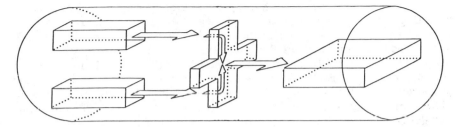

Fig. 8 Schematic representation of flow path through the "interaction chamber" of the Microfluidizer.

A comparative study of the efficiency various processing techniques on the production of parenteral feeding emulsions has been published by Washington and Davis [1]. They clearly showed that the Microfluidizer produced products with a similar droplet size and polydispersity to those of a commercially available product, Intralipid. They indicated that the droplet sizes and polydispersity of the emulsions produced by Microfluidizer technology were smaller than those produced by an ultrasonic probe and concluded that the Microfluidizer had several advantages over ultrasonication and would appear to be a useful technique for the preparation of intravenous lipid emulsions.

Although it has been a very short period of time since Microfluidizer processing technology has been introduced, it has become well accepted, with over 50 literature citations on record. Listing a detailed bibliography is not possible in this limited space, but a few references will be given as samples [18—22].

IV. PREPARATION OF LIPOSOMES BY MICROFLUIDIZER PROCESSING

Phospholipids swell upon hydration in aqueous media and then form bilayered vesicles by closing upon themselves. Their potential uses in pharmaceutics are the subject of a variety of reports and books [23, 24]. There are many ways by which one may produce liposomes. Before discussing the production methodologies, it is important to distinguish between mulilamellar vesicles (MLVs) and unilamellar vesicles (ULVs). MLVs consist of concentric spheres of bilayers. They were produced first in 1961 by Bangham using a method of solvent dissolution, film formation by evaporation, and rehydration by aqueous solutions of drugs/buffer [25]. These MLVs are heterogeneous in size and difficult to reproduce.

Small ULVs, on the other hand, consist of a single bilayer surrounding a central aqueous core. Since they have a discrete submicrometer particle size and uniformity, they can be reproduced and
can be most useful in drug delivery systems. ULVs were first
prepared from MLVs by sonication and separation techniques. Meyhew et al. [16] were the first to use Microfluidizer processing in the
preparation of ULV liposomes and showed that the Microfluidizer provides a practical and convenient way of preparing research and commercial quantities of liposomes on a reproducible basis. The liposomes produced by the Microfluidizer have a particle size of less than
200 nm with a narrow size distribution. Sizes in the 20—80 nm range
are usual.

Mayhew et al. [16] have shown that a capture or entrapment efficiency of 75% or higher can be obtained using ^{3}H-labeled Cytarabine
as a model aqueous soluble drug.

Beissinger et al. [27] have prepared liposome-encapsulated hemoglobin using a Microfluidizer. They concluded that liposome-encapsulated hemoglobin has adequate oxygen-carrying capacity, storage
stability, acceptable viscosity, and is filterable through a 0.22-μm
sterile filter. They used the Microfluidizer because of their need for
a commercially viable process and were satisfied with the results.

Koide and Karel [28] have utilized the Microfluidizer among other
techniques to encapsulate enzymes in liposomes and deduced that in
their case encapsulation efficiency will be higher at lower pressure
and one pass through the Microfluidizer.

Seltzer and his co-workers [29—31] have used the Microfluidizer
processing technique in the preparation and evaluation of radiograph-
ic contrast agents and showed that the entrapment capacity of liposomes prepared with this technique is much higher than other processing equipment.

V. ACKNOWLEDGMENT

I wish to thank Dr. Arthur Siciliano for his assistance in preparing
this chapter and Mary Kelliher for the typing of this manuscript.

VI. REFERENCES

1. G. E. Peck, H. G. DeKay, and G. S. Baker, *J. Amer. Pharm.
    Assoc. (Sci. Ed.)*, *49*:75 (1960).
2. R. Auerbach, *Chem. Tech.*, *15*:107 (1942).
3. B. B. Kudryavtsev, *Kolloidn. Zhur.*, *21*:58 (1959); through
    C.A. 53:16645b.
4. C. Washington, *Lab. Equip. Dig.*, *25*:69 (1987).
5. P. Becher, *Emulsions: Theory and Practice*, 2nd ed., R. E.
    Krieger Publishing Company, Malabar, Fla., 1977, p. 289.

6. B. J. Gaffney, Bias for Applied Ultrasonics, presented to Chemical Processing "Table-Top Show," Boston, Mass., reproduced by Sonic Corp., Statford, Conn.
7. W. W. McCarthy, *Drug & Cosmet. Ind.*, *94*:821 (1964).
8. *Homogenization and Emulsificaiton*, Technical Bulletin T.B. 67, Gaulin Corporation, Everett, Mass., 1982.
9. L. H. Rees, *Chem. Eng.*, *86* (May 13, 1974).
10. E. J. Cook, and A. S. Lagace, U.S. Patent 4,533,254 (1985).
11. H. Korstvedt, R. Bates, J. King, and A. Siciliano, *Drug Cosmet. Ind.*, November, 1984.
12. A. Siciliano and E. Tabibi, *J. Pharm. Sci.*, *76*:S98 (1987).
13. C. Washington and S. S. Davis, *Int. J. Pharm.*, *44*:169 (1988).
14. H. Korstvedt, G. Nikolopoulos, S. Chandonnet, and A. Siciliano, *Amer. Paint & Coat. J. 38* (January 1985).
15. R. Seva, J. Fieschko, R. Sachdev, and M. Mann, presented at the Society of Industrial Microbiology Annual Meeting, San Francisco, Calif., 1986.
16. E. Mayhew, R. Lazo, W. G. Vail, J. King, and A. M. Green, *Biochem. Biophys. Acta, 775*:169 (1984).
17. F. Koosha, R. H. Muller, and C. Washington, *J. Pharm. Pharmacol., 39(suppl.)*:136P (1987).
18. K. P. Oza, and S. G. Frank, *J. Disp. Sci. Tech.*, *7*:543 (1986).
19. R. T. Lostritto, S. Sylvestri, and L. Goei, *J. Parent. Sci. Tech.*, *41*:214 (1987).
20. R. T. Lostritto, and S. Sylvestri, *J. Parent. Sci. Tech.*, *41*: 220 (1987).
21. R. J. Prankerd, S. G. Frank, and V. J. Stella, *J. Parent. Sci. Tech.*, *42*:76 (1988).
22. D. L. Teagarden, B. D. Anderson, and W. J. Petre, *Pharm. Res.*, *5*:482 (1988).
23. D. Chapman, in *Liposome Technology*, Vol. I (G. Gregoriadis, ed.), CRC Press, Boca Raton, Fla., 1984, p. 1.
24. M. Ostro (ed.), *Liposomes*, Marcel Dekker, New York, 1983.
25. D. W. Dreamer, in *Liposome Technology*, Vol. I (G. Gregoriadis, ed.), CRC Press, Boca Raton, Fla., 1984, p. 29.
26. E. Mayhew, G. T. Nikolopoulos, J. J. King, and A. A. Siciliano, *Pharm. Manuf.*, *1*:18 (1985).
27. R. L. Beissenger, M. C. Farmer, and J. L. Gossage, *Trans. Amer. Soc. Artif. Intern. Organs.*, *32*:58 (1986).
28. K. Koide and M. Karel, *Int. J. Food Sci. Technol.*, *22*:707 (1987).
29. S. E. Seltzer, Contrast Carrying Liposomes: Current Status, presented at the Contrast Media World Symposium, France, 1987.
30. K. T Cheng, S. E. Seltzer, D. F. Adams, and M. Blau, *Invest. Radiol.*, *22*:47 (1987).
31. M. R. Zalutsky, M. A. Noska, and S. E. Seltzer, *Invest. Radiol.*, *22*:141 (1987).

Chapter 8

HYDROGELS FOR DRUG DELIVERY SYSTEMS

Stevin H. Gehrke

University of Cincinnati, Cincinnati, Ohio

Ping I. Lee

University of Toronto, Toronto, Ontario, Canada

I. INTRODUCTION

The term "gel" has long been used to describe states of matter that appear to be intermediate between solid and liquid. Common gels include soft contact lenses and gelatin desserts. As is the case with other imprecisely defined terms, many disparate substances have fallen under the umbrella of the term "gel," including:

Certain surfactant mesophases
Various inorganic colloids, including clays
Coagulated proteins
Solvent-swollen linear polymers
Network polymers

Over the decades, numerous authors have attempted to formulate more precise definitions of the term gel [1−3]. Each definition preserves the concept of a state intermediate between liquid and solid. What materials are included or excluded as "true" gels vary, depending on each author's perspective. Ultimately, the most appropriate definition is simply that which allows people to communicate a certain concept effectively.

In drug delivery, the term "hydrogel" is typically reserved for polymeric materials that can absorb a significant amount of water (>20% of its dry weight) while maintaining a distinct three-dimensional structure. This definition is normally taken to include dry polymers that will swell when placed in water, as well as the already-swollen elastic materials that inspired the original definition. The terms "aerogel" and "xerogel" are also used [4−6]: An aerogel is a dry, porous material that absorbs water into its pores without substantial swelling, while a xerogel is a nonporous material that absorbs water by swelling. This definition of hydrogel, however, does exclude hydrophilic polymers that are added to formulations as binders, disintegrants, or to increase viscosity. An elastic, not viscous, response to applied stress and maintenance of a distinct three-dimensional structure are integral characteristics of any gel [3]. While this implies that most hydrogels will be covalently crosslinked network polymers, this is not a requirement. Physical entanglements, crystallites, charge complexes, hydrogen bonding, and so forth, can all lead to materials that swell in water while maintaining a distinct structure.

Hydrogels thus defined are an important material in the design of specialized drug delivery systems. In recent years, there has been an explosion of interest in polymer-based delivery devices. Such systems can enhance drug stability by protecting labile drugs from denaturants in the body, control the release rate of therapeutic agents, and help target release to a chosen site in the body. In many cases, either natural or synthetic hydrogels are the most useful polymers.

Hydrogels are diverse: They can be made from a broad array of precursors in many different ways in order to match their properties to a given application. They can be made biodegradable, inert or reactive, derivatized with specialized groups such as enzymes, or grafted to other materials. Hydrogels can be formed in virtually any geometry from microspheres to bulk structures. Certain hydrogels can be made to respond to changes in their environment. Relatively low mechanical strength sometimes limits their biomedical applications, but this is not usually a concern for drug delivery applications.

Hydrogels have four key properties: swelling degree, biocompatibility, permeability, and swelling kinetics. Their high water content leads to good biocompatibility because impurities can be easily extracted; their soft, rubbery nature reduces mechanical irritation; and their hydrophilic character minimizes interfacial tension. The permeability of hydrogels to water, drugs, and other solutes is easily adjusted over a broad range by changing the gel precursor, crosslinker, or synthesis conditions. The reproducible, controllable swelling kinetics of hydrogels mean that the permeability of the gels can be made to vary with time, or even change in response to external conditions, enabling release of therapeutic agents in a prescribed fashion.

Hydrogels were studied by scientists long before the existence of polymers was recognized [7]. Wichterle and Lim proposed their use as contact lenses in 1960; this opened the door to other biomedical applications for hydrogels, including drug delivery [8]. The classic reference is *Hydrogels for Medical and Related Applications*, edited by Joseph Andrade [9]. The recently published three-volume series, *Hydrogels in Medicine and Pharmacy*, edited by Nikolaos Peppas, provides a thorough review (over 2000 references are cited) of the area

[10—12]. Volume I reviews the synthesis, swelling, and solute
permeation of hydrogels. Volume II examines the most important
hydrogels for drug delivery, including such materials as poly(2-
hydroxyethylmethacrylate) (PHEMA) and poly(vinyl alcohol) (PVA).
Various biomedical applications of hydrogels, including drug delivery, are covered in Volume III. The annual symposium proceed-
ings published by the rapidly growing Controlled Release Society
give a valuable look at the state of the art in hydrogel application
to drug delivery. A number of other recent reviews covering different aspects of gels are also available [3, 13—18]. The problem of
producing hydrogels for drug delivery on a commercial scale is relatively new, and information is mostly proprietary. As a result, little
has been published on scale-up of hydrogel-based drug delivery systems.

This chapter provides an introduction to the properties and production of hydrogels for drug delivery. It beings with a discussion
of the key properties of hydrogels, the variables that influence these
properties, and how experimental data are obtained and correlated.
Next, the various syntheses of hydrogels and the basic principles of
their production are reviewed. At this point, commercial production
of hydrogels is examined. The chapter concludes with a discussion
of special considerations for producing pharmaceutical-grade hydrogels, how monolithic hydrogel devices are loaded with bioactive compounds, and a brief review of current and potential drug delivery
systems that use hydrogels.

II. PROPERTIES OF HYDROGELS

A. Equilibrium Swelling

Theory

While permeability characteristics and biocompatibility make hydrogels
useful and although low mechanical strength can limit some applications, the single most important characteristic of a hydrogel is its
swelling degree in water. The amount of water absorbed is a function
of the hydrophilicity of the polymer, the network structure, and the
number of ionized groups on the polymer. Because swelling is central to any application of hydrogels, it is important to examine the
theory behind gel swelling.

The basic thermodynamic description for a gel in equilibrium with
a solvent was developed in the 1940s [19, 20]. Since that time,
other researchers have modified this basic theory to make it more
rigorous, striving for quantitative prediction of swelling effects [21—
36]. These enhanced theories retain the basic approach described
by Flory [37], which assumes that the swelling of gels is the result
of several independent free-energy changes that occur when the gel
is mixed with the solvent:

$$\Delta G_{tot} = \Delta G_{mix} + \Delta G_{elas} + \Delta G_{ions} + \Delta G_{elec} \tag{1}$$

where

ΔG_{tot} = total free energy change; ΔG_{tot} = 0 at equilibrium

ΔG_{mix} = mixing of polymer chains with solvent molecules

ΔG_{elas} = elastic response to changes in the configuration of the polymer network

ΔG_{ions} = mixing of ions from solution and from the polymer with solvent

ΔG_{elec} = changes in electrostatic interactions of ionized groups upon swelling

Only ΔG_{mix} and ΔG_{elas} need to be considered for nonionic gels; polyelectrolyte gels use all four terms. It is conceptually convenient to convert the free-energy terms to osmotic swelling pressures, Π, using the thermodynamic relation

$$\Pi = -\frac{1}{\tilde{V}_i} \left(\frac{\partial(\Delta G)}{\partial(n_i)} \right)_{P,T,n_j} \tag{2}$$

where

$\tilde{V}_i$ = molar volume of species i

n_i = moles of species i

n_j = moles of species j

P = pressure

T = absolute temperature

Then Eq. (1) becomes:

$$\Pi_{tot} = \Pi_{mix} + \Pi_{elas} + \Pi_{ions} + \Pi_{elec} \tag{3}$$

Flory-Huggins theory calculates the enthalpy and entropy changes associated with laying out a polymer chain on a lattice [37]. This theory yields the following expression for Π_{mix}:

$$\Pi_{mix} = -\frac{RT}{\tilde{V}_1} [\ln(1 - \phi_2) + \phi_2 + \chi\phi_2^2] \tag{4}$$

where

R = gas constant

ϕ_2 = volume fraction of polymer

χ = polymer-solvent interaction parameter

The key parameter in this expression is the Flory-Huggins interaction parameter, χ, which is indicative of the interactions between the solvent and the polymer. Interaction parameters are generally between 0 and 1; when $\chi < \frac{1}{2}$, polymer-solvent interactions dominate, and dissolution is favored; when $\chi > \frac{1}{2}$, polymer-polymer interactions dominate, discouraging dissolution. When $\chi = \frac{1}{2}$, termed the *theta state*, there are no net interactions. The behavior of χ, its theoretical formulation and estimation, and its experimental measurement have been reviewed by Barton [38].

While χ is widely used as an indicator of the quality of a solvent for a polymer, whether good, moderate, or poor, it does have theoretical and practical limitations, including:

1. χ is not a constant, but is a function of temperature, concentration, and molecular weight.
2. χ is strongly affected by specific interactions such as hydrogen bonding.
3. χ characterizes a particular polymer-solvent pair; the concept cannot be easily extended to multicomponent systems.
4. Empirical behavior of χ often deviates from theoretical predictions.

The interactions between water and hydrogels are usually complex. Extensive hydrogen bonding exists, polar interactions are significant, and water structuring usually occurs around the gel. While χ can be modified to include such effects, the resulting expressions are clumsy and of limited predictive value. Research groups are working to improve prediction of Π_{mix} [31, 39–42].

The next swelling pressure term in Eq. (3), Π_{elas}, accounts for the retractive force exerted by the network. This force is entropic in origin: As the chains are extended, the number of conformations that can accommodate this elongation is reduced. Only one conformation allows full chain extension, so this is a state of minimum entropy; if the extending force was removed, entropy-increasing randomization would cause contraction. Thus Π_{elas} opposes any tendency of a cross-

linked polymer to swell. Flory derived the following expression for
a network of freely jointed, random-walk polymer chains [37]:

$$\Pi_{elas} = \frac{RT\nu_e}{V_0}\left(\phi_2^{1/3} - \frac{1}{2}\phi_2\right)$$

$$= -RT\rho_x\left(\phi_2^{1/3} - \frac{1}{2}\phi_2\right) \tag{5}$$

where

ν_e = number of elastically effective polymer chains (those that
are deformed by stress)

V_0 = unswollen gel volume

ρ_x = ν_e/V_0 = effective crosslink density relative to the solid
state

This expression assumes:

1. Isotropic swelling.
2. Tetrafunctional crosslinks of zero volume (four chains are
   connected at a point).
3. Polymer chains are crosslinked in the solid state.
4. There is a Gaussian distribution of chain extensions.

The first two assumptions normally model hydrogels satisfactorily.
The third must be modified if the chains are crosslinked in solution
[28]. The last assumption is violated for highly swollen polymer gels.
A Gaussian chain distribution exists only when the average end-to-
end distance of the polymer chains is much less than the contour
length of the chain. In this case, the chains display Hookean
elasticity, with stress proportional to strain. For highly swollen
gels, a non-Gaussian distribution develops as chains begin to approach their maximum extension. Highly extended chains display non-
Hookean elasticity: stress increases faster than strain. Thus, for
highly swollen gels, a more complex expression must be used to account for the finite extensibility of the polymer chains [30, 37, 43].

For a nonionic gel in equilibrium with a solvent, subject to the
restrictions discussed above:

$$\Pi_{tot} = \Pi_{mix} + \Pi_{elas} \tag{6}$$

or

$$\ln(1 - \phi_2) + \phi_2 + \chi\phi_2^2 + \frac{\tilde{V}_1\nu_e}{V_0}\left(\phi_2^{1/3} - \frac{1}{2}\phi_2\right) = 0 \tag{7}$$

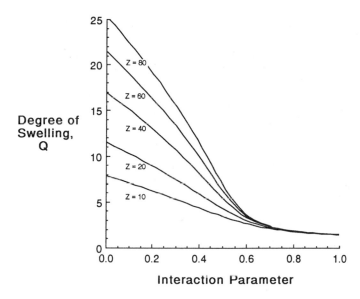

Fig. 1 Theoretical swelling curves for nonionic gels, assuming a Gaussian distribution of chain extensions [Eq. (7)] and $\tilde{V}_m/\tilde{V}_1 = 5$. Z is the number of monomeric units between crosslinks ($Z \approx 1/\rho_x \tilde{V}_m$) [44].

Thus the key parameters that determine the swellling of a nonionic gel in a solvent are the crosslink density and the χ-parameter. Figure 1 demonstrates that the degree of swelling Q (= $1/\phi_2$) for a gel falls as χ increases [44]. Highly crosslinked gels swell less than lightly crosslinked gels, though this difference becomes minimal in poor solvents ($\chi > 0.7$). For highly swollen hydrogels, however, the elasticity expression (Eq. 5) is inadequate. If the exact distribution of chain extensions [45] is used instead of the Gaussian approximation, the predicted swelling degree falls. Figure 2 demonstrates that assumption of a Gaussian network becomes poorer in good solvents ($\chi < 0.5$) [44].

If the gel contains ionizable groups, such as —RCOOH, the additional ion-related terms in Eq. (3) should be included. Polyelectrolyte gels normally swell much more than nonionic gels. The increased swelling arises primarily in the term π_{ions}; π_{elec} is often insignificant. In a qualitative sense, this means that Donnan ion exclusion is the dominant effect, while electrostatic repulsion of like charges on the polymer network can generally be ignored. This is fortuitous, since inclusion of the electrostatic term greatly complicates the problem [22, 26, 36].

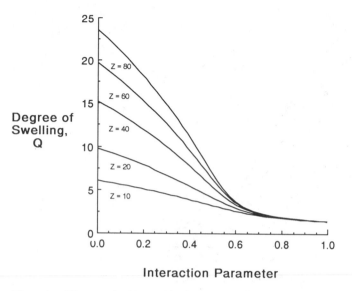

Interaction Parameter

Fig. 2 Theoretical swelling curves for nonionic gels, assuming the exact distribution of chain extensions [43] and $\bar{V}_m / \tilde{V}_1 = 5$. Each monomeric unit is assumed to behave as a link in a freely jointed chain [44].

Assuming that the ions form an ideal solution, the expression for the ionic swelling pressure is simple [37]:

$$\Pi_{ions} = RT(c - c^*) \tag{8}$$

where

    c = molar concentration of mobile ions in the solution inside the gel

    c* = molar concentration of mobile ions in the solution outside the gel

The ions inside the gel arise from two sources: dissociation of ionic groups bound to the network, and ions that diffuse into the gel from the surrounding solution. The concentration inside the gel is typically very much greater than the external solution, so Π_{ions} can be quite large. As a result, water flows into the gel to dilute the ions, causing the gel to swell.

It is useful to express Eq. (8) in terms of the ions in the gel arising from the dissociation of the gel's ionogenic groups (typically 1:1 electrolytes) and any additional ions contributed by the external solution:

$$\Pi_{\text{ions}} = RT \left[\frac{i\phi_2}{\tilde{V}_m} + \nu(c_s - c_s^*) \right] \tag{9}$$

where

i = the fraction of monomeric units on the gel that are ionized
$\tilde{V}_m$ = molar volume of a monomeric unit
ν = the number of ions into which a dissolved salt dissociates
c_s = molar concentration of electrolyte in the gel originating in the external solution
c_s^* = molar concentration of electrolyte in the external solution

The internal ion concentration is greater than the external concentration because electroneutrality must be maintained inside and outside the gel. Thus, while the counterions that arise upon dissociation of ionogenic groups can freely diffuse within the gel, they cannot diffuse out into the solution (unless ion exchange occurs). Were they to do so, the gel and the solution would become highly charged. The resulting distribution of ions between the gel and solution is governed by the theory of Donnan exclusion [24, 45]. Because Π_{ions} is a dominant effect in polyelectrolyte gels, the volume of such gels can change sharply with changes in the pH or ionic strength of the surrounding solution. In fact, these changes have been successfully predicted on the basis of osmotic swelling pressure changes governed by Donnan ion exclusion [36, 46, 47]. Predicting the degree of swelling a priori for a polyelectrolyte gel is more difficult because of the problems with quantifying Π_{net} and Π_{elas}.

Thus, for polyelectrolyte gels, the equation for the equilibrium swelling pressure (neglecting the electrostatic term) becomes:

$$\frac{i\phi_2}{\tilde{V}_m} + \nu(c_s - c_s^*) - \left(\frac{1}{\tilde{V}_1}\right)[\ln(1 - \phi_2) + \phi_2 + \chi\phi_2^2]$$

$$- \frac{\nu_e}{V_0}\left(\phi_2^{1/3} - \frac{1}{2}\phi_2\right) = 0 \tag{10}$$

This equation is sufficiently complex that its implications for gel swelling are not easily discerned. Changing the surrounding electrolyte solution affects c_s and c_s^*, which are related by Donnan equilibria. Figure 3 demonstrates how the degree of ionization i affects swelling in the absence of any added electrolyte [44]. The most unusual parts of this figure are the local maxima and minima that exist for ionized gels in poorer solvents. It can be demonstrated that these

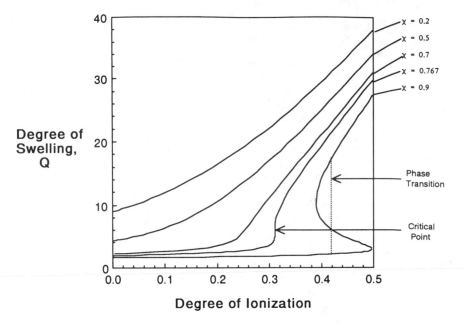

Fig. 3 Theoretical swelling curves for ionic gels, assuming a Gaussian distribution of chain extensions [Eq. (10)], Z = 20, and $\tilde{V}_m/\tilde{V}_1$ = 5. Phase transitions (discrete changes in volume at constant degrees of ionization) are predicted in sovlents with $\chi > 0.767$ [44].

bends are not thermodynamically stable and should be replaced by the straight lines shown (a Maxwell construction) [26, 27]. These states are thermodynamically analogous to vapor-liquid phase transitions. Here, polymer-dense gels (corresponding to the liquid state) expand by absorbing solvent to form a polymer-dilute phase (corresponding to the vapor state) at a distinct degree of ionization (corresponding to the vapor pressure). Gel systems that display only continuous volume changes are analogous to supercritical fluids. Phase transitions in gels were first noted by Tanaka in 1978 [32]; since then, phase transitions have been induced in both natural and synthetic gels by changes in the solvent [15, 32], temperature [31, 39], electric field [33], pH [34], and ionic strength [35]. Because of the potential for inducing drastic but controlled and reversible changes in the volume and/or permeability of gels that display phase transitions, interest has developed in their application to drug delivery [47–51].

Since ionized gels swell much more than typical nonionic hydrogels, the use of a non-Gaussian chain distribution is even more important.

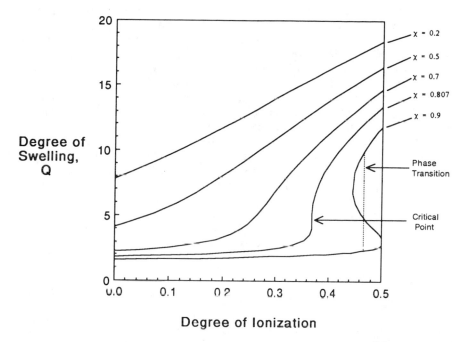

Degree of Ionization

Fig. 4 Theoretical swelling curves for ionic gels, assuming the exact distribution of chain extensions [43], Z = 20, and $\tilde{V}_m/\tilde{V}_1 = 5$. Each monomeric unit is assumed to behave as a link in a freely jointed chain [44].

As shown in Fig. 4, not only are the degrees of swelling reduced, but so are the locations and extents of the phase transitions [44].

Practical Considerations

Control of the degree of swelling of a hydrogel is often of central practical importance. The key adjustable parameters are the polymer-solvent interaction parameter χ, the crosslink density ρ_x ($= \nu_e/V_0$), and the degree of ionization i. Because drug delivery occurs in aqueous systems (though swelling in nonaqueous solvents is sometimes necessary for drug loading or leaching of impurities), χ must be adjusted through the polymer composition. Hydrogels of many diffferent types are available for use; an almost unlimited range of swelling degrees can be obtained by copolymerization of hydrophobic and hydrophilic monomers in appropriate ratios (Section III). The χ parameter is available for many polymer-solvent systems [38, 52]; a reasonable assumption is that χ is the same for a polymer, whether linear or lightly crosslinked. χ-Parameters have not been widely tabulated for hydrogels, however. Part of the reason for this is the relative lack of success of the theory in aqueous systems.

A related qualitative estimate of swelling is available through use of the solubility parameter δ. For a solvent, it is defined as the square root of the cohesive energy density of the solvent, with units of $(cal/cm^3)^{1/2}$ or $(MPa)^{1/2}$. For the polymer, δ is taken to coincide with that of the solvent in which it displays its maximum degree of swelling. Solubility parameters are widely available for polymers and solvents, and can be estimated for mixed solvents and copolymers [38]. The degree of swelling of a polymer in a solvent can be inferred from the match between the respective δ's. As for χ, the effectiveness of δ for aqueous hydrogel systems is often limited, despite efforts to make δ more responsive to specific interactions such as hydrogen bonding [38].

As seen in Figs. 1 and 2, the degree of swelling is also affected by the crosslink density, except in poor solvents. The crosslink density is generally fixed upon synthesis of the gel and can be measured in a number of ways, including tensile, compression, and swelling experiments [30]. The method of crosslinking, the nature of the crosslinking agent (functionality, chemical composition, etc.), and the phsyical structure of the gel (entanglements, inhomogeneities, phase-separation structures, etc.) also influence swelling, but their contributions are more difficult to predict or quantify. Whether the gel was synthesized in bulk or in solution also affects swelling. If the crosslinks were introduced in solution, the degree of dilution and the nature of the solvent also influence the swelling.

For polyelectrolyte gels, the degree of ionization is typically the key swelling parameter. This can be fixed through copolymerization of ionic and nonionic monomers or by chemical modification of a gel (e.g., hydrolysis of the amide groups of polyacrylamide gel, converting them to carboxylic acid groups). The number of ionic groups actually dissociated is typically a function of pH and ionic strength, except for strongly acidic or basic groups. Since changes in ionization lead to changes in swelling, as discussed earlier, polyelectrolyte gels can be undesirable for drug delivery applications. In some cases, however, control of swelling through pH is actively desired [46–51].

Solutes can have a variety of unpredictable effects on the swelling of both ionic and nonionic gels. For example, poly(ethylene glycol) (PEG) reduces the swelling of polyacrylamide gel, possibly by disrupting hydrogen bonding [53, 54]. Other solutes can also disrupt predicted swelling by enhancing or disrupting specific interactions between the solvent and the polymer.

Experimental swelling data are usually obtained by allowing a hydrogel to equilibrate with a solution, removing it and quickly blotting it dry, followed by weighing on a fast-response balance. For samples of well-defined geometry, microscopic measurement of dimensions can also be effective [55, 56]. The data are typically reported as either the volume degree of swelling Q, the mass degree of swelling q, or the equilibrium water content EWC, defined as follows:

Q = volume of swollen gel/volume of dry polymer
q = mass of swollen gel/mass of dry polymer
EWC = mass of water absorbed by gel/mass of swollen gel × 100%

It is possible for Q or q to range from 1.2 to over 1000; this translates to an EWC range of 20% to over 99%. The most commonly used hydrogel for drug delivery, poly(hydroxyethylmethacrylate) (PHEMA), has an EWC of about 40% or a q of about 1.7.

B. Permeability

Concepts

While equilibrium swelling may be the single most important characteristic of hydrogels, it is permeability that makes them useful for drug delivery. Hydrogels can be made impermeable, semipermeable, or fully permeable to virtually any class of solute. Their permeability can be made to change with time and to respond to external stimuli. Thus their diverse permeability characteristics make them applicable to a wide variety of drug delivery problems.

Hydrogels have been classified in three basic categories in terms of solute diffusion [57]:

1. Macroporous hydrogels—These hydrogels have pores in the range of 0.05 μm to 1.0 μm (50 nm to 1000 nm). Convective mass transfer of solutes may dominate diffusion in these gels.
2. Microporous hydrogels—The pore sizes of these hydrogels range from 40 Å to 500 Å (5 nm to 50 nm). Diffusion of solutes occurs in water-filled pores whose structure influences the mass transfer.
3. Nonporous hydrogels—The "pores" of these gels exist only on a molecular level. Solute diffusion must occur in the spaces between the network chains (the mesh). Convection is negligible in these gels.

The distinction between these types of gels is not sharp. Also, the pores are rarely well defined, especially for the nonporous gels. The physical dimensions of the interstitial spaces in the network may vary with time due to the thermal motion of the polymer chains. Nevertheless, a statistically averaged "pore" may be determined. In general, it can be assumed that the average pore size increases with degree of swelling. However, the details of the underlying network structure must be also considered [54].

Two basic mechanisms, the "pore" and "partition" mechanisms, have generally been assumed to explain solute diffusion through hydrogels. In the pore mechanism, the solute moves only through the water-filled regions of the gel. In the partition mechanism, solute transport is assumed to involve thermodynamic dissolution into the polymer phase. In most cases, the pore mechanism is sufficient to interpret the data.

Numerous models have been proposed to interpret diffusion through polymer networks. One prominent semiempirical equation that can be used to estimate a solute's diffusion coefficient within the gel is [58]:

$$D_g = D_0 \exp\left[-\frac{(5 + 10^{-4}M)}{q} \right] \tag{11}$$

where

D_g = diffusion coefficient of the solute in the hydrogel
D_0 = diffusion coefficient of the solute in the solvent
q = mass degree of swelling
M = solute molecular weight

Perhaps the most successful and widely used model has been that of Yasuda et al. [59, 60]. Theirs is a free-volume theory which assumes that the solute moves only within water-filled regions within the gel. The diffusion coefficient is proportional to $[\exp(-V_s/V_f)]$, where V_s is the characteristic volume of the solute and V_f is the free volume inside the gel. The free volume V_f is assumed to be linearly related to the weight fraction of water inside the gel. Combining these relations leads to:

$$\log(D_g) = \log(D_0) - \frac{k}{q - 1} \tag{12}$$

where k = constant related to the characteristic solute volume and the free volume of water, and q, D_g, D_0 are as defined above.

An example of this theory's success is illustrated in Fig. 5 [61]. In both models, the only parameter specifically related to the polymer itself is the degree of swelling. The absence of other parameters results from the assumption that transport occurs primarily in water-filled channels of the gel, as opposed to cooperative diffusion through the polymer mesh. These simple theories are not always successful, however; gels with the same degree of swelling can display quite different diffusive characteristics [62]. The most complete theories consider details of the network structure (such as average polymer mesh size, molecular weight between crosslinks, or degree of cross-

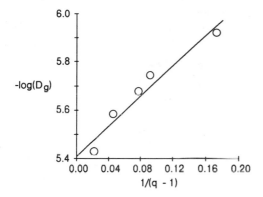

Fig. 5 The theory of Yasuda et al. [59, 60] successfully correlates data for the diffusion of vitamin B-12 in different swollen poly(acrylamide-co-sodium methacrylate) gels [54, 61].

linking), organization of water within the gel (whether bound or bulk), and dimensions of the solute, in addition to the degree of swelling [62–67]. The main disadvantage of the more sophisticated models is that they require additional data, which are not always available.

Measurement of Solute Diffusion Coefficeints

Solute diffusion coefficients in swollen hydrogels can be measured fairly easily by either the membrane permeation method or the sorption/desorption method. While the membrane permeation time-lag experiment has been widely used, it is not always the most practical method. This method requires that boundary-layer resistances be eliminated, that the hydrogel be cast as a strong membrane, and that steady state be established within a reasonable time period. The first problem can be minimized with careful experimental design. The second can be difficult or impossible to achieve, especially if the hydrogel is highly swollen; such gels typically have poor mechanical strength. The last can be a problem for drugs with high molecular weights and small diffusion coefficients, especially if the membrane must be thick to overcome limited mechanical strength.

A simpler way to obtain drug diffusion coefficients in hydrogels is to measure the rate of desorption of a drug dissolved in a hydrogel sheet of thickness L into an infinite reservoir. The drug diffusion coefficient D can be extracted from the slope of a plot of the fractional amount of drug desorbed M_t/M_∞ versus $t^{1/2}$ using the following equation [68]:

$$\frac{M_t}{M_\infty} = \left(\frac{4}{L}\right) \left(\frac{Dt}{\pi}\right)^{1/2}$$ (13)

This equation is accurate to within 1% for $M_t/M_\infty < 0.6$.

If the drug is dispersed, not dissolved, in the hydrogel sheet, the slope of a plot of M_t versus $t^{1/2}$ also yields D, though the equation is more complex [69]:

$$M_t = C_s(1 + H) \left(\frac{Dt}{3H}\right)^{1/2}$$ (14)

where

$H = C_s^{-1}[5A + (A^2 - C_s^2)^{1/2}] - 4$
C_s = drug solubility in the hydrogel matrix
A = initial drug loading per unit volume

This equation is valid to within 1% of the exact solution over the first 60% of release for values of A/C_s down to 1.04 (a situation that occurs for drugs with high water solubility).

Another effective method of determining drug diffusion coefficients in hydrogels is to measure the change of concentration in a constant, finite bath as the drug is absorbed or desorbed by a hydrogel sample. In this simple experiment, a hydrogel sample is immersed in a well-stirred solution whose volume is of the same order as the sample's. The concentration change with time can yield both D and the drug partition coefficient K. The method can be adapted to any gel sample, regardless of mechanical strength, and most geometries, including slabs, disks, cylinders, and spheres.

Although the solution to this problem has been known for many years [68], the mathematics made extraction of the diffusion coefficient from data tedious. Recently, Lee provided simple, accurate approximate solutions for spheres, cylinders, and slabs that are much more convenient to use [70]. For absorption of drug by a flat sheet, the equation is

$$F(C_t) = \left[\frac{C_0^2 - C_t^2}{2C_t^2} + \ln\left(\frac{C_t}{C_0}\right)\right]\left(\frac{3\lambda^2}{16}\right)$$ (15a)

$$F(C_t) = Dt/L^2$$ (15b)

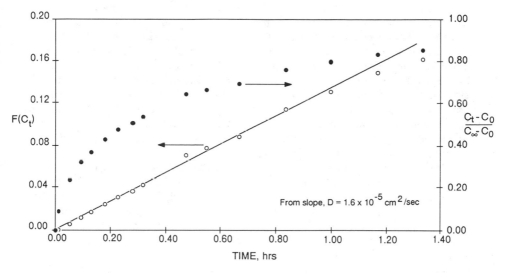

Fig. 6 The diffusion coefficient of D_2O in swollen poly(acrylamide-co-sodium methacrylate) gel is determined from a finite-volume sorption experiment using Eq. (15) [54, 61].

where

C_t = concentration of drug in the external solution at time t
C_0 = initial concentration of drug
λ = the effective volume ratio = $C_\infty / (C_0 - C_\infty)$
L = sheet thickness

The concentration change data are used to determine the values of $F(C_t)$ via Eq. (15a); the diffusion coefficient is then found from the slope of a plot of $F(C_t)$ versus t, as given by Eq. (15b). An example of the use of this equation is given in Fig. 6 [54]. Equation (15) is accurate for values of $\lambda < 10$. Larger values of λ correspond to nearly constant solution concentrations, the limit satisfied by Eq. (13). This procedure is easily adapted for desorption from gels, in addition to sorption.

C. Kinetics of Swelling

Concepts

The third key property of hydrogels is their controllable swelling kinetics. Because the solute permeability is directly related to the swelling degree, control of the swelling means control of the solute permeability, and therefore of drug release. Both glassy and rubbery

gels have characteristic swelling kinetics which can be exploited
for drug delivery devices. In glassy gels, a solvent front normally
develops that moves into the gel at a characteristic rate, causing
swelling behind the front. Drug can be immobilized in a glassy hydrogel; when placed in an aqueous environment, the drug will be
liberated from the rubbery, swollen (and therefore permeable) portion of the gel that exists behind the front—thus the release rate is
controlled by the swelling kinetics of the gel. Rubbery gels made
to swell or contract in response to environmental changes (e.g., temperature or pH) also show permeability changes that can be used to
release drugs in a prescribed fashion [71].

The swelling kinetics of glassy and rubbery gels are quite different, primarily due to the fact that rubbers have nearly instantaneous responses to applied stresses, while glasses generally exhibit
time-dependent responses. This difference in response time, or
relaxation, is a source of deviation from Fick's law of diffusion. In
this context, "relaxation" is a deliberately vague term, but is understood to be a measure of a polymer's mean or characteristic time of
response to stress [72, 73]. The relative rates of Fickian diffusion
and polymer relaxation determine the sorption behavior observed.

The relative importance of relaxation and diffusion can, in principle, be estimated with the Deborah number, De [72, 74—76]. De is
defined as the ratio of a characteristic relaxation time, λ, to a characteristic diffusion time, θ ($\theta = L^2/D$, where L = characteristic
length):

$$De = \frac{\lambda}{\theta} \tag{16}$$

Thus, when De << 1, relaxation is much faster than diffusion, and
Fickian diffusion is observed. This occurs well above T_g (the glass
transition temperature), where gels are rubbery, and the diffusion
coefficient D is generally a strong function of concentration. Fickian
diffusion with a constant diffusion coefficient is usually observed for
De >> 1. This corresponds to diffusion in a glassy polymer well
below T_g, where polymer relaxation is so slow that its structure is
unchanged by the diffusion process (thus the gel does not swell in
this region). When De $\approx$ 1, relaxation and diffusion interact, leading
to complex transport behavior that cannot be modeled by Fick's law
of diffusion with constant boundary conditions. Hence, such transport is termed "non-Fickian." When swelling causes De to change
from one range to another over the course of an experiment, non-
Fickian behavior is usually observed. Thus non-Fickian transport
is common in glassy hydrogels that become rubbery upon swelling.

Three basic categories of solvent sorption by polymer gels are
usually distinguished:

1. *Case I transport or Fickian diffusion.* Here molecular relaxation is either much faster than diffusion (well above T_g, De << 1) or so slow that it is not observed on the time scale of the experiment (well below T_g, De >> 1). It can be characterized by a single parameter, the diffusion coefficient D.
2. *Anomalous transport.* Here diffusion and relaxation occur at comparable rates (De $\sim$ 1) and thus interact in complex fashions. This category includes all forms of non-Fickian transport exclusive of case II.
3. *Case II transport.* This special case of non-Fickian transport is distinguished by the development of a solvent front that moves at a relaxation-controlled, constant velocity "v." Here relaxation occurs at an observable rate in the glassy part of the swelling gel, but this rate is much slower than diffusion in the rubbery part.

Fickian transport is reasonably easy to analyze, due to the relatively simple mathematics involved and the existence of a large body of solved Fickian-type equations [e.g., 68, 77]. For a sorption experiment, a plot can be made of the fractional approach to equilibrium, $M(t)/M(\infty)$, against $\sqrt{t}/L$, where

M(t) = mass of penetrant sorbed at time t
$M(\infty)$ = mass of penetrant sorbed at equilibrium
L = characteristic sample dimension.

If the sorption is Fickian, the plot will display the following characteristics [68, 78]:

1. The curve should be linear in its initial portion: generally up to 60% of equilibrium, depending on the geometry (higher for a slab, lower for a sphere or cylinder) and the concentration dependence of D (higher if D increases with C, lower if D decreases with C).
2. Above the linear portion, the curve is concave to the time axis, regardless of the concentration dependence of D.
3. The curves for different thicknesses superimpose for otherwise identical experiments.

Failure of any of these criteria classifies the sorption process as either anomalous or case II. An example of this type of Fickian diffusion plot is given in Fig. 7. In this case, ionized hydrogel cylinders are shrinking in response to a pH change that causes them to become nonionic [54, 61].

That criterion (1) should arise from Fick's law with constant boundary conditions [see Eq. (17)] can be anticipated from the use of the Boltzmann similarity transform ($\zeta = x/\sqrt{4Dt}$), where x is the

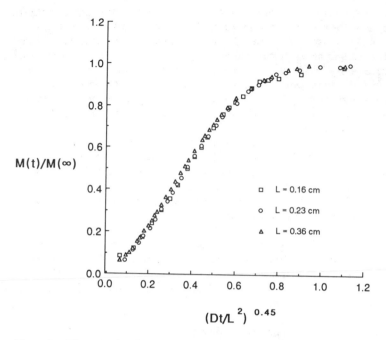

$M(t)/M(\infty)$

□   L = 0.16 cm

o   L = 0.23 cm

△   L = 0.36 cm

$$(Dt/L^2)^{\ 0.45}$$

Fig. 7 The shrinking rate in water of ionized poly(acrylamide-co-sodium methacrylate) gel cylinders of differing radii L in response to a reduction in pH meets the criteria for Fickian diffusion [54, 61]. The use of an of exponent 0.45 instead of 0.5 extends the linear portion of the curve for cylindrical geometries [105]. D = 7.4 × 10⁻⁷ cm²/sec.

spatial variable) to solve the semi-infinite slab problem [58, 79]. Any geometry will tend to appear as an infinite slab at short times, and the characteristic distance will scale with the square root of the characteristic time. The $\sqrt{t}$ dependence tends to be preserved by many geometries and boundary conditions (including sorption of a solute from a solution of limited volume), though this is not universal [58, 77]. Criterion 2 is based on widespread observation, though it has not been rigorously proven. Criterion 3 can be demonstrated by dimensional analysis of Fick's law, which creates the dimensionless time variable $\tau = Dt/L^2$ [80]. Thus, for every Fickian problem, time will always scale with the square of the characteristic linear dimension. This must hold over the entire range, not just for the initial portion as in criterion (1). Thus criterion (3) is the most stringent, but is not always applied, as it requires multiple experiments with samples of different dimensions. If criteria 1 and 2 hold, but not criterion 3, the transport is termed "pseudo-Fickian" [58, 78, 81].

Case II transport is a special case readily identified and characterized by the constant velocity of the moving solvent front and the resulting linear weight gain with time. However, its characteristics are not as well understood, nor are they as fundamental in origin as those of Fickian diffusion. Nonetheless, case II transport can serve as a useful limiting case of solvent transport. Its primary attributes are as follows [82]:

1. A sharp, advancing front exists between an inner glassy core and an outer rubbery shell.
2. This penetrant front moves at a constant velocity.
3. The rubbery gel behind the front is at an equilibrium degree of swelling. (Because the unswollen, glassy core restricts the swelling of the gel, this may be a stressed equilibrium, not the final, unstressed equilibrium.)
4. The weight gain is proportional to time for most of the process.

The most dramatic characteristic of case II transport is given by the moving penetrant front. However, since a strongly concentration-dependent diffusion coefficient can also lead to the development of a distinct front, criterion 2 is also required (the position of a diffusion-controlled front advances with $\sqrt{t}$, so its velocity continually decreases). Criteria 1–3 taken together lead to the development of criterion 4—the linear weight gain with time. If criterion 3 does not hold, there may be two moving fronts: a polymer/penetrant front and an equilibrium gel/nonequilibrium gel front. The linear weight gain is unlikely to occur if criterion 3 does not hold. The observation of the moving front and the measurement of a linear weight gain are often considered sufficient evidence of case II transport, though it is the constant velocity of the front that is crucial. It is also true that at very short times, the weight increases with $\sqrt{t}$, due to Fickian diffusion into the gel prior to establishment of the front [83–85].

In various proposed drug delivery devices, a constant velocity front and/or a constant sorption rate can lead to a constant rate of drug delivery. Thus there is much interest in developing a hydrogel that displays case II transport [14, 74–76]. While glassy hydrogels commonly display anomalous solvent transport, true case II water transport has yet to be reported.

Theoretical Modeling

Fick's law with constant boundary conditions can successfully describe much of the observed molecular transport in polymers. It is frequently a successful model for transport both above T_g (rubbery polymers) and well below T_g (for glassy polymers with invariant, defect-free structures). It also describes desorption in most cases, regardless

of the sorption mechanism [78]. In one dimension, the unsteady
state form of Fick's law at constant pressure and temperature is
simply:

$$\frac{\partial c}{\partial t} = \frac{\partial}{\partial x}\left[D(c)\ \frac{\partial c}{\partial x}\right]$$

(17)

The usual conditions are

$c = c_1$ at $x = 0$ and $t \geqslant 0$

$c = c_2$ at $x = L$ and $t \geqslant 0$

$c = f(x)$ for $0 < x < L$ and $t = 0$

$0 < D(c) < +\infty$

The choice of the frame of reference determines the solvent concentration unit and length unit to be used, and will determine the significance of the binary diffusion coefficient $D(c)$. When the polymer
swells, it is frequently convenient to choose a frame of reference
that expands with the polymer [68, 86, 87]. This leaves the mathematics unchanged, but alters the meaning of the diffusion coefficient.
Solutions to Eq. (17) and the analogous heat conduction problems
abound in numerous geometries with time-independent boundary conditions and diffusion coefficients [68, 77].

Scientists have found modeling non-Fickian transport an intriguing
challenge and have put a great deal of effort toward this end over
the past 40 years. Consequently, a plethora of models exist. Most
of these models are complex mathematically and are difficult to apply
to experiments. The purpose here is to provide an introduction to
the types of models proposed, focusing on those developed in the
past 10 years. Reviews include those by Peppas and Korsmeyer [76],
Frisch [80], and Rogers [81].

The various models usually modify either the boundary conditions
and diffusion coefficient defined above or the transport equation itself. Sometimes all of these are altered. These approaches have
been categorized as molecular relaxation models, "diffusion and convection" (or case I plus case II) models, and differential swelling
stress models [88, 89]. These distinctions are arbitrary, however,
as the models form a continuum more than they delineate separate
schools of thought.

All models introduce some sort of relaxation, but those termed
"molecular relaxation" models do so by introducing time dependence
to some part of Fickian problem statement, without altering the different equation itself. One approach is to use a time-dependent
diffusion coefficient [90, 91] or a time-dependent solubility coefficient

[92]. Another approach is to make the boundary condition time-dependent [93—95], so that the surface concentration slowly approaches (relaxes to) an equilibrium value. This approach is the only one that describes two-stage sorption—a phenomenon where a quasi-equilibrium develops for an intermediate period before reaccelerating toward a final, stable equilibrium value.

Perhaps the simplest models to grasp and utilize are the "diffusion plus convection" or "case I plus case II" models. These types are purely phenomenological. One type adds a pseudo-convective term ("-vc"), arising from the partial stress of the invading penetrant, to the basic Fickian equation (17) and assumes a certain propagating front velocity [83, 96—98]. A completely empirical model in this category [84, 85] simply combines a diffusion equation and a linear relaxation equation. While these models are easily grasped and applied, and can be successful, they suffer from their lack of a firm physical foundation. They are also inherently unable to deal with super-case II transport, which displays greater than linear time dependence.

The most successful models are the differential swelling stress models; the best can explain the broadest range of behaviors with the least empiricism, from Fickian to super-case II, as well as predict the front velocity. One approach is to use a stress-modified diffusion coefficient [82, 88, 90]. Another is to use the basic Fickian equations with a differential stress acting at the moving front; the key problem is prediction of the moving front velocity [99—101]. Thomas and Windle have proposed a comprehensive theory that requires two parameters, the penetrant diffusivity and the glassy polymer's flow viscosity [102]. They calculate an osmotic swelling stress at the front; the rate-controlling step becomes the mechanical resistance of the glass to deformation induced by this swelling.

Treatment of Experimental Swelling Data

Experimentally, the different modes of transport are generally distinguished by fitting sorption data over the first half (approximately) of the approach to equilibrium to the following empirical equation [68, 76, 80, 84, 85, 89, 90, 103, 104]:

$$\frac{M(t)}{M(\infty)} = Kt^n \qquad (18)$$

where

$M(t)$ = mass of penetrant sorbed at time t
$M(\infty)$ = mass of penetrant sorbed at equilibrium
K, n = curve-fitting constants

For Fickian diffusion, $n = \frac{1}{2}$; for anomalous transport, $\frac{1}{2} < n < 1$; and for case II transport, $n = 1$. When $n > 1$, the phenomenon is considered "super-case II." The existence of "super-case II" transport indicates both that case II transport is not a fundamental limiting case in the same sense as Fickian diffusion, and that the simple picture of diffusion-relaxation competition is inadequate.

It should be further noted that Eq. (18) does not account for the additional required dimensional dependence. A more rigorous test for the transport mechanism would be to write:

$$\frac{M(t)}{M(\infty)} = \frac{K't^n}{L} \tag{19}$$

where L is the characteristic sample dimension.

For different sample thicknesses, K' and n should be invariant for case I and case II transport. If they change, anomalous transport is indicated, even if $n = 1$ or $\frac{1}{2}$. This empirical equation holds strictly only for slabs, though it will tend to hold at shorter times for other geometries. It can be adjusted to apply to spheres, cylinders, and disks over longer time periods, as demonstrated in Fig. 7 [105].

The swelling of rubbery gels can normally be described with Fick's laws, although the diffusion coefficient is usually a strong function of concentration [68, 78, 80, 81, 104]. Normally, swelling is accounted for by using a frame of reference for diffusion fixed with the polymer instead of the laboratory. If the surface concentration slowly relaxes to an equilibrium value, two-stage sorption may be observed instead of monotonic Fickian sorption [68]. However, the surface concentration typically reaches equilibrium on a time scale much faster than diffusion for gels immersed in a solvent. Figure 8 is for a temperature-sensitive gel sheet swelling in response to a temperature change. Because the diffusion plot is initially linear, Fickian transport is indicated and a diffusion coefficient relative to the polymer-fixed frame of reference can be extracted form the data [54, 61]. However, the thickness effect should also be tested to verify Fickian kinetics. The swelling and shrinking kinetics of swollen, rubbery gels have not been extensively studied [107–110]. It is not yet clear what factors affect the rates most significantly. It has been shown that the rate of imposition of the driving force that induces the volume change can sometimes control the swelling/ shrinking rate [61].

Swelling kinetics have been studied more extensively for glassy hydrogels than for rubbery gels. However, the non-Fickian phenomena typically observed for glassy gels make the problem much more complex. There is much current activity in the area, driven primarily by drug delivery applications [14, 76]. Typically, a sharp

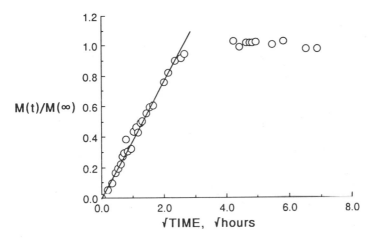

Fig. 8 The swelling rate in water of a rubbery sheet of poly(N-isopropylacrylamide) gel upon cooling from 27°C to 20°C is linear on a diffusion plot, a key criterion for Fickian transport [106].

moving front separating glassy from rubbery gel develops soon after immersion of the dry gel in water. In aqueous systems, this front has not been observed to lead to case II transport. We speculate that water molecules are small enough to penetrate the glassy gel with relative ease, thus plasticizing it and reducing the polymer relaxation time. As a result, various forms of anomalous transport result, instead of true case II sorption. Nonetheless, this sharp boundary between swollen and unswollen gel has an important impact on the swelling phenomena. Except for spheres, this sharp boundary requires anisotropic swelling of the sample, as the glassy core can resist swelling stresses. As a result, transport occurs only normal to the plane of the front. Once the core is gone, this constraint is removed. The result is that the polymer sample's dimensions change suddenly and drastically at nearly constant volume—that is, for a slab, the area increases suddenly at the expense of the thickness; and for a cylinder, the length suddenly increases at the expense of the diameter [74, 75]. An inflection point may develop in the plot of M_t/M_∞ versus $t^{1/2}/L$, as a result of the decreased diffusional path and the increased surface area, as shown in Fig. 9 [111]. The dimensional changes can be minimized if the gel is made with fixed, anisotropic internal stresses that resist changes in surface area, so that swelling occurs in only one dimension. The swelling curve for such a gel is shown in Fig. 10 [111].

The swelling kinetics may also be altered when drug is incorpora ted into the sample. Presence of the drug in the sample increases the

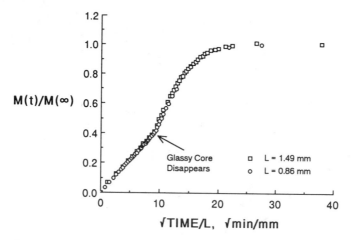

Fig. 9 The swelling rate in water of a glassy sheet of poly(2-hydroxyethylmethacrylate-co-sodium sulfopropylmethacrylate) gel meets the criteria for Fickian transport. An inflection point develops when the stress-resistant glassy core disappears, allowing the area to increase at the expense of thickness (a transition from one-dimensional to three-dimensional swelling) [111].

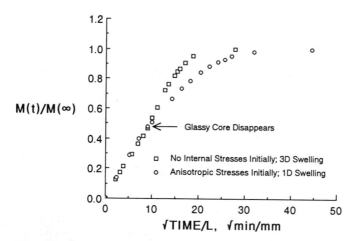

Fig. 10 A glassy hydrogel can be made with anisotropic internal stresses that force one-dimensional swelling (no increase in area). As a result, no inflection point is seen in the diffusion plot [111].

osmotic driving force for water transport. As a result, the gels go through swelling maxima that are functions of the incorporated drug properties and concentration [14, 112].

D. Biocompatibility

Biocompatibility is a requirement for any device or material placed in initmate contact with living tissue or biological fluids. Yet the term "biocompatibility" is not precisely defined but is used to describe a variety of biological responses. However, an ideally biocompatible material could be expected to avoid causing any of the following responses [113, 114]:

Thrombosis
Alteration or destruction of plasma proteins and enzymes
Depletion of electrolytes
Adverse immune responses
Damage to tissue
Toxic or allergic responses
Cancer

Hydrogels mimic living tissue more closely than any other nonnatural material. Their immediate resemblance to tissue is in their soft, flexible nature and high water content. This helps minimize mechanical irritation and damage to body tissues. While high water content in and of itself seems related to biocompatibility, it does not guarantee it. For example, some gelatin and polysaccharide gels cause inflammation despite water contents over 90% [9]. The connection between high water content and biocompatibility is indirect.

Of primary importance is the high permeability of hydrogels to low-molecular-weight solutes. This allows the leaching of initiators, monomers, and other impurities from the gels prior to use as or in drug delivery devices. Leaching of low-molecular-weight substances from biomaterials is known to be a leading cause of incompatibility. Less well understood, but possibly of equal importance, is the low interfacial tension typically displayed between water and a hydrogel surface. This tends to minimize interactions (e.g., adsorption) with the proteins in body fluids. However, the factors that affect this interfacial tension are compelx. Under certain conditions, hydrogels even appear to be hydrophobic [115]. This behavior is apparently due to the fact that the polymer chains have sufficient mobility to orient themselves with either hydrophilic or hydrophobic groups exposed, depending on the environment of the gel. Whether or not the surface of the hydrogel is hydrated with bulk or bound water also seems to affect the biocompatibility. Surface charge is also important; it is generally assumed that a negative surface charge enhances biocompatibility [116]. However, experimental results are ambiguous on this point [113, 117].

For oral dosage forms, it is usually sufficient to demonstrate that no significant amounts of impurities can leach from the gel. Thus any hydrogel that has been cleaned of extractable materials can usually be assumed biocompatible for this purpose. Implants and occular inserts would require more extensive testing to demonstrate biocompatibility.

E. Mechanical Strength

Though the definition is imprecise, the term "mechanical strength" has distinct implications—namely, that a material is capable of resisting structural failure in its designated application. Strength can be indicated by any combination of measurable properties, which may include [118]:

> Tensile strength
> Compressive strength
> Flexural strength
> Shear strength
> Toughness
> Rigidity
> Hardness
> Dimensional stability

Which of these properties are important for hydrogels depends on the specific application for the gel. Most dry hydrogels are hard, brittle materials, similar to poly(methyl methacrylate) (Plexiglas). In this glassy state, hydrogels can be tested by all the standard techniques designed for polymeric materials [118, 119]. For drug delivery applications, strength of glassy hydrogels is rarely a concern. Swollen, rubbery hydrogels are much less strong, and can be prone to breakage under mechanical or osmotic stress. Whether mechanical strength is a concern depends very much on the specific application. Chapters 8–10 in Rodriguez provide an excellent introduction to this area [118]. Questions of strength specifically related to hydrogels have also been discussed [30, 120–124].

Mechanical tests can also be used to determine the effective crosslink density ρ_x [30, 125]. This value of ρ_x is often lower than that obtained from swelling experiments (see Section II.A.1), because the effects of phsycial entangelements and interactions are minimized in the mechanical experiments. However, if χ is unknown or uncertain, mechanical measurements can provide a more meaningful measure of ρ_x (or ν_e).

There are a number of techniques that can be used to improve the strength of a swollen, rubbery hydrogel. One is to increase the degree of crosslinking, though this may strongly affect other properties. Different crosslinking agents can also improve the strength;

improved mechanical properties have been reported using polymeric crosslinkers [126]. Enhancement of physical interactions including ionic, polar, steric interchain forces, hydrogen bonding, and physical entanglements can also lead to enhanced performance. Unfortunately, these interactions are subject to ready disruption by changes in temperature, pH, ionic strength. The use of interpenetrating networks (IPNs) can also improve strength. IPNs are essentially networks within networks, and can be formed in a number of ways [127, 128]. For example, the hydrogel can be swollen in a monomer solution, which is then polymerized. Or two noninterfering polymerizations (e.g., step condensation and free-radical polymerization) can be initiated at the same time, leading to two distinct but intertwined gel networks.

Another common method is to bond the hydrogel to a much stronger underlying support. A film of high-strength polymer can be activated by the generation of free radicals on the polymer surface. An activated surface can be prepared in a number of ways, including bombardment by ionizing or ultraviolet radiation, or chemical treatment by peroxides or ceric IV ions [113]. Reactive polyester films are also commercially available (e.g., GelBond film from FMC, Inc.). The reactive solution is contacted with the sheet and polymerization is initiated. The gel forms with covalent bonds to the substrate. The composite will have the strength of the underlying polymer film but most of the desirable properties of the hydrogel.

III. PREPARATION OF HYDROGELS

Hydrogels comprise a surprisingly diverse group of materials. In certain respects, it is this diversity that makes them so valuable for drug delivery devices; their properties can be fine-tuned with ease by small modifications in their formulations. A hydrogel can be synthesized from any hydrophilic polymer that can be crosslinked to form an elastic three-dimensional network. Hydrophilicity is usually incorporated through side chains containing hydroxyl, amide, amine, ether, carboxylate, sulfonate, or similar groups. The crosslinks can be created by simultaneous polymerization of hydrophilic monomers and multifunctional crosslinking monomers, by causing chemical reactions between side chains of linear polymers, by bombardment of linear polymers with ionizing radiation, or through physical interactions such as entanglements or crystallites. Hydrogels can also be formed by chemical conversion of a preexisting gel (not necessarily hydrophilic). The gels can be made of natural polymers, synthetic polymers, or any combination of natural and synthetic materials to form semisynthetic gels. Hydrogels can be formed by most polymerization techniques, but bulk, solution, and suspension polymeriza-

tion are most common. This diversity can be a source of confusion
to the novice, intrigue to the research-oriented, and flexibility to
the development-minded. In this section, the range of hydrogel
types that are available will be discussed and the methods of synthesis explored.

A. Types of Hydrogels

Synthetic Hydrogels

Although hydrogels can be of either natural or synthetic origin,
covalently crosslinked synthetic hydrogels have gained the most
popularity for a variety of biomedical applications, spurred by the
development of soft contact lenses [8, 14, 123]. The most common
hydrogels are produced by the free-radical copolymerization of vinyl
monomers with a crosslinking agent. Equilibrium swelling has the
dominant influence on hydrogel properties; the key parameters that
affect swelling are the polymer-solvent interaction parameter χ, the
crosslinking density ρ_x, and degree of ionization i. Other influences
include the nature of the crosslinks, structural inhomogeneities
caused by phase separation, synthesis conditions, noncovalent interactions (hydrogen bonding, hydrophobic interactions, etc.), and so
forth. All of these properties can be adjusted by appropriate choice
of monomers and crosslinkers in an essentially endless variety of
combinations.

Tables 1 through 4 list a variety of monomers that have been used
to produce hydrogels. There are three categories of monofunctional
monomers—neutral hydrophilic (Table 1), neutral hydrophobic (Table
2), and ionic, including both anionic (acidic) and cationic (basic)
monomers (Table 3)—plus the polyfunctional crosslinking monomers
(Table 4). (Note: The neutral hydrophilic monomers produce water-
swellable or soluble homopolymers, while the neutral hydrophobic
monomers produce water-insoluble homopolymers.) Hydrogel properties can be adjusted through an appropriate mix of hydrophobic and
hydrophilic monomers (equivalent to adjusting χ), ionic monomers,
and crosslinks (type and concentration). To a lesser extent, reaction
conditions (temperature, solvent, etc.) also affect the properties. In
practice, differences between monomers in terms of solubility, reaction rate, and so forth will limit the combinations that can be achieved.
However, the number of combinations that may be obtained is truly
remarkable, and the tables provided here are by no means a complete
list of monomers and crosslinkers. The reviews by Kudela [13] and
by Ratner and Hoffman [113] provide further discussions of synthetic
hydrogels. Volume II of the series *Hydrogels in Medicine and Pharmacy* has chapters devoted to three of the most important synthetic
hydrogels: poly(vinyl alcohol), poly(2-hydroxyethylmethacrylate),
and poly(ethylene oxide) [11].

Table 1 Neutral Hydrophilic Monomers for Hydrogel Synthesis

Hydroxyalkylacrylates[a]	$CH_2=CH-C{\Large{\begin{smallmatrix}\\O\\OR\end{smallmatrix}}}$
Hydroxyalkylmethacrylates[a]	$CH_2=C(CH_3)-C{\Large{\begin{smallmatrix}\\O\\OR\end{smallmatrix}}}$
N-substituted acrylamides[b]	$CH_2=CH-C{\Large{\begin{smallmatrix}\\O\\N-R_1\\R_2\end{smallmatrix}}}$
N-substituted methacrylamides[b]	$CH_2=C(CH_3)-C{\Large{\begin{smallmatrix}\\O\\N-R_1\\R_2\end{smallmatrix}}}$
N-vinyl-2-pyrrolidone	$CH_2=CH-N{\Large<}$ (pyrrolidone ring)
2,4-pentadiene-1-ol	$CH_2=CH\text{-}CH=CH\text{-}CH_2OH$

---

[a] R groups include : $-CH_2CH_2OH$, $-CH_2\underset{OH}{CHCH_3}$, $-\underset{CH_3}{CHCH_2OH}$, $-CH_2\underset{OH}{CH}-\underset{OH}{CH_2}$,

$-CH_2\underset{O}{CH}-CH_2$, $-CH_2CH_2OCH_2OH$, $-CH_2CH_2OCH_3$, $-CH_2CH_2OCH_2CH_2OCH_3$

[b] R_1, R_2 groups include : $-H$, $-CH_3$, $-CH_2CH_3$, $-CH_2\underset{OH}{CHCH_3}$, $-\underset{CH_3}{CHCH_3}$

Table 2 Neutral Hydrophobic Monomers for Hydrogel Synthesis

Acrylics[a]	$CH_2{=}CH{-}C{\overset{O}{\underset{OR}{\diagup}}}$
Methacrylics[a]	$CH_2{=}\underset{CH_3}{C}{-}C{\overset{O}{\underset{OR}{\diagup}}}$
Vinyl acetate	$CH_3{-}C{\overset{O}{\underset{CH{=}CH_2}{\diagup}}}$
Acrylonitrile	$CH_2{=}\underset{CN}{CH}$
Styrene	$CH_2{=}CH$

[a] R groups include : $-CH_3$, $-CH_2CH_3$, $-CH_2CH_2CH_3$, $-CH_2CH_2CH_2CH_3$, $-(CH_2)_5CH_3$

The esters of acrylic and methacrylic acids provide the greatest diversity, as shown in Tables 1 and 2. The ester group determines the degree of hydrophilicity or hydrophobicity of the monomer. 2-Hydroxyethylmethacrylate (HEMA) is the most widely used and studied monomer for biomedical applications. N-substituted acrylamides and methacrylamides are also useful, but they lack hydrolytic stability unless they are doubly substituted. N-vinyl-2-pyrrolidone (NVP) interacts strongly with water, and is useful for increasing the swelling of a gel, though gels of crosslinked poly-NVP are difficult to prepare and have poor mechanical strength. Acrylic and methacrylic acids, shown in Table 3, are easily incorporated, producing anionic polyelectrolyte gels whose ionization is a function of pH. Incorporation of the sulfonates produce polyelectrolyte gels relatively insensitive to pH [13]. Cationic gels can be produced from the tertiary and quaternary amines shown in Table 3. Ethylene glycol dimethacrylate (EGDMA), tetraethylene glycol dimethacrylate (TEGDMA), and N,N'-methylenebisacrylamide ("bis" or MBAA) are the most widely used of the crosslinkers in Table 4. Other crosslinkers can be used to improve mechanical properties of the gels. Crosslinkers with more than two reactive groups are also available; triallylamine is one example.

Table 3 Ionic Monomers for Hydrogel Synthesis

Anionic, acidic monomers

Acrylic acid

$$CH_2{=}CH{-}C\diagup\hspace{-0.3em}{\overset{\displaystyle O}{\underset{\displaystyle OH}{\diagdown}}}$$

Methacrylic acid

$$CH_2{=}\underset{\displaystyle CH_3}{\overset{\displaystyle |}{C}}{-}C\overset{\displaystyle O}{\underset{\displaystyle OH}{}}$$

Crotonic acid

$$CH_3{-}CH{=}CH{-}C\overset{\displaystyle O}{\underset{\displaystyle OH}{}}$$

Sodium styrenesulfonate

$$CH_2{=}CH$$
(benzene ring)
$$SO_3Na$$

Sodium 2-sulfoxyethylmethacrylate

$$CH_2{=}\underset{\displaystyle CH_3}{\overset{\displaystyle |}{C}}{-}C\overset{\displaystyle O}{\underset{\displaystyle OCH_2CH_2OSO_3Na}{}}$$

Cationic, basic monomers

Vinylpyridine

$$CH_2{=}CH$$
(pyridine ring)

Aminoethyl methacrylates[a]

$$CH_2{=}\underset{\displaystyle CH_3}{\overset{\displaystyle |}{C}}{-}C\overset{\displaystyle O}{\underset{\displaystyle OCH_2CH_2N{\diagdown}^{R_1}_{R_2}}{}}$$

2-methacryloyloxy-trimethylammonium chloride

$$\cdot CH_2{=}\underset{\displaystyle CH_3}{\overset{\displaystyle |}{C}}{-}C\overset{\displaystyle O}{\underset{\displaystyle OCH_2CH_2\overset{\oplus}{N}(CH_3)_3\overset{\ominus}{Cl}}{}}$$

---

[a] R_1, R_2 groups include : -H, -CH$_3$, -CH$_2$CH$_3$, -CH$_2$CH$_2$CH$_2$CH$_3$

Table 4 Polyfunctional Crosslinking Monomers for Hydrogel Synthesis

N, N'-methylenebisacrylamide

$$CH_2=CH-C\overset{O}{\underset{NHCH_2NH}{\diagdown}}C-CH=CH_2$$

Ethylene glycol dimethacrylates

$$CH_2=\underset{CH_3}{\overset{|}{C}}-C\overset{O}{\underset{O(CH_2CH_2O)_x}{\diagdown}}\overset{O}{\underset{CH_3}{\diagup}}C-\underset{}{\overset{|}{C}}=CH_2$$

2,2'-(p-phenylenedioxy)diethyl dimethacrylate

$$CH_2=\underset{CH_3}{\overset{|}{C}}-C\overset{O}{\underset{OCH_2CH_2O}{\diagdown}}\langle\bigcirc\rangle OCH_2CH_2O\overset{O}{\diagup}C-\underset{CH_3}{\overset{|}{C}}=CH_2$$

Divinylbenzene

$$CH_2=CH\left\langle\bigcirc\right\rangle CH=CH_2$$

Triallylamine

$$\begin{array}{c}CH_2=CH\\ \diagdown\\ CH_2=CH\end{array}N-CH=CH_2$$

Methylenebis(4-phenyl isocyanate)

$$O=C=N-\langle\bigcirc\rangle-CH_2-\langle\bigcirc\rangle-N=C=O$$

Synthetic hydrogels can be produced by means other than co-polymerization-crosslinking. These methods include chemical conversion of one type of gel to another and the crosslinking of linear polymers. The most important gels of these types are poly(vinyl alcohol) (PVA) and poly(ethylene oxide) (PEO).

PVA cannot be prepared by the polymerization of vinyl alcohol, which rearranges to its more stable tautomer, acetaldehyde:

$$CH_2=\underset{}{\overset{OH}{\overset{|}{CH}}} \longrightarrow CH_3\overset{O}{\overset{\|}{CH}}$$

As a result, PVA must be prepared indirectly. Commercially, PVA is produced by the polymerization of vinyl acetate to form poly(vinyl acetate), which is then hydrolyzed to PVA:

$$n\ CH_2{=}CH \longrightarrow \ {+}CH_2CH{+}_n \longrightarrow \ {+}CH_2CH{+}_n$$

$$
\begin{array}{ccc}
| & | & | \\
O & O & OH \\
| & | & \\
C{=}O & C{=}O & \\
| & | & \\
CH_3 & CII_3 & \\
\end{array}
$$

Many different grades of PVA of different stereoregular structures (isotactic, syndiotactic, atactic, and mixtures) can be produced. The degree of hydrolysis can proceed up to 100% with either head-to-head or alternating hydroxyl groups:

$$
\begin{array}{cc}
{-}CH_2CH\ CHCH_2{-} \quad \text{or} \quad & {-}CH_2CH\ CH_2CH{-} \\
|\quad | & |\qquad | \\
OH\ OH & OH\qquad OH
\end{array}
$$

The synthesis and properties of PVA have been authoritatively reviewed by Peppas [129].

In a similar fashion, chemical reactions can be used to convert other polymers or gels from one type to another. For example, polyacrylonitrile can be converted to polyacrylamide, which can be converted to polyacrylic acid:

$$CH_2{=}CH \longrightarrow \ {-}CH_2CH{-} \longrightarrow \ {-}CH_2CH{-}$$

$$
\begin{array}{ccc}
| & | & | \\
CN & C{=}O & C{=}O \\
& | & | \\
& NH_2 & OH \\
\end{array}
$$

Gels can also be made from poly(ethylene oxide) (PEO) and poly(ethylene glycol) (PEG), which have the repeating units $-(CH_2CH_2)-$. The difference between these two polymers is that PEG chains terminate with hydroxyl groups at each end; also, PEGs tend to have lower molecular weights. The formation of hydrogels from these materials has been reviewed by Graham [6].

Linear polymers such as PVA, PEO, and PEG can be crosslinked to form gels in a number of ways, including radiation crosslinking, covalent chemical crosslinking, or molecular complex formation. Irradiation of linear polymers can lead to simultaneous chain scission and chain branching, forming a three-dimensional network of infinite molecular weight: a hydrogel. Radiation crosslinking will be discussed in Section III.B.2. Because many hydrophilic polymers contain hydroxyl groups, they can be easily crosslinked by any difunctional compound that will condense with —OH groups (Section III.B.1). It is more difficult to generalize systems of molecular complexes. In these systems, two different polymers form a network by noncovalent interactions. One type is the polyelectrolyte complex, stabilized via ionic bonds. An example is the hydrogel formed from a mixture of poly(vinylbenzyltrimethylammonium chloride) and poly(sodium p-styrenesulfonate) [13, 113]:

$$-CH_2CH- \qquad -CH_2CH-$$

$$^+N(CH_3)_3 \qquad SO_3^-Na^+$$
$$Cl^-$$

Another hydrogel-forming complex is the mixture of poly(ethylene oxide) and poly(methacrylic acid); the structure is stabilized by extensive hydrogen bonding [6]. Other types of noncovalent cross-linking that can be used to form hydrogels include the insoluble crystallites in semicrystalline polymers and the physical entangements of high-molecular-weight polymers [6, 129].

Natural and Semisynthetic Hydrogels

As important as natural and semisynthetic polymers are in various pharmaceutical applications, they have been overshadowed by the synthetic materials for use in drug delivery devices. This is a tribute to the great versatility and reproducibility of the synthetic gels, not a disparagement of the natural polymers. Because many types of natural polymers are very inexpensive, they are most valuable for high-volume uses such as absorbants and agricultural applications. This category of hydrogel has been recently reviewed by C. A. Finch [18].

Perhaps the most common gel of everyday experience is gelatin. Gelatin is a linear protein that can form helical strands bound together like rope fibers by extensive hydrogen bonding. Certain polysaccharides, such as carrageen, form similar gels. These structures are sometimes made more rigid by using aldehydes to covalently crosslink the polymers through their hydroxyl groups. Starch gels can be synthesized in a number of ways, including crosslinking with phosphoryl chloride ($POCl_3$) [130, 131].

For drug delivery systems, semisynthetic (modified natural polymer) gels are generally the most useful. Crosslinked dextran (Sephadex) and crosslinked agarose (Sepharose) are hydrogels that are widely used in chromatography; they also have biomedical applications [132]. The variety of water-soluble cellulose ethers available approaches that of the synthetic monomers [133]. Different substituents and degrees of substitution are available that give the polymers different degrees of hydrophobicity or hydrophilicity; they can also be

made anionic (as carboxymethylcellulose). Cellulose ethers are
also available in different molecular weights (sold as viscosity grades).
They can be crosslinked to form hydrogels by the reaction of epichlo-
rohydrin or divinylsulfone with the pendant hydroxyl groups, just
as the linear synthetic polymers are [134]. The various polysaccharides can be crosslinked in a similar fashion.

Semisynthetic gels can also be created by ceric ion-initiated polymerization of a solution of starch, acrylamide, and N,N'-methylene-
bisacrylamide [135]. Variants of this type of gel can absorb over a
thousand times their weight in water; they make highly effective ab-
sorbents.

B. Hydrogel Synthesis

There are two basic routes of hydrogel synthesis. One is to crosslink existing linear polymers, the other is to carry out simultaneous
polymerization of monofunctional monomers and crosslinking with polyfunctional monomers. Linear polymers can be crosslinked by chemical
reagents by ionizing radiation or by physical interactions. Copoly-
merization/crosslinking requires monomers, crossliners, and a source
of free radicals to initiate chain polymerization. With respect to
synthesis, hydrogels are typical polymers; information about reaction
rates, mechanisms, and so forth, can be found in textbooks on polymer chemistry. Peppas and Mikos recently discussed the basics of
hydrogel preparation [136]. Our goal here is to provide sufficient
information for the reader to appreciate the concerns that are basic
to hydrogel production.

Chemical Crosslinking of Linear Polymers

One of the major techniques for the synthesis of hydrogels is to
crosslink linear (or branched) polymers by using a relatively minor
amount of crosslinking reagent. As mentioned earlier, crosslinks
can be formed with many different difunctional compounds capable
of condensing with the pendant hydroxyl groups contained by most
hydrophilic polymers. Chemicals that have been used for this purpose include formaldehyde, glutaraldehyde, acetaldehyde, trimethylo-
melamine, polyacrolein, diisocyanates, oxalic acid, dimethyl urea,
divinyl sulfate, ceric redox systems, and so forth [129]. The reaction is normally carried in solution, though suspension polymerization can also be used to form crosslinked particles. The solvent is
typically water, but other solvents can be used, especially alcohols.
The extent to which the resulting gel is crosslinked is typically defined in terms of the nominal crosslinking ratio, X. This parameter
is defined as the ratio of moles of crosslinking agent used to moles
of polymer repeating units present. It is important to recognize that
the nominal crosslinking ratio X need not be directly related to the

effective crosslink density ρ_X, though ρ_X is generally assumed to be
proportional to X. Not all crosslinking molecules will react: Some
will react with only one chain, some will form loops or dangling ends
that do not contribute to the network (are not "elastically effective").
A nominal number-average molecular weight between crosslinks, M_c,
can be related to X as follows for difunctional crosslinkers:

$$M_c = \frac{M_r}{2X} \tag{20}$$

where M_r is the molecular weight of the repeating unit.

Another important concept is that of the gel point. At first,
when crosslinks are added to a solution of linear polymers, large,
branched molecules are produced. At a critical level of crosslinking—
the gel point—a three-dimensional structure of infinite molecular
weight and viscosity is formed, which spans the volume of the container. Those polymer chains that have been linked to the network
are considered part of the gel, while those molecules that are still
independent are considered part of the "sol." The crosslinking reaction continues past the gel point, as more and more of the sol become connected to the gel network. Statistical theories, including
percolation theories, exist that predict the gel point for different
types of crosslinking reactions [120, 136—139]. From a practical
point of view, knowledge of the gel point is critical if molds are
being filled with a solution of linear polymer and crosslinking reagents.
The solution can gel in midair if the gel point is reached before the
molds are filled!

Radiation Crosslinking of Linear Polymers

Radiation crosslinking of linear polymers is another important technique for producing hydrogels; it has been reviewed recently by
several authors [136, 140, 141]. Its key advantage is the lack of
any residual impurities in the product such as unreacted monomers,
crosslinkers, or initiators. Its main drawbacks are the expense and
inconvenience of working with sources of ionizing radiation, typically
high-energy electrons and γ-radiation. Electron beam are commonly
generated by a van de Graaff accelerator and γ-rays by a ^{60}Co
source.

Bombardment of linear polymers with ionizing radiation in either
bulk form or in solution leads to the formation of free radicals on the
polymer chain. These radicals can react to form crosslinks between
neighboring chains, or they may cause the polymer to split into
fragments. If the crosslinking rate is faster than the degradation
rate, a network polymer—a gel—will be produced. As a general
role of thumb, vinyl polymers with the structure

$$
\begin{array}{c}
H \\
| \\
-CH_2-C- \\
| \\
R
\end{array}
$$

tend to crosslink, while those with the structure

$$
\begin{array}{c}
R' \\
| \\
-CH_2-C- \\
| \\
R
\end{array}
$$

tend to degrade. Thus polyacrylamides and polyacrylates usually crosslink, while polymethacrylamides and polymethacrylates usually degrade. Other important hydrophilic polymers that can be radiation-crosslinked include poly(vinyl alcohol) and poly(N-vinyl-2-pyrrolidone). An important practical note is that since oxygen promotes degradation, it is important to irradiate polymers in oxygen-free environments, especially if the crosslinking occurs at slow irradiation dose rates. Another potential problem is the evolution of gases, expecially hydrogen, which can be trapped in the polymer. These gases arise from combination of the free radicals generated (e.g., the reaction $2H \cdot \rightarrow H_2$). Also, free radicals can linger inside solid polymers for several hours after the cessation of irradiation.

Physical Crosslinking of Linear Polymers

Physical crosslinking is less generally applicable as a method for producing useful gels for drug delivery, but it can be very important in certain cases. Physical crosslinks include entanglements, charge complexes, nonspecific (hydrophobic) or specific interactions, and crystallites. If a polymer is of sufficiently high molecular weight and of only modest hydrophilicity, it can absorb water and swell, but the entangelements will prevent dissolution of the chains, despite the absence of any covalent crosslinks. Ionic interactions or hydrogen bonding can also lead to stabilization of a three-dimensional network; typical examples were given in Section III.A.2.

Certain polymers can at least partially crystallize. These semi-crystalline polymers can be largely amorphous with small regions of crystallinity on the order of 10 nm (100 Å) thick. These crystallites serve as polyfunctional crosslink junctions that tie a number of chains together. Placed in an aqueous solution, the amorphous regions can imbibe water, but the insoluble crystallites prevent dissolution. Crystallite formation is a particularly important crosslinking technique for poly(vinyl alcohol) [129].

Copolymerization/Crosslinking Synthesis from Monomers

As discussed earlier, synthetic hydrogels synthesized by copolymerization/crosslinking techniques have received the lion's share of attention for drug delivery application. With this technique, monofunctional and polyfunctional monomers are mixed together and the polymerization is initiated; the crosslinks develop as polyfunctional monomers are incorporated into two or more different growing chains. While gels can be made by both step condensation and chain free-radical polymerization, the latter route is by far the most important for hydrogel production. The principles of condensation and free-radical polymerization can be found in any text on polymer chemistry [e.g., 37, 118, 142]. The gelation phenomenon is similar to that seen with linear polymers, though the statistical analysis is different. The advantage of this technique lies in the diversity of hydrogels that can be produced. Almost any combination of monomers can be copolymerized to form a gel if they are miscible or soluble in a common solvent. The caution to be added here is that copolymerization in practice is quite complex. Different monomers have different reactivities, so only in special cases will monomers be incorporated into the network in a random, evenly dispersed fashion. The gel may be produced with distinct regions of monomer A and distinct regions of monomer B; such gels are prone to phase separation, which can have a major impact on the properties of the gel. Also, since the reactions rarely go to completion, the composition of the network may differ significantly from that of the original, unreacted solution if one monomer is much more reactive than another. Thus it is important to anticipate whether a copolymer will be random (—ABBAAABABAABABBB—), alternating (—ABABABABAB—), or block (—AAAAAAABBBBBBB—). This estimate can be made using the simple, moderately successful Alfrey-Price "Q-e" scheme [118, 143, 144].

Once the desired monomers and crosslinker have been chosen and mixed, the reaction must be initiated by the generation of free radicals. Radicals may be produced by ionizing radiation, chemical initiators, or ultraviolet radiation in the presence of a photosensitive chemical. Regardless of initiation choice, oxygen must be scrupulously eliminated from the reacting mixture, as it inhibits the polymerization.

Chemical initiators that generate free radicals upon decomposition caused by elevated temperatures or dissolution are the most widely used. A wide variety of initiators can be used, including azo compounds, peroxides, and redox couples [145]. Common examples include azobisisobutyronitrile (AIBN), t-butyl peroctoate, benzoyl peroxide, diisopropyl percarbonate, and the ammonium persulfate-sodium metabisulfite redox couple. Since these initiators are incorporated into the gel network as chain ends, Gregonis et al. have proposed the use of azo initiators modified to resemble the repeating units of the gel [155]. The choice of an initiator and its concentration level are largely empirical. The initiator must be soluble in the monomer solution and initiate the reaction at a reasonable rate (too fast generates excessive heat, while gelation may not occur if the reaction is too slow). There is evidence that different initiators and concentrations can produce gels of differing character [146, 147]. These differences are often subtle and hard to predict. If no active hydrogens are present in the monomer or solvent, the reaction can also be initiated with anionic initiators such as n-butyl lithium or lithium t-butoxide. However, this is much less common. Certain compounds such as riboflavin as well as compounds such as AIBN generate free radicals upon exposure to ultraviolet light. Sometimes these can operate at lower concentrations than the thermally decomposed initiators discussed above. Ultraviolet initiation is also much easier to control, since it can be turned on and off at will. With most other types of initiation, reaction can begin as soon as the initiator is dissolved in the monomer solution, which can cause practical problems. Heating to cause initiation has built-in time lags due to the heat capacity of the solution and is more difficult to control.

Gamma-radiation can also be used to initiate free-radical polymerization. Its advantages over the chemical initiators are that it leaves no residual initiator in the gel that must be removed prior to use, and it does not cause undesired groups to be added to the hydrogel network. Hydrogels prepared both by ionizing radiation and by chemical initiation have been observed to have different swelling properties, apparently due to residual initiator effects [148].

The properties of the hydrogel also depend on the type and amount of solvent used. If the monomer is a liquid, bulk polymerization in the absence of solvent is also possible. If the polymerization is carried out in the presence of a good solvent for both the monomer and polymer, a transparent, homogeneous gel is usually formed. If the polymerization is carried out in a solvent that is a poor one for the resulting polymer, opaque, white, and heterogeneous gels are formed as a result of the ensuing phase separation. The opaque gels generally display mechanical properties that are inferior to those of the transparent gels. The quantity of diluent also affects the resulting gel properties. For example, crosslinking efficiency may be poor in dilute monomer solutions. The basic polymer structure will also vary with diluent concentration, as is seen in necessary corrections to the elasticity expression for networks [28, 29]. Other, more subtle effects have been observed when the monomer solution concentration is varied [149].

IV. POLYMERIZATION PROCESSES

The most important processes for the synthesis of hydrogels are
bulk, solution, and suspension polymerizations. These techniques
are in widespread use for many different kinds of polymeric materials; as a result, they have been well studied [118]. Here we will
provide an introduction to the topic with emphasis on the special
concerns of hydrogel production. A given type of hydrogel can often
be produced by any of these techniques, so it is important to understand their basic characteristics in order to select the most appropriate process for a given application. In general, bulk and solution
polymerization are the most appropriate for preparing hydrogels for
topical and implant applications or as membranes, since a gel of any
geometry can be prepared by casting in a suitable mold. In contrast,
suspension polymerization is the preferred technique for producing
uniform, spherical hydrogel particles.

A. Bulk/Solution Polymerization

Bulk and solution polymerization are the simplest and most common
techniques for producing hydrogels. With bulk polymerization, the
crosslinker and initiator are dissolved in the monomer before the solution is poured into the mold. Solution polymerization differs in that
the reactive species are dissolved in a suitable solvent. The solutions must be degassed under vacuum and/or sparged with an inert
gas (e.g., N_2 or Ar) prior to initiation, since oxygen inhibits polymerization. Metal ions and other species that interact with free
radicals must also be scrupulously removed from the system or irre-
producible inhibition or acceleration of the reaction may occur. Sometimes the mold itself may inhibit the reaction near the surface; thus
mold materials must be chosen with care. Typical molds are made of
nylon or polypropylene. Gels sometimes adhere to glass.

Table 5 provides a comparison of the advantages and disadvantages
of these two techniques. There are three major problems that commonly develop in bulk or solution polymerization: heat removal,
shrinkage, and incomplete monomer conversion. Heat removal is the
most serious and results from the combination of highly exothermic
heats of reaction (10 to 20 kcal/mole) with the low thermal conduc-
tivity of polymers. Since the reaction kinetics have exponential
temperature dependence, runaway reactions and localized hot spots
can develop. This frequently causes inhomogeneities, opacity, bubble
formation, and surface shrinking marks. As a result, uniform hydrogel samples are easily prepared only for thicknesses in the millimeter
range. Another problem that aggravates temperature control is the
Trommsdorff or gel effect. Since the termination rate of chain polymerization is controlled by the mobility of the growing polymer chains,

Table 5 Comparison of Bulk and Solution Polymerization

Advantages of Bulk Polymerization

Simplest technique: only monomer, crosslinker, and initiator are needed

Product is typically a dry, strong material

No chain transfer to solvent

Phase separation inhomogeneities are avoided if the polymer is soluble in the monomer

Advantages of Solution Polymerization

Monomers may be solid or liquid

No shrinkage in molds

Greatest flexibility: proper solvent choice can aid processing

Solvent serves as a heat sink, minimizing temperature control problems

Solvent choice and dilution factor can be used to alter gel properties

once the network is formed, largely immobilizing the polymer chains, the termination rate slows dramatically. The propagation rate, however, is determined by monomer mobility and slows much less upon gelation. Thus the overall reaction rate accelerates and heat build-up increases sharply. Thus, effective control of the reaction temperature requires a heating and cooling pattern that varies with conversion [118].

Upon conversion of monomer to polymer in bulk polymerization, the volume contracts about 20%. This shrinkage, which occurs mainly in the first stage of polymerization as the basic matrix is formed, can lead to problems in casting uniform pieces. However, this problem can be overcome, and has been extensively studied in contact lens manufacture [123]. These details are largely proprietary. The use of flexible molds and annealing of pieces at elevated temperatures after removal from the molds can improve uniformity. Dry, glassy hydrogels can be machined to precise tolerances, but the expense is much higher than molding, even assuming a much higher rejection rate of molded pieces.

The degree of monomer conversion is dependent on the specific monomer and the reaction conditions. Though it can be made to approach 100%, incomplete conversion is not necessarily a problem, since purification of the gels generally requires leaching extractable impurities from the gels prior to loading with drug or other use, anyway. It is possible to polymerize a gel in a drug solution, thereby trapping the drug in the matrix. However, possible side reactions between the drug and monomer and the inability to remove residual monomers, initiators, and other impurities make this method generally unsuitable for drug delivery. A better method of drug loading is to equilibrate the gel with a concentrated drug solution in a good swelling solvent for the polymer.

Chain transfer can be a problem in these reactions, especially in solution polymerization. Chain transfer involves abstraction of a free radicals from growing chains by monomer, solvent, or polymer. The result can be reduced molecular weights or unexpected crosslinking [136].

B. Suspension Polymerization

Suspension polymerization is the method of choice for producing hydrogel particles. Gel sheets or cylinders produced by bulk or solution polymerization would have to be ground or diced to produce particles. These irregularly shaped granules would be esthetically objectionable and have poor reproducibility for controlling drug release. In contrast, suspension polymerization can produce spherical beads with particle sizes ranging from about 0.1 to 5 mm in diameter. This technique has been widely used for producing polymer beads, including hydrogel beads, for ion exchange, gel filtration, and chromatography.

Hydrogels produced by suspension polymerization are in principle the same as those produced by bulk polymerization. In suspension polymerization, the monomer solution is simply mechanically dispersed into a nonsolvent, forming droplets. The droplets are stabilized by a protective colloid, though a true emulsion is not formed. Polymerization is induced by thermal decomposition of a free-radical initiator. Because the suspending phase acts as a heat sink and the particles are relatively small, temperature control during suspension polymerization is much easier than in bulk polymerization. The hydrogel beads can be easily recovered from the suspending phase and extracted with a good swelling solvent to remove any residual monomers and other impurities. Particle size, size distribution, and shape of the beads produced depends on the suspending agent, stirring rate, and impeller design, as well as more subtle details of the preparation procedure (see Section V.B) [118].

Production of hydrogel beads by suspension polymerization has been recently reviewed by Lee [14]. The shape of the particle is controlled by the interfacial tension between the monomer phase and the suspending phase. Suspending phases that have been used include silicone oil, mineral oil, xylene, and concentrated aqueous solutions of sodium sulfate. Water-soluble polymers such as poly(vinyl pyrrolidone), poly(vinyl alcohol), or hydroxyethylcellulose may be added as suspension stabilizers. An improved process for producing hydrogel beads as uniform spheres, not irregular blobs, was recently reported by Mueller et al. [150]. This technique made use of water-insoluble, gelatinous, strongly water-bonding inorganic hydroxides as suspending agents. The use of magnesium hydroxide allowed production of spherical, smooth-surfaced hydrogel beads based on copolymers of HEMA. A typical synthesis is described in the next section.

Although hydrogel beads produced by suspension polymerization should have the same properties as gels of the same nominal composition produced by bulk polymerization, differences may be observed in practice. This may be due differences in thermal history, initiation rates, specific interactions with the suspending agents, and so forth.

V. LARGE-SCALE PRODUCTION OF HYDROGELS

Despite the growing number of publications and patents on hydrogels and their applications, very little information is available in the literature addressing large-scale production of hydrogel devices. Most of the work done in this area is for commercial interests and therefore still proprietary. However, from published patents and associated examples, one can gain insight into the potential problems that may arise during large-scale production. In addition, based on a general knowledge of chemical engineering process development, one can draw parallels between the production of hydrogels and other chemical production processes. This is particularly true in the area of raw material purification, where standard separation processes such as filtration, extraction, ion exchange, and distillation are employed. A good example is in the purification of 2-hydroxyethyl methacrylate (HEMA) monomer. The degradation of HEMA monomer during transportation and storage at ambient temperature generally leads to increased levels of impurities such as methacrylic acid (MAA), ethylene glycol dimethacrylate (EGDMA), and ethylene glycol. The presence of an unknown and uncontrollable level of EGDMA, a cross linker formed by trans-esterification of two HEMA molecules, is undesirable since it will crosslink HEMA even when no crosslinker is added to the monomer. The MAA can also affect the properties significantly even at typical impurity levels on the order of 1% [151]. The batch purification is normally carried out in a reactor by first extracting the aqueous solution of HEMA with a nonpolar solvent such as carbon tetrachloride or hexane, followed by alumina treatment to remove polar impurities, and finally distilling under vacuum in the presence of a polymerization inhibitor such as hydroquinone [14, 146]. The removal of impurities from other raw materials such as the comonomer, initiator, and solvent is generally carried out by a similar type of unit operation in order to meet pharmaceutical quality standards acceptable to regulatory agencies.

A. Bulk/Solution Polymerization

Bulk/solution polymerization processes, where a mixture of monomer, initiator, and an optional solvent such as water is charged into a mold and subsequently polymerized, had been employed in the batch mode to produce soft contact lenses, implants, catheters, and other shaped articles [152—154]. Because of the exothermic nature of the polymerization process, the dissipation of heat of reaction, which can lead to the formation of bubbles and other inhomogeneities, is a major problem in production. Means of overcoming these problems include (a) degassing of the monomer mixture to eliminate dissolved gases; (b) reduction of sample thickness and construction of molds with thinner and highly thermoconductive materials to facilitate heat dissipation; and (c) introduction of larger driving forces (larger temperature gradient) for heat dissipation by carrying out the polymerization at a lower temperature (e.g., UV curing at ambient temperature).

   The only good example of large-scale bulk polymerization of hydrogels is soft contact lens manufacturing, where hundreds of solvent-free hydrogel buttons of about 1 to 1.5 cm in diameter and 0.5 to 0.8 cm in thickness are routinely produced by UV-initiated bulk polymerization at ambient temperature under a nitrogen blanket in thin molds. After time-consuming lathing and polishing steps, lenses of predetermined curvatures are obtained by swelling the finished pieces in water. One interesting way to overcome complicated production steps in soft contact lens manufacturing is by the use of a spin casting technique [152], which also offers an unexpected advantage in heat dissipation. In this process, a small amount of the monomer and initiator mixture is first charged into a concave lens mold under a nitrogen blanket, followed by rotating the mold about an axis transverse to the supporting surface at a speed sufficient to displace the solution radially under centrifugal force to form a lens shape. After the polymerization, activated either by heat or by UV radiation, a lens-shaped article is formed in situ. Because of the small lens thickness (<<1 mm), the spin casting technique results in a fast heat dissipation during hydrogel polymerization.

B. Suspension Polymerization

Suspension polymerization has been employed as a batch process to produce spherical hydrogel beads with particle sizes ranging from 0.1 to 5 mm in diameter [150, 155, 156]. The production process is normally carried out in a chemical reactor equipped with a condenser, nitrogen sparge, thermoregulator and, most important, a stirrer and baffle of a design that will ensure good mixing at low stirring speeds. Figure 11 shows the basic design of a reactor. For a typical production run, a saturated aqueous sodium chloride solution is first charged into the reactor together with a soluble magnesium or alumi-

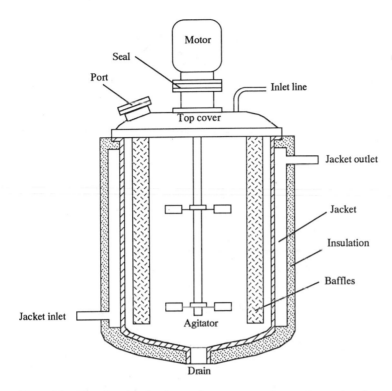

Fig. 11 The basic design of a suspension polymerization reactor.

num salt as the suspending agent. The solution is then heated to the polymerization temperature and the gelatinous metal hydroxide is precipitated by adding a prescribed amount of aqueous base with rapid stirring. Following this, the stirring speed is reduced to a predetermined value for a specific size range of beads. Subsequently, the monomer mixture containing dissolved initiator is charged into the reactor and the reaction kept at a constant temperature (typically 80–90°C) for at least 3 hr, followed by an optional 1 hr at 100°C with reflux. A nitrogen blanket is normally maintained at all times. The reaction mixture is then cooled to room temperature and the metal hydroxide is dissolved by adding HCl. The slurry in the reactor is then discharged through a filter to recover the beads. After washing free of surface salt, the wet beads are soaked overnight in an excess amount of ethanol or an ethanol/water mixture to extract unreacted monomer. Subsequently, the swollen beads are isolated again by batch filtration and dried in an industrial dryer. The dried hydrogel beads are then weighed and fractionated into

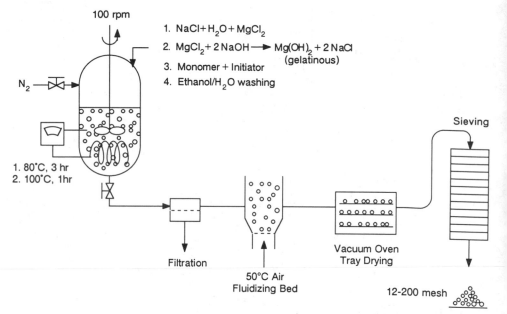

Fig. 12 A typical flowsheet for the production of PHEMA copolymer hydrogel beads by suspension polymerization.

different particle sizes by sieving. A sample flowchart for this suspension polymerization process is shown in Fig. 12.

Several process parameters affecting the suspension polymerization can be readily identified. First, the selection of suspending medium is important to the shape and surface roughness of the resulting beads. Mueller et al. [150] reported that only insoluble, gelatinous inorganic hydroxides such as magnesium hydroxide gave rise to uniform spherical beads with smooth surfaces when used in the suspension polymerization of their specific monomers. Second, the particle size and size distribution are affected by the viscosity of the monomer mixture, the stirring rate (rpm), and the amount of the suspending agent. The contribution from each of these factors may vary from case to case; however, as a rule of thumb, the particle size increases as the rpm decreases or viscosity increases. Finally, the sequence of addition of the monomer mixture into the reactor can also affect the particle size and bubble formation; e.g., the addition of monomer at full stirring speed versus the addition of monomer at a lower stirring speed followed by a gradual increase to full stirring speed. The reason for this is not clear; however, it may be attributed to the formation of dispersed monomer droplets containing multiple phases under the right surface tension and stirring conditions.

Other large-scale production processes involve drying and sieving the hydrogel beads. Immediate vacuum drying of wet beads after separation generally created a dried, glassy outer shell around each bead, which retards subsequent solvent transport from inside the bead and slows down the drying process. A more efficient drying process involves initial drying of wet beads in a fluidized bed with hot air to remove most of the swelling solvent, quickly followed by vacuum drying at moderate temperature to remove the residual solvent. As to the sieving process, static buildup in the dry beads can cause considerable problems in the particle size determination. This is best avoided by retaining a small amount (1–2%) of residual water in the beads before sieving.

C. Quality Control and Batch Testing

Quality control of hydrogels produced by either bulk/solution suspension polymerization processes generally involves the measurement of equilibrium swelling properties of the hydrogel batch. Other tests may be appropriate for specific applications; for example, in the case of soft contact lenses, additional optical tests are needed. As we emphasized earlier, the equilibrium swelling is the single most important properties of a hydrogel, since it has a profound impact on the mechanical, drug loading, and release properties of the material. For drug delivery applications, the quality control procedure generally goes beyond just measuring a single water or ethanol swelling of the hydrogel. Instead, hydrogel swelling in a series of ethanol/ water mixtures covering the range from 0 to 100% ethanol is obtained (Fig. 13). From this, the maximum swelling of a specific hydrogel batch is determined and the solubility parameter of this hydrogel batch is then calculated from the solubility parameter of the solvent composition at the swelling maximum (Section II.A.2). The magnitude and location of the maximum swelling as well as the full swelling spectrum are generally used as quality control criteria to spot batch-to-batch variations. The range and peak in particle size distribution and other gross physical defects such as bubbles and localized inhomogeneities are also important parameters for quality control purposes. The specifications and variabilities on the swelling parameters for quality control are generally established based on experimental limitations.

VI. PROCESSING OF HYDROGELS FOR DRUG DELIVERY

From a safety standpoint, the drug of interest cannot be incorporated into the monomer mixture because of the possible reactions between the drug and the monomer, and the inability to remove residual mono-

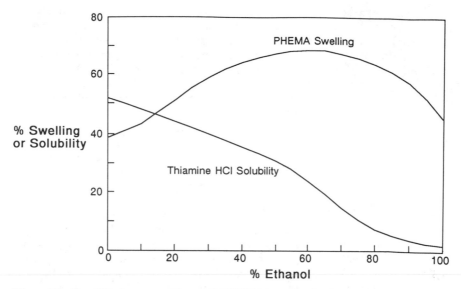

Fig. 13 Equilibrium swelling of PHEMA and thiamine HCl solubility in ethanol/water mixtures [14].

mer and initiator while keeping the entrapped drug intact. The most practical approach at this time is to extract the hydrogel in a good swelling solvent to remove all leachable by-products and residual monomers in order to make hydrogels acceptable for drug delivery applications. The drug loading can then be achieved by equilibrating the cleaned hydrogel in a concentrated drug solution prepared in a good swelling solvent [14].

A. Purification and Drying of Hydrogels

The purification of either bulk, solution, or suspension polymerized hydrogels is normally carried out in batches by soaking the hydrogel in an excess amount of ethanol or ethanol/water mixtures for an extended period of time, usually 12 to 24 hr, to remove the extractables. The extracting solvent is generally replaced several times during the purification process, and the level of extractables in the extracting solvent is assayed by gas chromatography (GC) or high-performance liquid chromatography (HPLC).

For handling and storage purposes, purified hydrogels are generally dried before the drug loading step. Occasionally, the drying step can be bypassed when it is certain that the hydrogel meets quality control specifications. The drying of bulky hydrogel articles such as sheets, cylinders, or disks is best carried out initially in an

oven with continuous air stream flowing over the hydrogel surface.
For hydrogel beads, this can best be accomplished in an air suspension column. This air drying process can remove a major portion
(70—80%) of the moisture in a short period of time without creating
a dried, glassy shell around hydrogel articles, which can slow down
the drying process considerably. After this initial drying, the
residual moisture can be removed effectively in a vacuum oven (see
Fig. 12).

B. Drug Loading Properties

The loading of hydrogels with drug, particularly beads, is usually
carried out in batches by equilibrium absorption from concentrated
drug solution. When there are no substantial variations of drug
solubilities over the solvent composition range, the loading solution
is normally prepared in an ethanol/water composition that gives rise
to a maximum hydrogel swelling. However, when there is a substantial difference in drug solubilities over the ethanol/water composition range, the ethanol/water composition at maximum hydrogel
swelling may not be the optimum loading solvent due to lower drug
solubility (see Fig. 13). In this case, the ethanol/water composition that results in a maximum in the product of drug solubility and
equilibrium swelling is selected as the loading solvent.

The volume of the loading solution is generally kept in excess of
the volume of the hydrogel (e.g., larger than 10:1) in order to ensure that the external drug concentration remains relatively constant.
The loading equilibrium is usually reached within 24 hr. Subsequent
filtration, rinsing, and drying result in glassy, dehydrated hydrogels containing uniformly dissolved or dispersed drug. The drying
process involved here is similar to that described in the previous
section. The resultant drug loading is determined by dividing the
weight gain after loading and drying by the dry weight of the
loaded hydrogel.

C. Quality Control and Batch Testing

The quality control of drug-loaded hydrogels generally involes the
assay of drug loading and the measurement of release profiles. The
drug loading in a quality control test is typically determined by extracting a known amount of drug-loaded hydrogel in a fixed amount
of solvent such as methanol or ethanol followed by assaying the drug
concentration in the extracting solvent. The drug release profile is
generally measured in a thermostated USP dissolution apparatus using
either an HPLC or a UV-visible spectrophotometer for the monitoring
of drug concentration. The drug diffusion coefficients are calculated
from release data based on Eqs. (13)—(15). The specifications and
variabilities on the drug loading level as well as on the release t_{50}

(time for release of 50% of the loaded drug) and t_{90} (time for release of 90% of the loaded drug) are usually established based on regulatory requirements and experimental limitations.

VII. APPLICATIONS OF HYDROGELS FOR DRUG DELIVERY

No drug delivery systems based on chemically crosslinked hydrogels have yet been commercialized; however, a physically crosslinked poly(vinyl alcohol) gel has been used in a transdermal nitroglycerin product (Nitro-Dur, Key Pharmaceutical), and morphine suppositories and prostaglandine E_2 vaginal pessaries based on PEO hydrogels have been clinically evaluated [157, 158]. Based on available patents and publications, it is apparent that several pharmaceutical companies, including CIBA-GEIGY and Squibb, have been working actively in this area. Judging by the work of Mueller et al. [150, 159–161] and Lee [14, 112, 162, 163], CIBA-GEIGY appears to be the most advanced in developing suspension-polymerized hydrogel beads for oral drug delivery applications. In fact, Lee has reported a controlled-extraction process to immobilize a sigmoidal, nonuniform initial drug profile in glassy hydrogel beads, which gives rise to a zero-order drug release behavior previously obtainable only from a membrane-reservoir delivery system [14, 112, 162, 163]. If properly developed, this process can potentially be utilized to develop rate-programmed dosage forms to meet a variety of therapeutic needs.

Hydrogels responsive to changes in their environment (e.g., pH, temperature) are also being applied to drug delivery problems. Here the control of solute permeability through the gel is often the key. Kim et al. are using temperature-sensitive gels as on-off switches for drug release: The expanded network is permeable to drugs, the shrunken network is not [164]. Horbett, Ratner, and co-workers have combined glucose oxidase and pH-sensitive gels to create a device that will release insulin in response to rising glucose levels [49, 165, 166]. Firestone and Siegel have proposed a related idea [167]. Kou and Amidon are using a pH-sensitive gel to design a pH-controlled oral dosage form [51]. Hoffman and co-workers have proposed an oral dosage form using temperature-sensitive gels [168, 169]. Heller has reviewed a number of other proposed applications of reversible swelling/shrinking hydrogels with promise for drug delivery applications [170].

The only topic that has not been addressed so far is cost. Admittedly, the raw material and the processing costs may be initially prohibitive when compared with other conventional dosage forms; however, as one optimizes the process design, automates key processes, and starts with lower-grade raw material, the cost factor for hydrogel systems can be substantially reduced.

VIII. ACKNOWLEDGMENTS

The authors would like to express their thanks to Ming-Chien Yang and Lii-Hurng Lyu for their help with compiling references and creating figures. The authors also gratefully acknowledge the financial support of the National Science Foundation (Grant CBT-8809271) [SHG], a State of Ohio Research Challenge Grant [SHG], and the Faculty of Pharmacy of the University of Toronto [PIL] in preparing this chapter and in performing the previously unpublished work cited.

IX. REFERENCES

1. J. D. Ferry, *Viscoelastic Properties of Polymers*, 3rd edition, John Wiley, New York, 1980, p. 529.
2. P. J. Flory, *Disc. Farad. Soc.*, 57:7 (1974).
3. P. Russo, in *Reversible Polymeric Gels and Related Systems* (P. Russo, ed.), ACS Symposium Series 350, American Chemical Society, Washington, D.C., 1987, pp. 3–5.
4. H. Determann, *Gel Chromatography*, Springer-Verlag, New York, 1984, p. 4.
5. L. Fischer, *Gel Filtration Chromatography*, 2nd ed., Elsevier/ North-Holland Biomedical Press, New York, 1980.
6. N. B. Graham, in *Hydrogels in Medicine and Pharmacy, Volume II, Polymers* (N. A. Peppas, ed.), CRC Press, Boca Raton, Fla., 1987, p. 98.
7. H. R. Proctor and J. A. Wilson, *J. Chem. Soc.*, 109:307 (1916).
8. O. Wichterle and D. Lim, *Nature*, 185:117 (1960).
9. J. D. Andrade (ed.), *Hydrogels for Medical and Related Applications*, ACS Symposium Series 31, American Chemical Society, Washington, D.C., 1976.
10. N. A. Peppas (ed.), *Hydrogels in Medicine and Pharmacy, Volumn I, Fundamentals*, CRC Press, Boca Raton, Fla, 1986.
11. N. A. Peppas (ed.), *Hydrogels in Medicine and Pharmacy, Volume II, Polymers*, CRC Press, Boca Raton, Fla, 1987.
12. N. A. Peppas (ed.), *Hydrogels in Medicine and Pharmacy, Volume III, Properties and Applications*, CRC Press, Boca Raton, Fla., 1987.
13. V. Kudela, in *Encyclopedia of Polymer Science and Engineering*, Vol. 7, 2nd ed., (H. F. Mark, N. M. Bikales, C. G. Overberger, G. Menges, and J. I. Kroschwitz, eds.), John Wiley, New York, 1987, pp. 783–807.
14. P. I. Lee, in *Controlled Release Systems: Fabrication Technology*, Vol. II (D. Hsieh, ed.), CRC Press, Boca Raton, Fla., 1988, pp. 61–63.
15. T. Tanaka, *Sci. Ameri.*, 224:124 (1981).

16. T. Tanaka, in *Encyclopedia of Polymer Science and Engineering*, Vol. 7, 2nd ed. (H. F. Mark, N. M. Bikales, C. G. Overberger, G. Menges, and J. I. Kroschwitz, eds.), John Wiley, New York, 1987, p. 514–531.

17. J. Kalal, in *Chemistry and Technology of Water Soluble Polymers* (C. A. Finch, ed.), Plenum Press, New York, 1981, pp. 71–80.

18. C. A. Finch, in *Chemistry and Technology of Water Soluble Polymers* (C. A. Finch, ed.), Plenum Press, New York, 1981, pp. 81–111.

19. D. Vermaas and J. J. Hermans, *Rec. Trav. Chem. Pays-Bas*, *67*:983 (1948).

20. P. J. Flory and R. Rehner, Jr., *J. Chem. Phys.*, *11*:521 (1943).

21. K. Dusek and D. Patterson, *J. Polym. Sci. A-2*, *6*:1209 (1968).

22. H. Hasa, M. Ilavsky, and K. Dusek, *J. Polym. Sci., Polym. Phys. Ed.*, *13*:253 (1975).

23. J. Hasa, M. Ilavsky, *J. Polym. Sci., Polym. Phys. Ed.*, *13*:263 (1975).

24. F. Helfferich, *Ion Exchange*, McGraw-Hill, New York, 1962.

25. I. Michaeli, A. Katchalsky, *J. Polym. Sci.*, *23*:683 (1954).

26. M. Ilavsky, *Polymer*, *22*:1687 (1981).

27. M. Ilavsky, *Macromolecules*, *15*:782 (1982).

28. N. A. Peppas and W. W. Merrill, *J. Polym. Sci. Polym. Chem.*, *14*:441 (1976).

29. N. A. Peppas and L. M. Lucht, *Chem. Eng. Commun.*, *30*:291 (1984).

30. N. A. Peppas and B. D. Barr-Howell, in *Hydrogels in Medicine and Pharmacy, Volume I, Fundamentals* (N. A. Peppas, ed.), CRC Press, Boca Raton, Fla., 1986, pp. 27–56.

31. S. Hirotsu, Y. Kirokawa, and T. Tanaka, *J. Chem. Phys.*, *87*:1392 (1987).

32. T. Tanaka, *Phys. Rev. Lett.*, *40*:820 (1978).

33. T. Tanaka, I. Nishio, S. T. Sun, and S. Ueno-Nishio, *Science*, *218*:467 (1982).

34. T. Tanaka, D. Fillmore, S. T. Sun, I. Nishio, G. Swislow, and A. Shah, *Phys. Rev. Lett.*, *45*:1636 (1980).

35. I. Ohime and T. Tanaka, *J. Chem. Phys.*, *11*:5725 (1982).

36. J. Ricka and T. Tanaka, *Macromolecules*, *17*:2916 (1984).

37. P. J. Flory, *Principles of Polymer Chemistry*, Cornell University Press, Ithaca, N.Y., 1953.

38. A. F. M. Barton, *Handbook of Solubility Parameters and Other Cohesion Parameters*, CRC Press, Boca Raton, Fla, 1983.

39. R. F. S. Freitas and E. L. Cussier, *Chem. Eng. Sci.*, *41*:97 (1986).

40. I. C. Sanchez and R. H. Lacombe, *Macromolecules*, *11*:1145 (1978).

41. A. C. Balazs and I. C. Sanchez, *Polym. Prepr.*, *29*:456 (1988).

42. M. S. Jhon, S. M. Ma, S. Hattori, D. E. Gregonis, and J. D. Andrade, in *Hydrogels for Medical and Related Applications*

(J. D. Andrade, ed.), ACS Symposium Series 31, American Chemical Society, Washington, D.C., 1976, pp. 60—68.

43. A. Galli and W. H. Brumage, *J. Chem. Phys.*, *79*:2411 (1983).

44. S. H. Gehrke, unpublished work, University of Cincinnati, 1988.

45. C. Tanford, *Physical Chemistry of Macromolecules*, John Wiley, New York, 1961, pp. 221—227.

46. S. H. Gehrke, G. P. Andrews, and E. L. Cussler, *Chem. Eng. Sci.*, *41*:2153 (1986).

47. R. A. Siegel and B. A. Firestone, Ionic strength and buffer effects on swelling in polyelectrolyte hydrogels, *Proc. 15th Int. Symp. Controlled Release of Bioactive Materials*, Basel, Switzerland, 1988.

48. A. M. Weiss, A. J. Grodzinsky, and M. L. Yarmush, in *Recent Advances in Separation Techniques—III* (N. N. Li, ed.), *AIChE Symp. Ser. No. 250*, *82*:85 (1986).

49. G. Albin, T. A. Horbett, and B. D. Ratner, *J. Controlled Release*, *2*:153 (1985).

50. B. A. Firestone and R. A. Siegel, Dynamic pH-dependent swelling properties of a hydrophobic polyelectrolyte gel, *Polymer (Commun.)*, *29*:204 (1988). *Toronto*, 1987, pp. 81—82.

51. J. H. Kou and G. L. Amidon, Mechanism of drug release from a dynamically swelling hydrogel matrix, *Proc. 14th Int. Symp. Controlled Release of Bioactive Materials*, Toronto, 1987, pp. 79—80.

52. R. A. Orwell, *Rubber Chem. Technol.*, *50*:451 (1977).

53. I. Iliopoulos, R. Audebert, and C. Quivoron, in *Reversible Polymeric Gels and Related Systems* (P. Russo, ed.), ACS Symposium Series 350, American Chemical Society, Washington, D.C., 1987, pp. 72 86.

54. S. H. Gehrke, *The Kinetics of Gel Volume Change and Its Interaction with Solutes*, University of Minnesota, Minneapolis, MN, 1986.

55. P. I. Lee, *Polymer (Commun.)*, *24*:45 (1983).

56. E. L. Cussler, M. R. Stokar, and J. E. Varberg, *AIChE J.*, *30*:578 (1984).

57. N. A. Peppas and S. R. Lustig, in *Hydrogels in Medicine and Pharmacy, Volume I, Fundamentals* (N. A. Peppas, ed.), CRC Press, Boca Raton, Fla., 1986, pp. 57—83.

58. B. K. Davis, *Proc. Natl. Acad. Sci. USA*, *71*:3120 (1974).

59. H. Yasuda, C. E. Lamaze, and A. Peterlin, *J. Polym. Sci. A-2*, *9*:1117 (1971).

60. H. Yasuda, C. E. Lamaze, and L. D. Ikenberry, *Macromol. Chem.*, *118*:19 (1968).

61. S. H. Gehrke and E. L. Cussler, *Chem. Eng. Sci.*, *44*:559 (1989).

62. N. A. Peppas and H. J. Moynihan, in *Hydrogels in Medicine and Pharmacy, Volume II, Polymers* (N. A. Peppas, ed.), CRC Press, Boca Raton, Fla., 1987, p. 59.

63. N. A. Peppas and C. T. Reinhardt, *J. Membr. Sci.*, *15*:275 (1983).

64. R. W. Korsmeyer, S. R. Lustig, and N. A. Peppas, *J. Polym. Sci.*, *Polym. Phys. Ed.*, *24*:395 (1986).

65. R. W. Korsmeyer, E. Von Meerwall, and N. A. Peppas, *J. Polym. Sci.*, *Polym. Phys. Ed.*, *24*:409 (1986).

66. N. A. Peppas, R. Gurny, E. Doelker, and P. Buri, *J. Membr. Sci.*, *7*:241 (1980).

67. S. R. Lustig and N. A. Peppas, *Polym. Prepr.*, *26*:72 (1985).

68. J. Crank, *The Mathematics of Diffusion*, 2nd ed., Oxford University Press, London, 1975.

69. P. I. Lee, *J. Membr. Sci.*, *7*:255 (1980).

70. P. I. Lee, in *Controlled Release of Bioactive Materials* (R. W. Baker, ed.), Academic Press, New York, 1980, pp. 135–153.

71. A. S. Hoffman, *J. Controlled Release*, *6*:297 (1987).

72. J. S. Vrentas, C. M. Jarzebski, and J. L. Duda, *AIChE J.*, *21*:894 (1975).

73. S. Joshi and G. Astarita, *Polymer*, *20*:827 (1979).

74. G. W. R. Davidson, III, and N. A. Peppas, *J. Controlled Release*, *3*:243 (1986).

75. G. W. R. Davidson, III, and N. A. Peppas, *J. Controlled Release*, *3*:259 (1986).

76. N. A. Peppas and R. W. Korsmeyer, in *Hydrogels in Medicine and Pharmacy, Volume III, Properties and Applications* (N. A. Peppas, ed.), CRC Press, Boca Raton, Fla., 1987, pp. 109–135.

77. A. S. Carslaw and J. C. Jaeger, *The Conduction of Heat in Solids*, 2nd ed., Clarendon Press, Oxford, 1959.

78. H. Fujita, in *Diffusion in Polymers* (J. Crank and G. S. Park, eds.), Academic Press, London, 1968, pp. 75–104.

79. E. L. Cussler, *Diffusion: Mass Transfer in Fluid Systems*, Cambridge University Press, Cambridge, 1984, pp. 32–35.

80. H. L. Frisch, *Polym. Eng. Sci.*, *20*:2 (1980).

81. C. E. Rogers, in *Physics and Chemistry of the Organic Solid State*, Vol. II (D. Fox, M. M. Labes, and A. Weissberger, eds.), Interscience, New York, 1965, pp. 509–635.

82. T. Alfrey, E. F. Gurnee, and W. G. Lloyd, *J. Polym. Sci.*, *C12*:249 (1966).

83. A. Peterlin, *Polym. Eng. Sci.*, *20*:238 (1980).

84. D. J. Enscore and H. B. Hopfenberg, *Polym. Eng. Sci.*, *20*:102 (1980).

85. A. R. Berens and H. B. Hopfenberg, *Polymers*, *19*:489 (1978).

86. J. Crank, in *Diffusion in Polymers* (J. Crank and G. S. Park, eds.), Academic Press, London, 1968, pp. 1–37.

87. J. L. Duda and J. S. Vrentas, *AIChE J.*, *17*:464 (1971).

88. J. H. Petropoulos and P. P. Roussis, *J. Membr. Sci.*, *3*:343 (1978).

89. P. I. Lee, *J. Controlled Release*, 2:277 (1985).
90. J. Crank, *J. Polym. Sci.*, 11:151 (1953).
91. P. I. Lee, in *Controlled Release Technology: Pharmaceutical Applications* (P. I. Lee and W. R. Good, eds.), ACS Symposium Series 348, American Chemical Society, Washington, D.C., 1987, pp. 71–83.
92. J. H. Petropoulos, *J. Polym. Sci., Polym. Phys. Ed.*, 22: 1885 (1984).
93. D. Richman and F. A. Long, *J. Amer. Chem. Soc.*, 82:509 (1960).
94. F. A. Long and D. Richman, *J. Amer. Chem. Soc.*, 82:513 (1960).
95. A. Kishimoto and T. Kitahara, *J. Polym. Sci. A1*, 5:2147 (1967).
96. T. T. Wang, T. K. Kwei, and H. L. Frisch, *J. Polym. Sci. A2*, 7:2019 (1969).
97. N. A. Peppas and J. L. Sinclair, *Colloid and Polym. Sci.*, 261:404 (1983).
98. A. Peterlin, *J. Res. NBS*, 81A:243 (1977).
99. C. Gostoli and G. C. Sarti, *Polym. Eng. Sci.* 22:1018 (1983).
100. G. C. Sarti, *Polymer*, 20:827 (1979).
101. C. Gostoli and G. C. Sarti, *Chem. Eng. Commun.*, 21:67 (1983).
102. N. L. Thomas and A. H. Windle, *Polymer*, 23:529 (1982).
103. J. H. Petropoulos and P. P. Roussis, *J. Polym. Sci.*, C22: 917 (1969).
104. J. S. Vrentas and J. L. Duda, in *Encyclopedia of Polymer Science and Engineering*, Vol. 5, 2nd ed. (H. F. Mark, N. M. Bikales, C. G. Overberger, G. Menges, and J. I. Kroschwitz, eds.), John Wiley, New York, 1987, pp. 36–68.
105. P. L. Ritger and N. A. Peppas, *J. Controlled Release*, 5:23 (1987).
106. L. H. Lyu and S. H. Gehrke, unpublished data, University of Cincinnati, 1988.
107. T. Tanaka, E. Sato, Y. Hirokawa, S. Hirotsu, and J. Peetermans, *Phys. Rev. Lett.*, 55:2455 (1985).
108. T. Tanaka and D. J. Fillmore, *J. Chem. Phys.*, 70:1214 (1979).
109. A. Peters and S. J. Candau, *Macromolecules*, 19:1952 (1986).
110. N. Yoshio, N. Hirohito, and M. Matsuhiko, *J. Chem. Eng. Japan*, 19:274 (1986).
111. B. Kabra, *Controlling Hydrogel Swelling Kinetics*, M.S. thesis, University of Cincinnati, 1988.
112. P. I. Lee, *Polymer*, 25:973 (1984).
113. B. D. Ratner and A. S. Hoffman, in *Hydrogels for Medical and Related Applications* (J. D. Andrade, ed.), ACS Symposium Series 31, American Chemical Society, Washington, D.C., 1976, pp. 1–36.

114. S. D. Bruck, *Biomat. Med. Dev., Artif. Organs,* 1:79 (1973).

115. B. D. Ratner, in *Hydrogels in Medicine and Pharmacy, Volume I, Fundamentals* (N. A. Peppas, ed.), CRC Press, Boca Raton, Fla., 1986, pp. 85–94.

116. E. W. Merrill, R. W. Pekela, and N. A. Mahmud, in *Hydrogels in Medicine and Pharmacy, Volume III, Properties and Applications* (N. A. Peppas, ed.), CRC Press, Voca Raton, Fla., 1987, pp. 7–8.

117. E. H. Schacht, in *Recent Advances in Drug Delivery Systems* (J. M. Anderson and S. W. Kim, eds.), Plenum Press, New York, 1984, pp. 259–278.

118. F. Rodriguez, *Principles of Polymer Systems,* 2nd ed., McGraw-Hill, New York, 1982.

119. N. G. McCrum, C. P. Buckley, and C. B. Bucknall, *Principles of Polymer Engineering,* Oxford University Press, Oxford, 1988, pp. 72–88.

120. S. B. Ross-Murphy and H. McEvoy, *Brit. Polym. J.,* 18:2 (1986).

121. J. Janacek, *J. Macromol. Sci.—Revs. Macromol. Chem.,* C9: 1 (1973).

122. N. A. Peppas and E. W. Merill, *J. Appl. Polym. Sci.,* 21:1763 (1977).

123. B. J. Tighe, in *Hydrogels in Medicine and Pharmacy, Volume III, Properties and Applications* (N. A. Peppas, ed.), CRC Press, Boca Raton, Fla., 1987, pp. 53–82.

124. N. Sarkar, *J. Appl. Polym. Sci.,* 24:1073 (1979).

125. V. F. Janas, F. Rodriguez, and C. Cohen, *Macromolecules,* 13:977 (1980).

126. W. R. Good and K. F. Mueller, in *Controlled Release of Bioactive Materials* (R. W. Baker, ed.), Academic Press, New York, 1980, p. 155.

127. K. F. Mueller and S. J. Heiber, *J. Appl. Polym. Sci.,* 27: 4043 (1982).

128. H. L. Frisch, *Brit. Polym. J.,* 17:149 (1985).

129. N. A. Peppas, in *Hydrogels in Medicine and Pharmacy, Volume II, Polymers* (N. A. Peppas, ed.), CRC Press, Boca Raton, Fla., 1987, pp. 1–48.

130. W. Jarowenko, in *Encyclopedia of Polymer Science and Technology,* Vol. 12 (H. F. Mark and N. G. Gaylord, eds.), John Wiley, New York, 1970, pp. 787–862.

131. F. H. Otey and W. M. Doane, in *Starch: Chemistry and Technology* (R. L. Whistler, J. N. BeMiller, and E. F. Paschall, eds.) Academic Press, New York, 1984, pp. 389–415.

132. M. V. Sefton, in *Hydrogels in Medicine and Pharmacy, Volume III, Properties and Applications* (N. A. Peppas, ed.), CRC Press, Boca Raton, Fla, 1987, pp. 17–52.

133. E. Doelker, in *Hydrogels in Medicine and Pharmacy, Volume II, Polymers* (N. A. Peppas, ed.), CRC Press, Boca Raton, Fla., 1987, pp. 115–160.
134. D. Harsh and S. H. Gehrke, unpublished data, University of Cincinnati, 1988.
135. G. F. Fanta and W. M. Doane, in *Modified Starches: Properties and Uses* (O. B. Wurzburg, ed.), CRC Press, Boca Raton, Fla., 1986, pp. 148–178.
136. N. A. Peppas and A. G. Mikos, in *Hydrogels in Medicine and Pharmacy, Volume I, Fundamentals* (N. A. Peppas, ed.), CRC Press, Boca Raton, Fla., 1986, pp. 1–26.
137. A. G. Mikos, C. G. Takoudis, and N. A. Peppas, *Macromolecules, 19*:2174 (1986).
138. A. Charlesby, *Proc. R. Soc. London, Ser. A., 222*:542 (1954).
139. O. Saito, *Polym. Eng. Sci., 19*:542 (1979).
140. A. S. Hoffman, *Radiat. Phys. Chem., 9*:207 (1977).
141. Y. Ikada, T. Mita, F. Horii, I. Sakurada, and M. Hateda, *Radiat. Phys. Chem., 9*:633 (1977).
142. G. Odian, *Principles of Polymerization*, 2nd ed., Wiley-Interscience, New York, 1981.
143. T. Alfrey, Jr., and L. J. Young, in *Copolymerization* (G. E. Ham, ed.), Wiley-Interscience, New York, 1964, Chap. 2.
144. L. J. Young, in *Polymer Handbook*, 2nd ed. (J. Brandrup, E. H. Immergut, with W. McDowell, eds.), Wiley-Interscience, New York, 1975, pp. 387–404.
145. H. G. Elias, *Macromolecules*, Vol. 2, 2nd ed., Plenum Press, New York, 1984, Chap. 20.
146. D. E. Gregonis, C. M. Chen, and J. D. Andrade, in *Hydrogels for Medical and Related Applications* (J. D. Andrade, ed.), ACS Symposium Series 31, American Chemical Society, Washington, D.C., 1976, pp. 88–104.
147. N. Weiss and A. Silberberg, *Brit. Polym. J., 9*:144 (1977).
148. M. Wood, D. Attwood, J. H. Collett, *Int. J. Pharm., 7*:189 (1981).
149. M. Ilavsky and J. Hrouz, *Polym. Bull., 9*:159 (1983).
150. K. F. Mueller, S. J. Heiber, and W. L. Plankl, U.S. Patent 4,224,427 (1980).
151. L. Pinchuk, E. C. Eckstein, and M. R. Van De Mark, *J. Appl. Polym. Sci., 29*:1749 (1984).
152. O. Wichterle, U.S. Patents 3,408,429 (1968); 3,496,254 (1970); 3,660,545 (1972); 3,699,089 (1972).
153. B. D. Ratner, *Biocompatibility of Clincial Implant Materials, Vol. 2—CRC Series in Biocompatibility* (D. F. Williams, ed.), CRC Press, Boca Raton, Fla., 1981, p. 145.
154. D. G. Pedley, P. J. Skelly, and B. J. Tighe, *Brit. Polym. J., 12*:99 (1980).

155. P. Speiser, U.S. Patent 3,390,050 (1968).
156. M. T. DeCrosta, N. B. Jain, and E. M. Rudnic, U.S. Patent 4,575,539 (1986).
157. M. E. McNeil and N. B. Graham, J. Controlled Release, 1:99 (1984).
158. M. E. McNeil and N. B. Graham, in Controlled Release Technology: Pharmaceutical Applications (P. I. Lee and W. R. Good, eds.), ACS Symposium Series 348, American Chemical Society, Washington, D.C., 1987, p. 158.
159. K. F. Mueller, in Controlled Release Technology: Pharmaceutical Applications (P. I. Lee and W. R. Good, eds.), ACS Symposium Series 348, American Chemical Society, Wsahington, D.C., 1987, p. 139.
160. K. F. Mueller and W. R. Good, U.S. Patent 4,192,827 (1980); 4,277,582 (1981); 4,304,591 (1981).
161. K. F. Mueller and S. J. Heiber, U.S. Patent 4,423,099 (1983).
162. P. I. Lee, J. Pharm. Sci., 73:1344 (1984).
163. P. I. Lee, U.S. Patent 4,624,848 (1986).
164. S. W. Kim, T. Okano, Y. H. Bae, R. Hsu, and S. J. Lee, Hydrophilic-hydrophobic balanced polymers for controlled delivery of drugs, Proc. 14th Int. Symp. Controlled Release of Bioactive Materials, Toronto, 1987, pp. 37–38.
165. J. Kost, T. A. Horbett, B. D. Ratner, and M. Singh, J. Biomed. Mat. Res., 19:1117 (1985).
166. T. A. Horbett, J. Kost, and B. D. Ratner, in Polymers as Biomaterials (S. W. Shalaby, A. S. Hoffman, B. D. Ratner, and T. A. Horbett, eds.), Plenum Press, New York, 1984, pp. 193–207.
167. B. A. Firestone and R. A. Siegel, Swelling equilibrium and kinetics in pH-sensitive hydrophobic copolymer membranes, Proc. 14th Int. Symp. Controlled Release of Bioactive Materials, Toronto, 1987, pp. 81–82.
168. A. S. Hoffman, A. Afrassiabi, and L. C. Dong, J. Controlled Release, 4:213 (1986).
169. L. C. Dong and A. S. Hoffman, J. Controlled Release 4:223 (1986).
170. J. Heller, in Polymers as Biomaterials (S. W. Shalaby, A. S. Hoffman, B. D. Ratner, and T. A. Horbett, eds.), Plenum Press, New York, 1984, pp. 167–179.

Chapter 9

MANUFACTURING OF A MULTILAYER MATRIX SYSTEM FOR TRANSDERMAL DRUG DELIVERY

Jürgen Maass

LTS Lohmann Therapie-Systeme GmbH & Co., KG, Neuwied,
Federal Republic of Germany

I. INTRODUCTION

Matrix systems contain the drug dispersed in a polymeric matrix.
They are pressure-sensitive self-adhesive devices, which guarantee
a controlled release of the drug during application. Their stickiness
has to be adjusted to provide sufficient contact between the drug
delivering surface of the transdermal therapeutical systems (TTS)
and the skin, so it cannot be lost during the period of application.
On the other hand, it must not damage the skin upon removal of the
system. These properties can be achieved by single- or multilayer
matrix systems. In contrast to single-layer systems, in multilayer
systems the drug content in the individual layers may vary in concentration and saturation.

In this chapter the manufacturing procedure for a multilayer matrix
system (Fig. 1) will be described. This multilayer matrix system is
distinguished by an increasing drug content from the surface layer
to the main reservoir layer and it is known for its properly controlled
drug release.

The art of manufacturing is basically derived from known coating
technologies for medical adhesive tapes or wound patches. For transdermal systems the manufacturing technology had to be adapted to
Good Manufacturing Practice (GMP) standards common in the pharmaceutical industry.

The manufacturing procedure can roughly be devided into steps
as shown in Fig. 2.

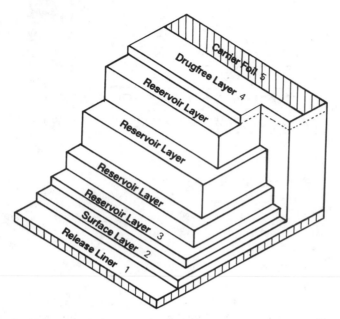

Figure 1   Model of a multilayer matrix system.

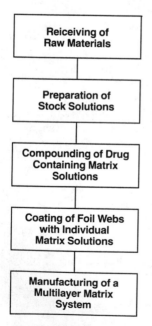

Figure 2   Manufacturing procedure for a multilayer matrix system.

II. PREPARATION OF MATRIX SOLUTIONS

One way the prepare drug-containing matrix solutions is based on
stock solutions of the different raw materials in organic solvents.
Preferably the different matrix solutions for a multilayer system consist of the same basic ingredients, such as base polymers, softening
agents, tackifiers, inert fillers, dyes, etc. The individual stock
solutions can be compounded as formulated to a matrix solution. The
active ingredients normally are added separately.

Necessary equipment such as kneaders for base polymers and
dissolvers for other solid or liquid raw materials, as well as pumps,
filters, storage tanks, and piping, are employed for only one raw
material or stock solution.

While most raw materials can normally be dissolved directly without
further processing, the base polymer has to undergo a pretreatment.
Polymers are delivered in blocks of approximately 25 kg weight. To
reduce dissolving times the surface of these compact blocks has to be
increased either by chopping them into small pieces or by milling the
blocks into flat sheets in a two-roller mill (see Fig. 3).

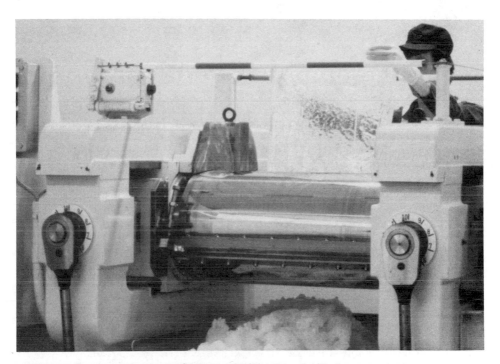

Figure 3 Calandering of base polymers.

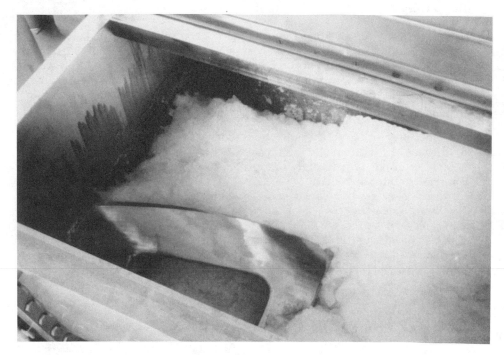

Figure 4 Kneading of base polymers with organic solvent.

In a double Z kneader (Fig. 4), the chopped or milled polymer sheets are overlaid with organic solvents and allowed to swell before they are kneaded. This is done in intervals—swelling, kneading, etc., until a homogeneous, colorless, and clear polymeric solution is obtained. This solution is pumped via a filter into storage tanks. All these procedures have to be performed under controlled conditions in a validated process to guarantee the molecular integrity of the polymer.

Preferably, two storage tanks are used for each stock solution (see Fig. 5). While the content of one tank is released for production by the quality assurance laboratory, the content of the other tank is under quarantine.

Each matrix solution has its own formulation, depending on the design of the multilayer matrix system. The matrix solutions are compounded from different amount of the polymeric stock solutions according to these formulations. The active principle generally is added separately as a solution or as crystals, or adsorbed to an inert bulking agent such as, for example, nitroglycerol adsorbed to lactose. The batch size for a matrix solution or suspension depends

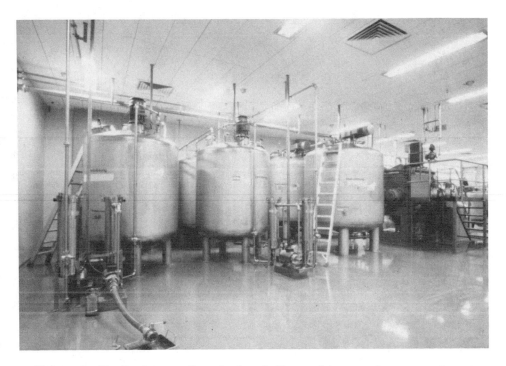

Figure 5 Tank storage for stock solutions of base polymers and other raw materials.

on the planned thickness of the layer, its content of solid material, and the area of substratum planned to become coated in one production step. Figure 6 shows a typical compounding room. The final matrix solution is checked for its content of active substance, solid content, and viscosity before it is released for further processing. To manufacture a multilayer matrix system as described in the following, five different matrix solutions are necessary. For each matrix solution a separate container should be used, which is reserved for only one solution formulation (see Fig. 7).

III. COATING PROCEDURE

Coating is performed in a specially designed coating machine, which consists basically of three units: the coating head, the drying tunnel, and the laminating device (see Fig. 8). These main units are complemented by helper units such as winders.

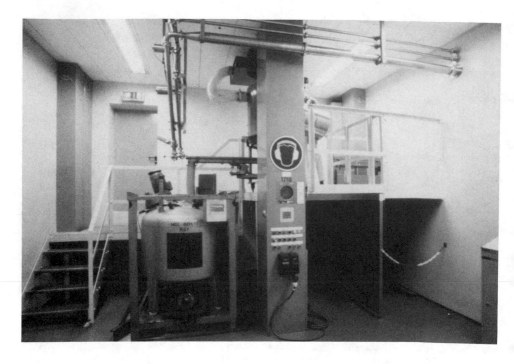

Figure 6 Compounding room.

During production, foil or paper webs as substrata are covered
with layers of the matrix solution or suspension. The organic solvent
is evaporated by heat and removed by intensive ventilation.

Because each matrix layer is manufactured individually, the order
of coating depends on the design of the multilayer matrix system.
The coating procedure thus may begin with the layer next to the
skin and all following layers are laminated one upon the other.

The coating head is constructed as a reverse-roller coater that
has to work very precisely. The working principle of this type of
coater can be described as follows (Fig. 9). Two rollers of different diameters with polished surfaces are required. The bigger main
roller is partly surrounded by the web. The smaller roller is
equipped with a knife. Both rollers form a trough with a gap that
can be adjusted to an accuracy of 0.01 mm. The trough is filled with
the matrix solution or suspension. The main roller is synchronized
with the drive of the coating engine. The reverse roller rotates
in the same direction but at a different speed. Through the gap a
defined amount of matrix solution or suspension is spread over the
substratum. Due to its viscosity the solution or suspension does
not form drops, an even layer is achieved.

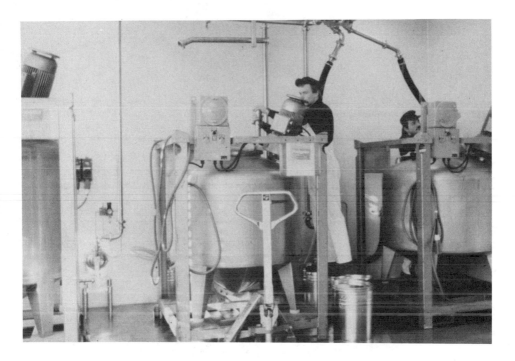

Figure 7 Stirring container for matrix solutions or suspensions.

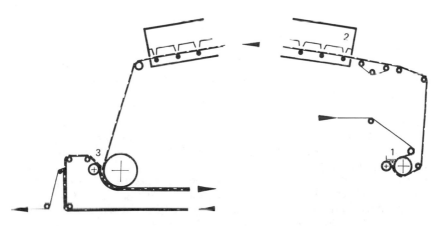

Figure 8 Coating machine working principle: (1) coating head; (2) hot-air dryer; and (3) laminating device.

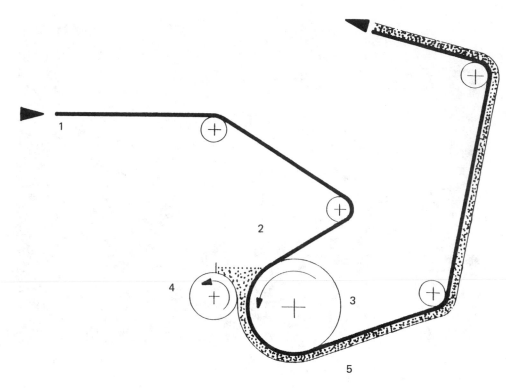

Figure 9 Coating head: (1) foil web; (2) matrix solution; (3) main roller; (4) reverse roller; and (5) coated foil web.

In practice, for a multilayer system with a total matrix weight of 300 g/m^2, a coating accuracy of ± 5 g/m^2 is necessary to obtain the requested release profile.

As mentioned previously, the described multilayer system consists of five individually made layers of different weights from 20 g/m^2 to 200 g/m^2. For each layer, the coating gap has of course to be adjusted again. Because evaporation of organic solvents and even of active substances may take place in the coating unit, the unit is completely cased and thus hermetically closed to the surrounding environment. The casing of the coating unit is connected directly with the drying system.

The individual matrix layers are dried by removing the organic solvents of the matrix solution or suspension by evaporation. This is achieved by running the coated web through a drying tunnel or drying oven (see Fig. 10).

Different systems of drying tunnels exist. Most common is a system known as a high-performance air-nozzle dryer, which works ac-

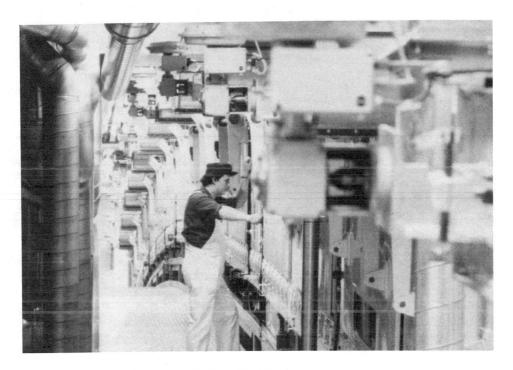

Figure 10 Drying tunnel (length 48 m).

cording the following principle (see Fig. 11). Cleaned, conditioned
air is blown through air nozzles onto the surface of the freshly manufactured matrix layer. The fresh air is loaded with vapors or organic solvents and is removed afterwards. To prevent environmental
pollution with organic solvents, the air from the drying oven is
cleaned by incineration.

To achieve optimal drying of matrix layers, i.e., to achieve the
specified content of residual organic solvent in the layer without
affecting the content of the active ingredient, the dryer should be
divided into sections that can be controlled individually. Such a
drying tunnel normally consists of several (e.g., 12) sections, which
are connected directly to each other. To prevent contact of the
matrix with any part of the drying tunnel, it is arched. The coated
foil web is moved through the drying tunnel by a system of driven
idler rollers. To meet GMP requirements the dryer is internally
made completely from stainless steel and can be taken to pieces and
cleaned easily.

In each section of the dryer, several parameters can be adjusted
individually and are controlled by a sophisticated system of control

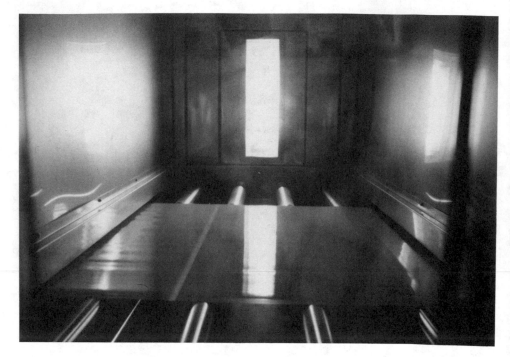

Figure 11 View into the drying tunnel.

and recording mechanisms. The following parameters are controlled and recorded:

Temperature
Air flow
Percentage of organic solvent in the air
Speed of the engine
Tension of the foil web

These technical features are necessary to develop "drying profiles," which are optimized for the drug, the individual matrix solutions, and coating weights (see Fig. 12). Thus a comprehensive validation procedure for each matrix layer is necessary. Besides these production data, safety regulations concerning the drug and organic solvents have to be considered. For example, the amount of organic solvents in the air must not exceed 50% of the lower explosion limit, and the temperature of any part of the drying tunnel must not exceed 54°C because nitroglycerol is an active ingredient.

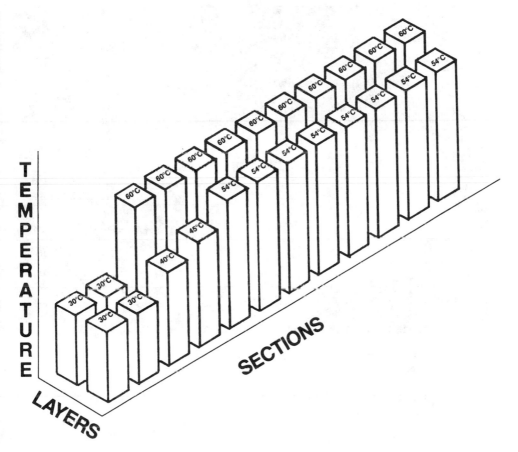

Figure 12 Drying profiles of two different layers.

To allow continuous running of the coating machine the substratum is available in big rolls—so-called jumbo rolls (see Fig. 13). Depending on the thickness of substratum, the jumbo roll consists of webs of approximately 3.000 to 5.000 m in length.

The web is wound off from the rolls in the unwinding stand (Fig. 13). It is then put through the coating and drying system to a winding stand at the end of the drying channel where the coated web is wound up.

As the matrix is self-adhesive, special precautions must be taken to avoid hazards to the matrix. There are two techniques for winding substrata coated with a self-adhesive matrix: Wind it in itself, and wind the matrix covered with an intermediate protective foil web.

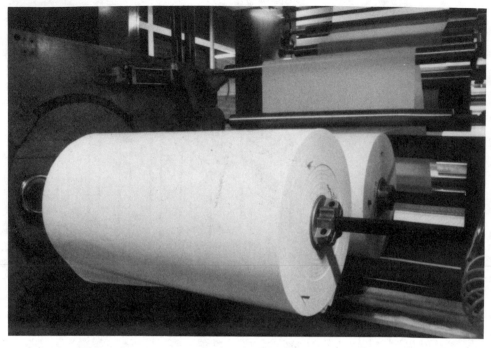

Figure 13   Jumbo roll in an unwinding stand.

To wind a coated web in itself, both surfaces of the web have to be provided with releasing properties of different strength. In this way an unwanted transfer of the adhesive layer to the reverse side of the foil web is prevented.

Another way to prevent unwanted transfer of an adhesive layer is to apply an intermediate protective foil. This method is more expensive, but it is safer. If production starts with the layer next to the skin, the substratum serves as a final covering foil and has to be removed prior to application. Therefore it has to be provided with a dehesive silicone film. The releasing properties of the substratum and the protective foil web have to be adjusted carefully to prevent unwanted transfer of the matrix from the substratum to the covering foil.

IV.   LAMINATING PROCEDURE

In this section a procedure will be described that starts with the matrix layer next to the skin, to so-called skin layer. It is on a foil web that is aluminized to prevent unwanted uptake of the drug.

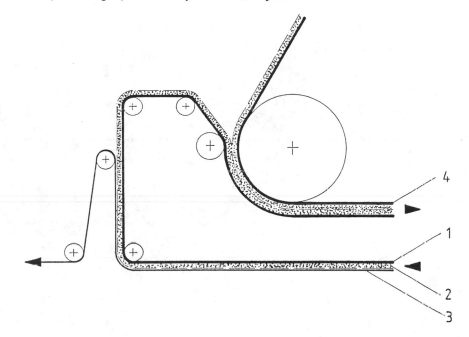

Figure 14 Laminating unit: (1) partly built-up multilayer system; (2) removed protective web; (3) coated and dried web; and (4) multilayer system.

The skin layer is covered with an intermediate protective foil, which is removed when the lamination procedure begins.

The second layer is laminated to the skin layer after removing the protective foil. The substratum of the second layer then serves as a protective foil. This procedure is continued; the third layer is laminated to the surface of the two-layer matrix after removing the protective foil, and so on until a matrix of six or more layers is built up.

These production steps are performed in the laminating unit (Fig. 14). Two rollers—one coated with rubber, the other made from steel with a polished surface—are pressed together with the laminate in between.

The line pressure of the two counter-rotating roller can be adjusted. The sensitive matrix layers, only a few micrometers thich, can be destroyed easily if the pressure is too high. If the pressure is too low, poor adhesion between the two layers will result. In both cases the laminate cannot be used.

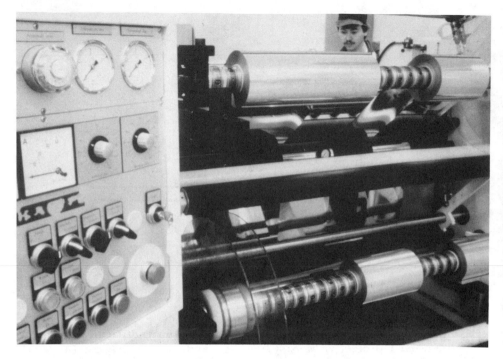

Figure 15 Slitting machine.

The speed of all units of the coating machine must be synchronized carefully in order to prevent varying web tensions. After completing the laminating procedure, a bulk product is received that is
wound up in the form of big rolls—so-called jumbo rolls.

With increasing thickness of the multilayer matrix, the weight
increases correspondingly. At a certain matrix weight, gravity may
destroy the matrix if it is stored in jumbo rolls. In this case the
jumbo roll has to be cut into smaller rolls, which can be stored lying
on the flat side. This is performed in a slitting machine (Fig. 15).

The width of the small rolls is product-specified, which means
that it is determined by the size of the final product.

V. SEPARATING AND PACKING OF
   TRANSDERMAL SYSTEMS

The individual TTS are punched or cut from the small rolls. For
this production step, specially designed, custom-made machines are
used, which punch patches with surfaces of high precision to guar-

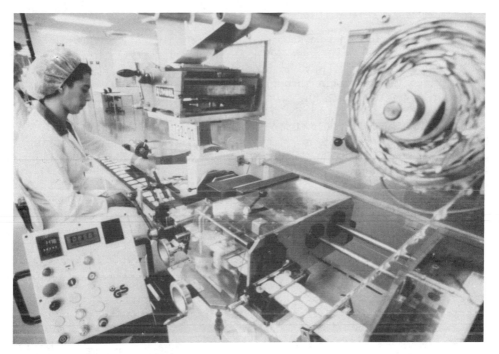

Figure 16   Machine to punch out the systems.

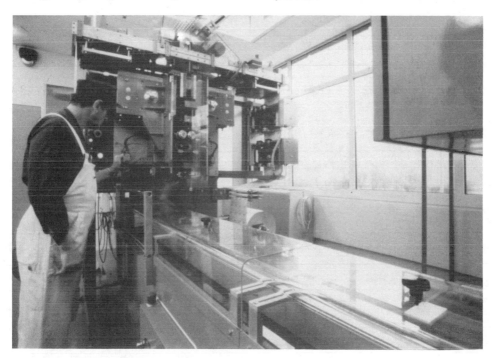

Figure 17   Sealing machine for four-cornered pouches.

antee the requested release rate. The protective foil of the last layer normally is exchanged for a skin-colored carrying foil.

There are several ways to produce single systems. One way is to punch the size right through the matrix and the foil webs. Another way is to punch the size of the system only through the carrying foil and the matrix and make a pre-cut into the protective foil. In that case, laminate in the form of a ladder around the system has to be removed. The isolated systems lay on the backing foil, which is cut to single patches. The backing foil then serves as a release liner. Figure 16 shows a machine used to punch out the systems.

Following separation of the TTS into single patches, they are sealed into four-cornered pouches and packed into cardboard boxes. These production steps are done with machines such as the one shown in Fig. 17.

Chapter 10

SOFTGELS: MANUFACTURING CONSIDERATIONS

Paul K. Wilkinson

Mediventure, Inc., Ann Arbor, Michigan

Foo Song Hom

R. P. Scherer Corporation, Ann Arbor, Michigan

I. THEORY AND HISTORICAL PERSPECTIVE

The need for encapsulation of liquids, semisolids, and pastes within
a gelatin shell in such a way as to preclude uncontrolled leakage has
resulted in the development of a very functional dosage form: the
soft gelatin capsule. The first version was developed in the middle
of the nineteenth century. While an arduous and not particularly
accurate process initially, the current manufacture is fully automated,
with a high degree of precision. In modern times the manufacture
of what were formerly known as soft elastic gelatin (SEG) capsules
has been championed by specialist companies.

The *softgel* [the currently accepted nomenclature adopted by the
SoftGel Association (SGA)] is a one-piece, hermatically sealed soft
gelatin shell containing a liquid, a suspension, or a semisolid [1].
The name change for this specialized dosage form was made to em-
phasize the differences between the soft gelatin capsule dosage form
and the conventional two-piece, hard-shell gelatin capsule. The
methodology for forming, filling, and sealing the capsule, a continuous process, is most cost-effective for contract manufacturers that
produce the product to the exacting standards of the client company.
The growth of this support industry is due in part to economics:
"[T] the volumes of softgels marketed [by a given company] often
does not justify [the] capital expenditure for equipment, facilities
and support personnel. Additionally, due to the nature of the production of softgels, a continuous operation of . . . [three
shifts]. . . , seven days a week is most efficient" [1].

The unique manufacturing processes involved in the preparation

lends itself to the establishment of manufacturing specialists to service the growing drug and health care industries. The earliest
patent was issued in May 1834 to two pharmacists, Mothes and Du-
Blanc, "for a capsule prepared by dipping a mercury-filled leather
sac into a solution of molten gelatin" [1]. Following solidification of
the resultant gelatin shell, the mercury-filled sac was removed (probably by pouring the mercury out of the sac). Selected medicaments
would then be instilled into the empty soft elastic gelatin shell via a
dropper. The patient-ready soft gelatin dosage form was hand-
sealed by applying molten gelatin.

Later, iron molds were developed, but this one-at-a-time manufacturing continued to be "tedious with fill variation of some 20 to
40% and yield losses of up to 20%" [1]. Even though this manufacturing method provided flexibility in therapeutics because the empty
shells could be filled with patient-specific medication, the soft gelatin
capsule was not a particularly commercially viable dosage form.

A. Plate Method

The first methodology to make softgels a vaible commercial entity was
the plate method. This method, utilizing a matched set of metallic
plates with multiple cavities, is a batch process. Each capsulation
machine consists of two stations. The operators must coordinate
their movements and speed, since each has to complete the capsulation process started by the other [2]. Briefly, the Unicap manufacturing process shown in Figs. 1 through 8 is as follows:

> As gelatin mass passes over a large cooled drum, a 0.034" gel
> sheet is formed. This sheet is lubricated and cut to fit capsule
> molds. Vacuum draws half of the gel sheet into 312 capsule mold
> cavities and each cavity is filled with vitamin mixture, or "fill."
> Operators then fold the gel sheet on top of itself and machine
> pressure seals and cuts out the completed capsules for washing
> and drying [3].

New equipment for this process is no longer available, requiring
refabrication if parts are damaged. This manufacturing method has
most recently (1/89) been phased out by The Upjohn Company in
favor of current (rotary die) methods [2].

B. Continuous Methods

In 1933 the method for softgel manufacture that was to become the
international benchmark was invented by a young engineer, Robert
Pauli Scherer. His idea for the unique delivery system was sound:
"the capture of a liquid in a soluble and pliable membrane" [4].
The rotary die machine, a continuous (automatic) process of encap-

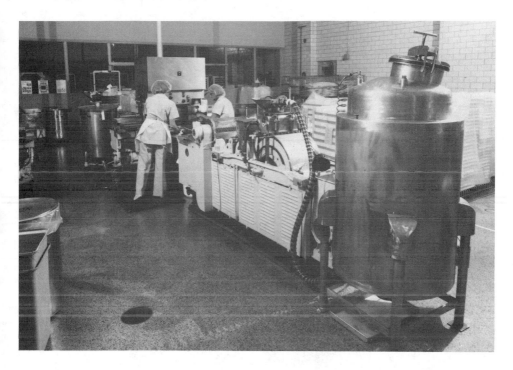

Fig. 1 Plate method: A capsulation line with the gelatin mass tank at the near end and the fill tank at the far end on the right. (Courtesy of The Upjohn Company, Kalamazoo, Mich.)

sulation, permitted for the first time large-scale commercial manufacture of soft gelatin capsules with liquid centers (fills). The original R. P. Scherer rotary die encapsulation machine (Fig. 9) is on permanent loan to the Smithsonian Institute in Washington, D.C.

In 1948 another rotary die machine was invented by Lederle Laboratory pharmaceutical scientist Dr. Frank Stern and associates. This apparatus, the Accogel machine, which is still in use, represents an expansion of the R. P. Scherer machine in that it permitted the filling of *dry* powders into softgels formed via a rotary die mechanism [5]. Figure 10 shows the Accogel machine. The manufacturing process is as follows:

Capsules are manufactured by this equipment, using three separate rotating rolls, a measuring roll, a die roll, and a sealing roll in four continuous but distinctly separate steps:
1. Two gelatin ribbons are prepared automatically and continuously and are fed to the die roll and sealing roll. At the same time the powder blend to be capsulated is fed to the mea-

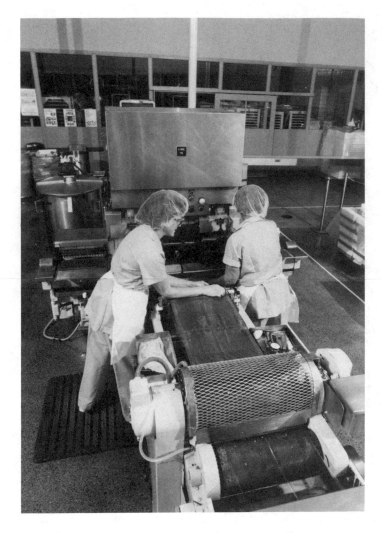

Fig. 2 Plate method: Formation of the gelatin sheet. (Courtesy
of The Upjohn Company, Kalamazoo, Mich.)

suring roll, which is accurately machined to form powder plugs
or pellets of uniform weight.

    2. The gelatin ribbon fed to the die roll is drawn into the
die pockets by means of a vacuum, thus forming one half of
the capsule. The measuring roll, geared to the die roll, deposits
the powder plug into the gelatin pocket.

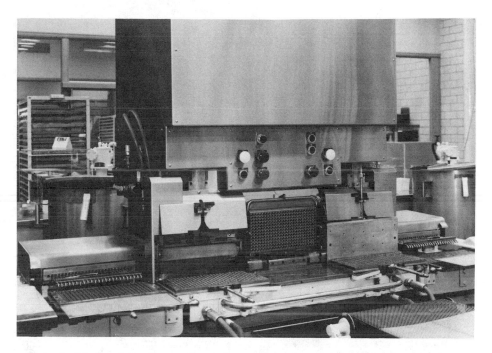

Fig. 3 Plate method: The encapsulation machine. There are two filling heads, two brushing stations, and one pressure sealing station. The filling heads, the pressure sealer, and one of the roller brushes are visible. The mesh belt bringing the gelatin sheet is seen in the lower right-hand corner. (Courtesy of The Upjohn Company, Kalamazoo, Mich.)

3. The filled die rotates immediately to the unrecessed sealing roll where the second gelatin ribbon becomes the upper half of the capsule and the capsules are then formed, sealed, and "cut out." The resulting gelatin netting is collected for possible reuse.

4. The resulting capsules are then tumbled to help shape them and treated with stearyl alcohol to prevent their sticking together. The capsules are then spread on trays for drying [6].

In 1949 the Norton Company, Worchester, Massachusetts, developed a reciprocating die machine for the continuous preparation of softgel capsules. The rights to this machine were sold to Revlon in 1975. Figures 11 and 12 show this machine and its operating sequence. "This process is again similar to the Scherer process ex-

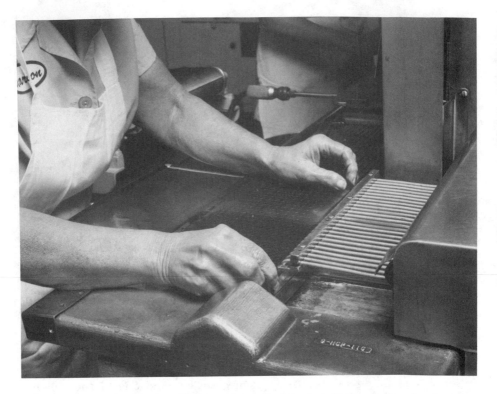

Fig. 4 Plate method: The operator is placing the gelatin sheet over
the mold cavities. (Courtesy of The Upjohn Company, Kalamazoo,
Mich.)

cept that the softgels are formed, sealed and cut out by vertically
positioned reciprocating dies. The dies first form open sheets in
the gelatin ribbon. These are filled with medicament. As the softgels pass through the dies a second time, the dies seal and cut the
softgels out of the ribbon" [1]. This machine is also suitable for
the encapsulation of metered doses of dry pelleted materials [5].

The Scherer rotary die method (Fig. 13) is one in which two
gelatin ribbons pass between twin rotating dies. As the ribbons
meet, the liquid to be encapsulated is precisely injected between
them. The capsule halves are sealed and ejected by the continuous
rotation of the dies [4]. This methodology is the basis for greater
than 90% of the encapsulating machines utilized in the worlwide production of seamed softgels.

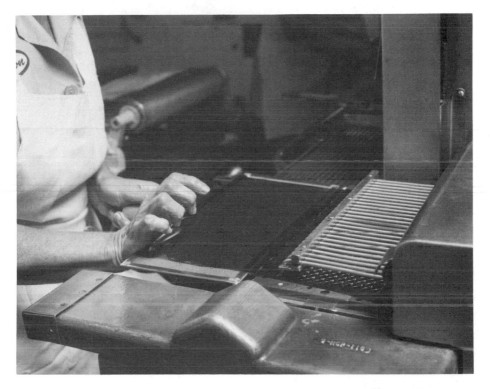

Fig. 5 Plate method: A vacuum line is attached to the mold and sucks the gelatin sheet into the cavities. The operator then pushes the mold under the filling head. Filling starts, one row at a time. The mold advances automatically as each row is filled. (Courtesy of The Upjohn Company, Kalamazoo, Mich.)

Numerous manufacturers of rotary die machines exist to support this worldwide industry. Machines are available in mini, standard, and maxi orientations with regard to die size (e.g., number of pockets across the die) and rotational speed. Examples of encapsulation equipment are often demonstrated at industrial trade shows such as Interphex USA. A partial listing of rotary die machine makers is presented in Table 1. In general, these same companies will manufacture and maintain the ancillary equipment required for support functions for softgel manufacture. Scherer machines *are not* sold, rather, self-maintained in a world-wide network of factories.

Table 1 Partial List of Rotary Die Encapsulation Machine Manufacturers

Company	Country
Banner	United States
Capsulation Services	India
Chang Saij Co.	Korea
Chang Yaij Co.	Taiwan
Cosdan	Belgium
Freund Industries	Japan
Kamata	Japan
Leiner	
Nippan Pharmaceutical Machine Works	Japan
Ped	China
Pharmacaps	United States
Pharmagel	Italy
Pharmatronics	India
Procaps	United States
R. P. Scherer	United States
Sankyo Co.	Japan
Shanghai Yenon Pharmaceutical	China

II. MANUFACTURING

A. Plant Layout

Due to the moisture sensitivity of some of the raw materials that are
utilized in the manufacture of softgels, all phases of the process—
from receiving to shipping—are under strict air quality (temperature
and relative humidity) control. Figure 14 presents a schematic layout of a typical softgel encapsulation factory as envisaged by Pharmagel spa (Italy). Figures 15 and 16 present typical air handling/dry-
ing setups used to maintain the comfort (35—50% RH) and low (20%
RH)-humidity air required in a softgel manufacturing site.

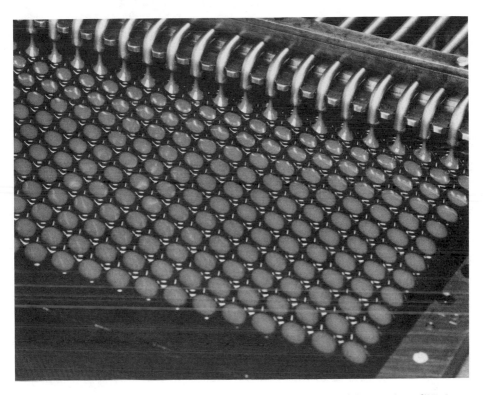

Fig. 6 Plate method: A close-up showing the cavities being filled. (Courtesy of The Upjohn Company, Kalamazoo, Mich.)

B. Materials Flow

In compliance with current Good Manufacturing Procedures, all incoming materials (actives and excipients) are placed into a quarentine area until Quality Control/Assurance (QC/A) has qualified and released them to general warehouse storage. Since most softgel manufacturing is on a contract basis, many of the incoming actives are shipped by the client and thus are known as customer-owned. The specifications (as supplied by the client) for these customer-owned raw materials are verified by the softgel manufacturer's QC/A function. Additionally, the client may choose to undertake the preparation of the medicine mixture (fill). Upon receipt, these mixtures would also enter the quarantine area. QC/A release activity may be reduced, with qualification based solely on the client's documentaiton. Bulk (tank car) shipments of critical fluids (fill oils, polyethylene

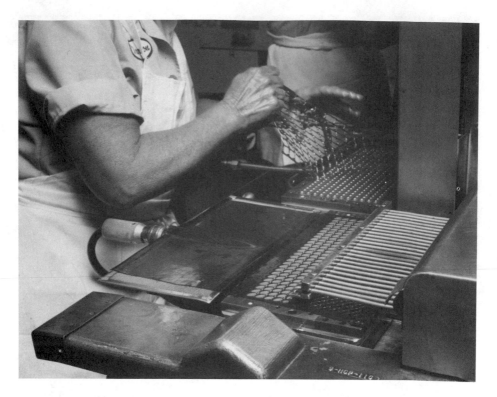

Fig. 7 Plate method: As the filling proceeds on one side of the machine, the adjacent operation is completed. This operator removes the trim from the completed capsules. (Courtesy of The Upjohn Company, Kalamazoo, Mich.)

glycol, propylene glycol, etc.) will also be evaluated. Tanker transfer (off-loading) into suitable holding tanks within the temperature/ humidity-controlled environment of the raw materials store will be permitted once the QC/A release is obtained. Smaller quantities of raw materials and excipients are stored in such fashion to ensure appropriate inventory (first-in, first-out) control as well as security control.

In response to a manufacturing master order, materials are transfered to either the gelatin preparation or medicine mix (fill) preparation areas of the plant. These two processing areas are physically separated to prevent cross-contamination and product mix-up.

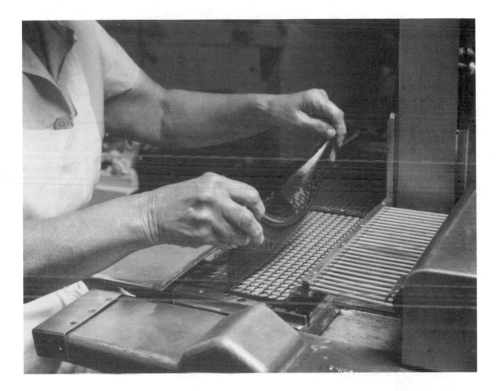

Fig. 8 Plate method: When all the cavities are filled, the operator rolls the other half of the gelatin sheet over the top of the filled cavities. The mold is pushed to the center of the machine, the top plate brought down, and the mold pushed into the pressure sealer. When the capsules are sealed, the top plate is flipped up, the vacuum is disconnected, the mold with the completed capsules is tipped up into the brushing station. The capsules are automatically brushed off and collected on trays for washing and drying. (Courtesy of The Upjohn Company, Kalamazoo, Mich.)

C. Gelatin Preparation

Various gelatin shell masses may be prepared, depending on the fill properties, climatic conditions, and end use. Alterations of the formula result in varying degrees of plasticity [7] as well as moisture level (at the time of encapsulation). While each softgel manufacturer will have its own set (highly confidential) of gelatin formulas, the basic ingredients are the same: gelatin, plasticizer(s), and water ± preservatives. The preformulation aspects of gelatin shells are

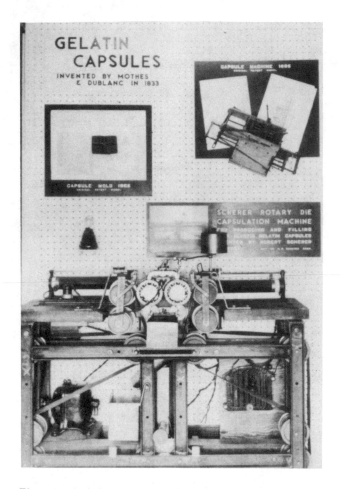

Fig. 9 Original rotary die encapsulation machine on display with other inventions of the field at the Smithsonian Institute, Washington, D.C. (Courtesy R. P. Scherer Corp., Troy, Mich.)

detailed elsewhere [1, 6−9] and are usually accomplished in consultation with a specific client.

Gelatin, a partially hydrolyzed collagen derived from the skin, white connective tissue, and bones of cattle and/or swine [10, 11], is obtained by extraction, neutralization, drying, and grinding. The physical and chemical characteristics of the gelatin are determined largely by the type of collagen used, method of extraction, pH, thermal history, and electrolyte content [1]. Compendial specifications are supplemented by such manufacturer requirements as

Table 2 Typical Shell "Hardness" Ratios and Their Uses

Hardness	Ratio dry glycerin/ dry gelatin	Usage
Hard	0.4/1	Oral, oil-based, or shell-softening products and those destined primarily for hot, humid areas
Medium	0.6/1	Oral, tube, vaginal oil-based, water-miscible-based, or shell-hardening products and those destined primarily for temperate areas
Soft	0.8/1	Tube, vaginal, water-miscible-based or shell-hardening products and those destined primarily for cold, dry areas

bloom (gel strength), viscosity (of a known concentration in water at a set temperature), iron or other heavy metals content, and microbiological status.

Hom and Jimerson [1] describe the methodology, developed by O. T. Bloom in 1925, which is still used worldwide to evaluate the strength of the crosslinking between gelatin molecules. Iron content, in the raw gelatin (collagen) or in the process water supply, is an important factor with respect to reactivity with reducing agents in the medicine mixture and the FD&C dyes used to color the shell. The bacteriological status is likewise critical, since gelatin is an excellent growth medium when stored at suitable moisture and temperature levels. Many shell formulas contain a suitable preservative (i.e., methyl and propyl parabens), while others, especially designed for the health food industry, are preservative-free.

Without a plasticizer, the gelatin shell would be too brittle. Therefore, various amounts [20—30% (w/w)] of plasticizer (e.g., glycerin, sorbitol, propylene glycol) are added to obtain the degree of plasticity desired [7]. Table 2 [9] summarizes capsule hardness as a function of the ratio of dry glycerin to dry gelatin. To ensure adequate viscosity and flexibility of the cast ribbon, the ratio of water to dry gelatin in the moltent gelatin mass is approximately 1:1 (0.7:1 to 1.3:1). Stanley [9] has grouped "other capsule additives" into three categories: (a) the amount required to produce the desired effect, (b) their effects on capsule manufacture, and (c) eco-

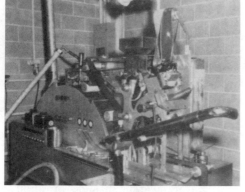

(a)

Fig. 10 Accogel machine for making softgel capsules. (a) Overview. (b) Close-up of equipment. Key: A, gelatin ribbon casting drum; B, gelatin ribbon feed; C, medicine tank; D, measuring roll; E, die roll; F, sealing roll. (Courtesy of Lederle Labs. Div., American Cyanamid Co., Pearl River, N.Y. (a) From Ref. 7 and (b) from Ref. 6, with permission.)

Table 3 Additional Components of the Gelatin Mass

Ingredient	Concentration	Purpose
Category I:		
Methylparaben, 4 parts; propylparaben, 1 part	0.2%	Preservative
FD&C and D&C water-soluble dyes, certified lakes, pigments, and vegetable colors, alone or in combination	q.s.	Colorants
Titanium dioxide	0.2–1.2%	Opacifier
Ethyl vanillin	0.1%	Flavoring for odor and taste
Essential oils	to 2%	Flavoring for odor and taste
Category II:		
Sugar (sucrose)	to 5%	To produce chewable shell and taste
Fumaric acid	to 1%	Aids solubility reduces aldehydic tanning of gelatin

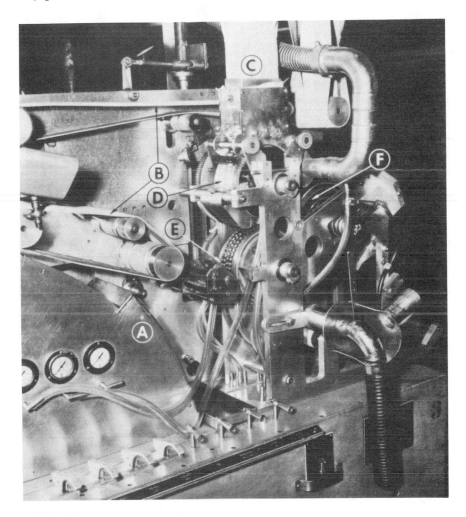

(b)

Fig. 10 (Continued).

nomic factors. Table 3 presents examples of ingredients from the first two catagories.

The preparation of a suitable encapsulation mass entails the blending of chilled (7°C) water, the desired plasticizer(s), and gelatin using immersion-type (e.g., Pony) mixers. For greatest efficiency at this mixing stage, a fairly uniform particle size (20–100 mesh) gelatin is required. If the brittle flakes of gelatin are too large, the hydration process is prolonged. A mincer (Fig. 17)

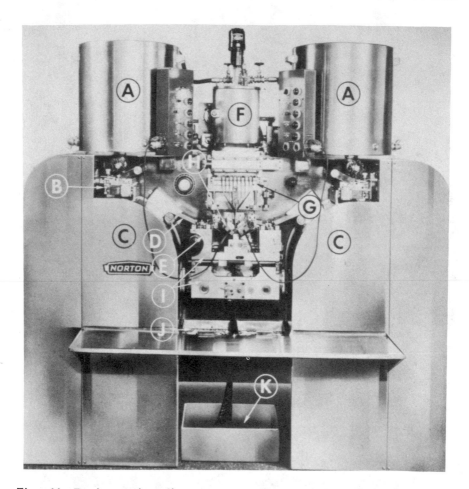

Fig. 11 Reciprocating die process equipment. A, gelatin tank; B,
spreader box; C, gelatin ribbon casting drum units; D, gelatin ribbon; E, mineral oil lubricant bath; F, medicine tank; G, filling pump
and tubes; H, gelatin ribbon heaters; I, encapsulating mechanism;
J, capsule receiving pans; K, gelatin net receiver. (Courtesy of
Machine Tool Div., Norton Company, Worcester, Mass. (From Ref.
6, with permission.)

is often used to provide a uniform particle size. The mixture is
blended (usually for 15 to 30 min for a 150-kg batch) until a light,
fluffy consistancy is obtained. When an appropriate "fluff" state is
reached, the mixture is transferred to a melter. The ultimate
product (shell) characteristics are determined by the quality of the

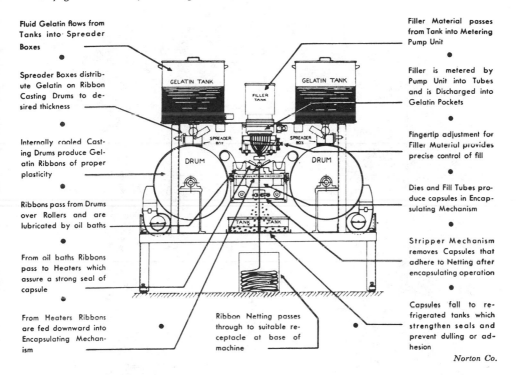

Fluid Gelatin flows from Tanks into Spreader Boxes

Spreader Boxes distribute Gelatin on Ribbon Casting Drums to desired thickness

Internally cooled Casting Drums produce Gelatin Ribbons of proper plasticity

Ribbons pass from Drums over Rollers and are lubricated by oil baths

From oil baths Ribbons pass to Heaters which assure a strong seal of capsule

From Heaters Ribbons are fed downward into Encapsulating Mechanism

Filler Material passes from Tank into Metering Pump Unit

Filler is metered by Pump Unit into Tubes and is Discharged into Gelatin Pockets

Fingertip adjustment for Filler Material provides precise control of fill

Dies and Fill Tubes produce capsules in Encapsulating Mechanism

Stripper Mechanism removes Capsules that adhere to Netting after encapsulating operation

Capsules fall to refrigerated tanks which strengthen seals and prevent dulling or adhesion

Ribbon Netting passes through to suitable receptacle at base of machine

Norton Co.

Fig. 12 Reciprocating die machine. Schematic view of the operating sequence. (Courtesy of Machine Tool Div., Norton Company, Worcester, Mass. From Ref. 5, with permission.)

"fluff." The melting of the fluffed mixture is performed in heated (electric or steam), jacketed tanks under vacuum (750 mmHg). In the melter (Figs. 18 and 19) the encapsulation mass fluff is placed onto a heated (95°C) stage that resembles an inverted colander. As the fluff melts, the entrained air is evacuated (2 to $2\frac{1}{2}$ hr at 750 mmHg), and the resultant air-free liquid drips through the holes of the plate into the receiving portion of the melter, which is maintained at 57–60°C with continuous stirring. The moltent encapsulation base is then ready for use or further processing. Visual examination of the molten fluid determines its suitability by comparison against color standards. The natural gelatin mass has an amber hue at this bulk mixing stage.

Only about 50% of the gelatin ribbon is actually formed into capsules. Reuse of the ribbon net is common and is an economic factor. The ribbon net quality is evaluated after a production run. If gross contamination is apparent, it is discarded. If suitable, the net is reprocessed by chopping (see the mincer in Fig. 17) and washing

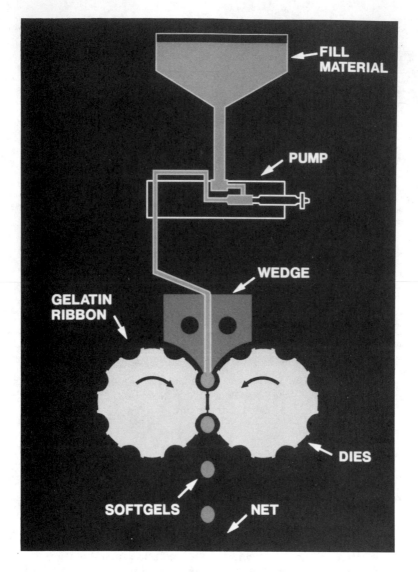

Fig. 13 R. P. Scherer rotary die process. Schematic view of the operating principles. See text for details. (Courtesy of R. P. Scherer Corp., Troy, Mich.)

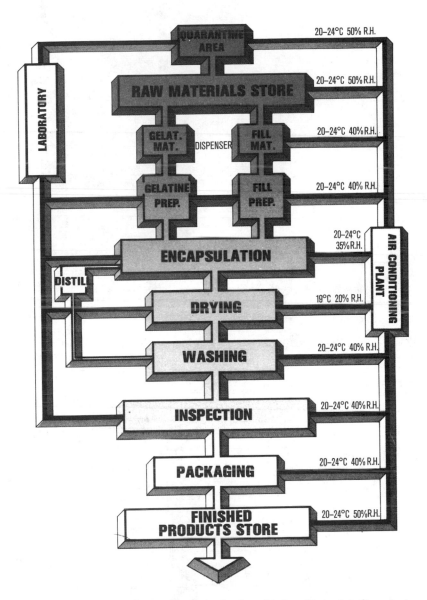

Fig. 14 Layout of a softgel capsule plant. Material flow between departments is one-way. Temperature and humidity of comfort and process air in the department is noted on the right (outflow of air-conditioning plant.) (Courtesy of Pharmagel s.p.a., Italy.)

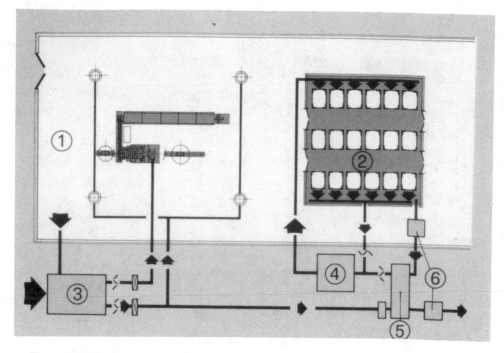

Fig. 15 Air-handling layout for a softgel capsule plant. Key: 1, encapsulating room; 2, capsule drying; 3, air-handling unit (8000 m^3/hr); 4, fan unit (12,000 m^3/hr); 5, dryer; 6, fan unit. (Courtesy of Pharmagel s.p.a., Italy.)

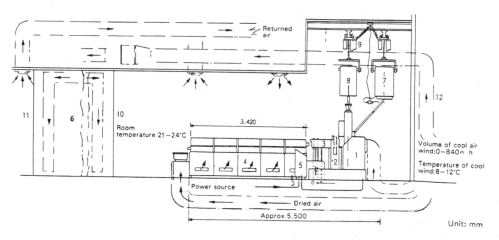

Fig. 16 Air-handling layout for encapsulation area of a softgel capsule plant. Key: 1, encapsulation machine; 2, capsule conveyer; 3, capsule washer; 4, rotary drier; 5, regulating panels; 6, drying room; 7, gelatin tank; 8, medicine tank; 9, winch; 10, air-conditioning equipment room; 11, air return filter; 12, incoming air supply. (Courtesy of Nippon Pharmaceutical Machine Works, Japan.)

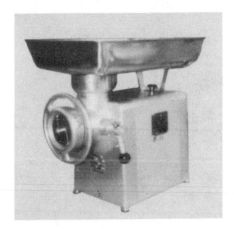

Fig. 17 Mincer for gelatin. Stainless stell blade and plate with 8-mm holes. For size reduction of raw gelatin and gelatin netting. (Courtesy of Pharmagel s.p.a., Italy.)

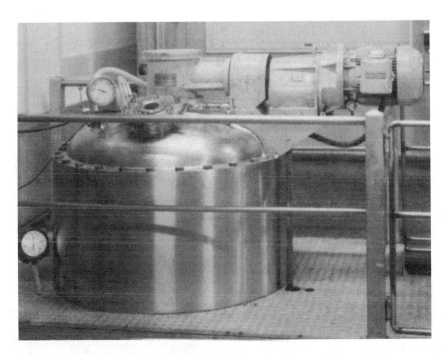

Figure 18 Melter for capsule base production. Large-volume capacity (500 liters). (Courtesy of Pharmagel s.p.a., Italy.)

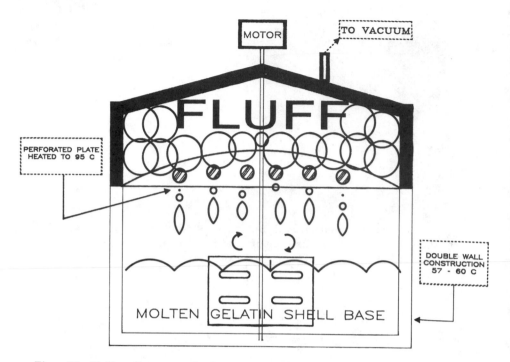

Fig. 19 Melter for capsule base production.   Schematic of melter.
Gelatin base "fluff" is added to perforated conical plate (heated to
95°C) for melting.   De-aerated gelatin base is stirred in receiver,
which is heated to 57–60°C.

with solvents such as naphtha to remove the lubricant oil (usually
mineral oil) applied during the encapsulation process.   A centrifuge
washer with solvent recovery (Fig. 10) may be used at this stage.
The clean, chopped netting can be remelted, cooled, and stored as
blocks in inventory for a short period of time (expiration dated)
until needed.   The percentage of reprocessed netting used may be
as high as 66% but is usually in the 33–50% (by weight) range
basis of the new galatin mass.   The use of reworked netting is not
usually permitted in preservative-free capsule masses.
    Depending on the needs of the operation, the gelatin mass prepa-
ration may be on a batch basis—that is, only enough capsule base
(40 to 150 liters) is prepared to satisfy a production order—or
large orders (ca. 500 liters) are prepared and subdivided to gelatin
receivers as needed.   Pigments, opacifiers, and flavorings may be
incorporated into the liquid capsule base at this stage.   High-torque
mixers placed off-center provide efficient blending without vortex

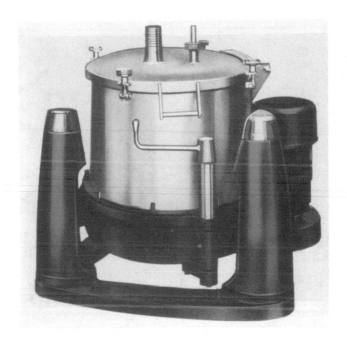

Fig. 20 Centriguge of net washing. Large-capacity (50-kg) washer
rotates at 1200 rpm to clean (naphtha wash) mineral oil from ribbon
netting prior to reworking. (Courtesy of Pharmagel s.p.a., Italy.)

and result in minimal air entrapment. The de-aerated gelatin mass
is maintained at 57–60°C in thermostated gelatin receivers until
needed in the manufacturing (encapsulation) area.

D. Medicine Mix Preparation

With the exception of the Accogel process, in which dry powders can
be encapsulated, the typical rotary die process requires a flowable
liquid. This "liquid" may be a single-phase liquid active, a mixture
of miscible liquids, or a solution or suspension of solid(s) in
liquid(s). Since the optimal sealing temperature of gelatin ribbons
(to each other) is 37–40°C, the liquid to be encapsulated should
have acceptable flow characteristics at a temperature not exceeding
35°C. If possible, the fill material should be able to flow (preferably at room temperature) by gravity. However, viscosity alone is
not the sole criterion for suitability of a fill. Glycerin (954 cP at
25°C) flows freely but is quite tacky, a property that often causes
sticking valves and pumps. High-viscosity (>3000 cP at 25°C) adhesives can be successfully encapsulated (with active pumping of
the fluid).

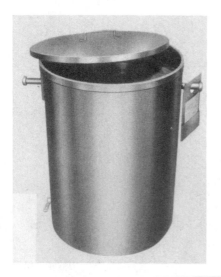 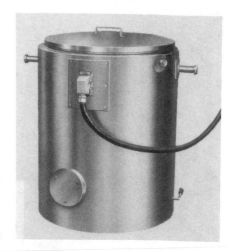

Fig. 21 Medicine tanks for use in encapsulation. These tanks are
hoisted above encapsulation machine where medicine mix is charged
(bottom discharge valve not seen) to injection pump. A, not
heated; B, with thermoregulator. (Courtesy of Pharmagel s.p.a.,
Italy.)

    Since the normal medicine mix is a free-flowing liquid or semisolid
(paste), all the normal concerns and constraints of solution, suspension, and paste manufacture must be delt with. Following blending
in a suitable vessel (e.g., 40 to 2000 liter jacketed, glass-lined or
stainless steel vessels with agitator) to ensure the wetting of all incorporated solids, milling, and/or homogenizing to break up agglom-
erates if needed, the medicine mix undergoes a special treatment not
normally applied to oral or topical liquids. The mixture is de-
aerated—much like the gelatin mass—to ensure uniformity of capsule
fill via the positive (volume)-displacement pump. Most liquids and
suspensions are de-aerated while being gently stirred to continuously expose a fresh layer of material to a vacuum (750 mmHg). This
operation may be combined with the transfer of material into the
holding tanks. If the medicine mix contains volatile liquids or agents
subject to foaming upon evacuation, passive de-aeration may be
achieved by controlled heating (without vacuum) to about 60°C for
a period sufficient to achieve the desired effects. Once de-aerated,
the medicine mix is transfered to a medicine tank (with or without
thermal regulation) (Fig. 21) and held until encapsulation is initiated.
    Consistent with in-process control procedures, samples of both
the gelatin mass and the medicine mix can be obtained for QC/A

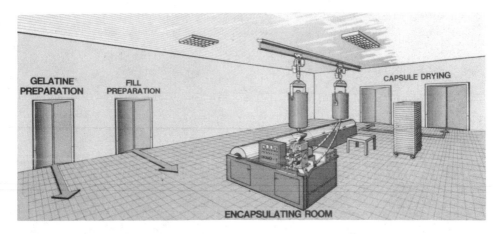

Fig. 22 Encapsulating department. Schematic of encapsulating area with orientation of incoming activity (gelatin and medicine mix) and outgoing activity (capsule drying). (Courtesy of Pharmagel s.p.a., Italy.)

evaluation. The frequency of testing should reflect the inherent stability of the formulations. To ensure traceability and confirmation of the formula, all additions (solid and liquid) should be accomplished on printomatic electronic (or PC)-controlled scales.

E. Encapsulation: Scherer Rotary Die Process

Following QC/A release of the gelatin mass and the medicine mix, the appropriate tanks are transported into the encapsulation room. Figure 22 shows the physical layout of the encapsulation room with respect to incoming material flow (gelatin and medicine mix) and outgoing material flow (capsule drying operation). Figures 23 and 24 show a typical encapsulation room during a manufacturing run.

Figure 25 presents a keyed photograph of the encapsulation process, while Fig. 26 gives a (keyed to Fig. 25) schematic. A close-up of the encapsulation mechanism (also keyed to Fig. 25) is presented in Fig. 27. The flow of the gelatin mass and medicine mix through the encapsulation process is described.

A heated receiver (A) of gelatin is suspended above the encapsulation machine. The gelatin flows through heated tubes (A1) to two spreader boxes (B) on either side of the machine. The distance of the spreader box from the casting drum (C) determines the thickness of the resultant gelatin ribbon. This micrometer-controlled distance determines (±10%) the thickness, and therefore the weight, of the dry capsule shell. The heated (57−60°C) gelatin mass is

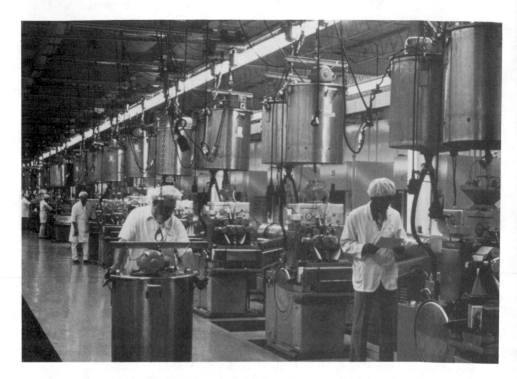

Fig. 23 Encapsulating department. Encapsulation production line.
Note hoist operator preparing medicine mix receiver for placement
above encapsulation machine. (Courtesy of R. P. Scherer Corp.,
Troy, Mich.)

metered onto the rotating, air-cooled (13–14°C) drums, where the
gelatin cools and a ribbon forms. The cast ribbon lifts off the casting drum and passes through a mineral oil lubricating bath (D),
which deposits a film of oil on both sides of the gelatin as the ribbon
advances over a series of rollers. The ribbon moves forward up
and over feed rolls and is fed between the injector wedge (G1) and
the rotating dies (G2) of the encapsulation mechanism (G).

Simultaneously with the gelatin ribbon formation, the medicine
mix receiver (E) delivers the fluid for encapsulation through a
hopper or manifold mechanism into the positive-displacement filling
pump (F). Medicine mix is metered by pump action through a
series of leads (F1) through the injection wedge (G1). Finished
softgel capsules, formed, sealed, and ejected by the action of the
rotating dies (G2), are dropped onto a capsule chute (H1), which
delivers the capsules onto a conveyor (H). The conveyor moves the

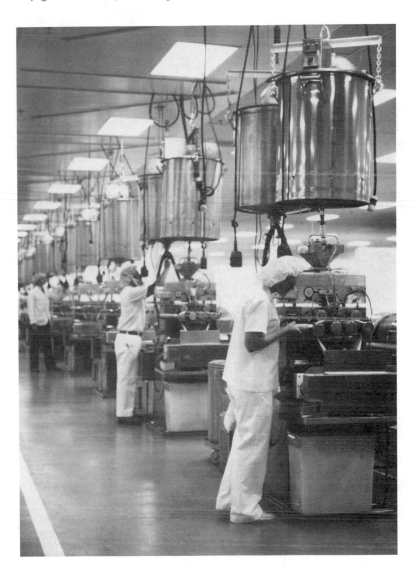

Fig. 24 Encapsulation department. Note position of gelatin receiver (rear tank) and medicine mix receiver (forward tank) at each encapsulation machine. The operator at second machine is connecting the heated gelatin tubes to the gelatin receiver. (Courtesy of R. P. Scherer Corp., Troy, Mich.)

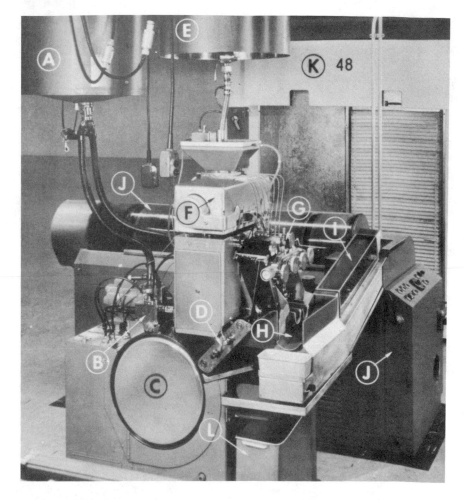

Fig. 25 R. P. Scherer rotary die encapsulation machine. See text for key and description of operation. (Courtesy of R. P. Scherer Corp., Troy, Mich. From Ref. 6, with permission.)

capsules to the dryer mechanism (J–K) after passage through a washing mechanism (I).

F. Capsule Washing

The washer (I) depicted in Figs. 25, 27, and 28 is an ascending trough partially filled with a solvent (usually naphtha) that will degrease [mineral oil lubricant added at (D)] the external surface of

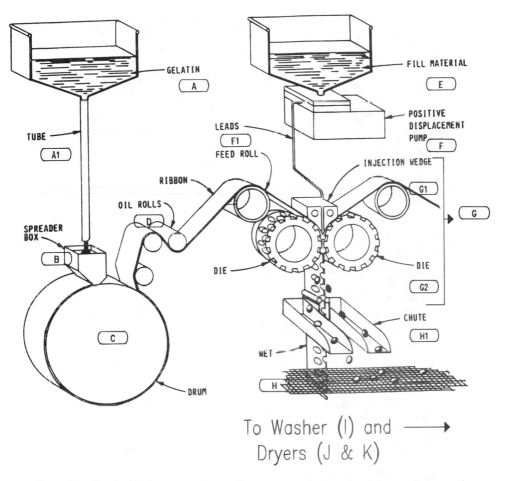

Fig. 26 R. P. Scherer rotary die encapsulation machine. Schematic
view. See text for key (same as Fig. 25) and description of operation. (Courtesy of R. P. Scherer Corp., Troy, Mich.)

the formed capsules. The capsules are transported up this incline
in a series of rotating baskets much as a ship moves through a series
of locks. The two uppermost baskets are above the solvent level and
thus permit the excess solvent to drain back into the trough before
the capsules are transported into the tumble-drying apparatus (J).
Alternative solvents (often subject to local regulatory concerns) or
mechanical degreasing (lint-free rags in a tumble drum) can be incorporated at this stage.

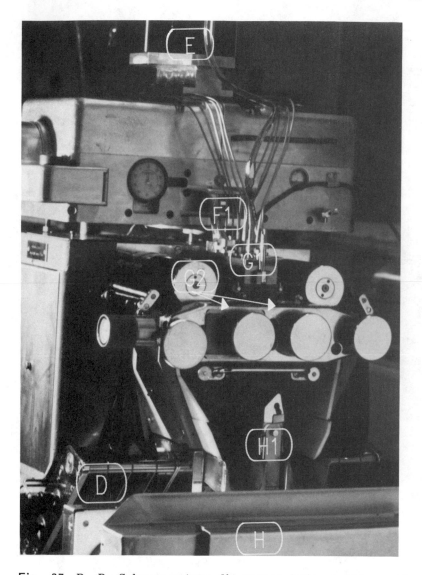

Fig. 27 R. P. Scherer rotary die encapsulation machine. Close-up of encapsulation mechanism. See text for key (same as Fig. 25) and description of operation. (Courtesy of R. P. Scherer Corp., Troy, Mich.)

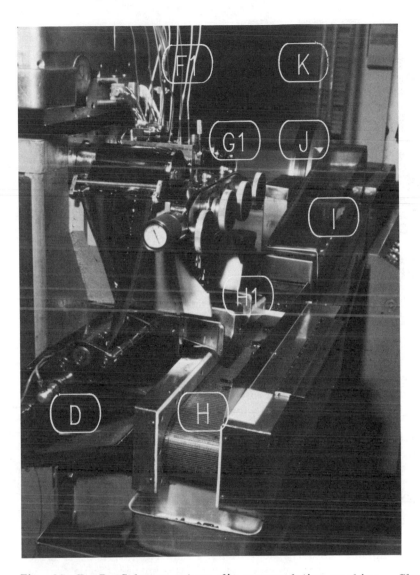

Fig 28 R. P. Scherer rotary die encapsulation machine. Close-up view of encapsulation machine with orientation of washer and driers. See text for key (same as Fig. 25) and description of operation. (Courtesy of R. P. Scherer Corp., Troy, Mich.)

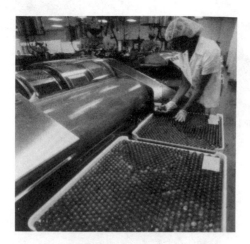

Fig. 29 Rotary die encapsulation. Softgel capsules are placed into shallow trays following removal from tumble dryer apparatus. Operator is performing visual inspection of capsules as they are being placed into trays for the drying tunnels. (Courtesy of R. P. Scherer Corp., Troy, Mich.)

G. Capsule Drying

The tumble-drying apparatus (J) traditionally is a series (four to six) of hollow drum with perforated walls. Dry air is continuously pumped through the rotating drums, and heat (air temperature < 35°C) via heat lamps may or may not be utilized as required. The warm air being blown onto the capsules appears to penetrate the shell and cause it to dry from the inside by moving the water outward to the surface of the capsule [6]. Even though the air in the forward drums is heated, the tumbling capsules never become overheated due to the evaporation of the shell moisture.

The capsules move through the drums by centrifigal force as spring-loaded half-doors are opened and closed between the rotating drums. First the doors distal to the washing trough are opened to empty the capsules into the next drum. This (distal) door is closed and the proximal door is opened to permit the entry of capsule from the adjacent drum. By the time the capsules exit this process, all of the solvent used in washing has been evaporated, and a large proportion (50–60%) of the water in the gelatin shell has been removed. Recent developments in drying have been evaluated as alternatives to the serial drums. In some instances the drum drying stage is bypassed and the capsules are prepared directly for the drying tunnel.

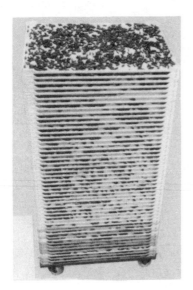

Fig. 30 Fiberglass-reinforced plastic drying trays for capsule drying. Corners of trays interlock to permit stable stacking while maintaining air flow across the surface of each tray. (Courtesy of Pharmagel s.p.a., Italy.)

As the capsules exit the last drying drum (after 90 to 180 min), they are spread on shallow drying trays lined with absorbent paper These "shallows" (Figs. 29 and 30) are constructed in such a way that air flow is possible through the stacked, interlocking trays. The final drying phase for softgel capsules is accomplished in drying tunnels (K). These tunnels are often the dividing wall between the production area and the finishing area (see Fig. 22). The stacks of shallow trays are inserted into the drying tunnels, in which controlled-temperature (21—24°C) and low-humidity (20—30%) air is continuously circulated. Warmed air (≥30°C) may also be used. Softgel capsules permitted to come to equilibrium in this controlled environment are considered "dry." The gelatin shell contains 6—10% water (depending on the specific gelatin formula used).

"Dry" capsules are obtained, depending on the fill nature, gelatin formula, and efficiency of the tumble-drying stage, within several hours (16 to 24 hr following heated tumble drying) to 3 days or more (if not tumble-dried or if "case-hardened" capsules were obtained due to inappropriate tumble-drying conditions). In-process testing of shell moisture content is performed by appropriate methods (loss on drying, Karl Fischer, toluene distillation, etc.) to ensure that the capsules have achieved the target dryness. These

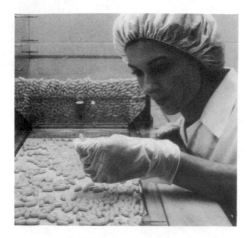

Fig. 31 Inspection of tunnel-dried capsules as they are removed from shallow trays. (Courtesy of R. P. Scherer Corp., Troy, Mich.)

tests permit the identification of "case-hardened" capsules in which a high level of shell mositure is retained even though the surface of the shell is "dry."

H. Inspection

The stacks of "dry" capsules are next transfered to the inspection area, where the "shallows" are subjected to 100% inspection. The most obvious defect detectable at this inspection is the presence of "leakers" (see Fig. 31). As the capsules are spread in a single layer on paper (prior to tunnel drying), any capsules that leak will mark the paper. As long as the shallows are handled properly and not shaken, the observation of wet spots on the paper liner correspond to leaking capsules. Any defective capsules can be easily removed for examination.

The location of the leak can be used to help determine if the capsule failed to seal properly (leak along long axis) or if there is a defect in the matched set of dies (usually end leakers). Capsule sealing results from the mechanical pressure of the die rolls (pressing the two gelatin ribbon tegether) and the heat form the wedge [1]. As noted above, the optimal sealing tempeature is 37—40°C. If the wedge temperature is too low and the roll pressure is insufficeint due to roller aligment, a poor seal will result. If the wedge temperature exceeds about 40°C, the gelatin begins to melt and becomes sticky, and clean capsule release is not achieved. Likewise, poor maintenance of the precision-tooled dies may result in unequal cutting of the capsule from the ribbon as the twin dies rotate. This will result in a leak at a point other than normal capsule sealing.

Other physical abnormalities detectable in this inspection include color or hue, soft spots (uneven drying or contact with other capsules during drying), and seam continuity. QC/A laboratory testing may include physical measurements of seal thickness, total and/or shell moisture, capsule fragility or rupture tests, and freeze and high-temperature effects as specified by the client. Hom and Jimerson [1] discuss in detail some of the more prevalent physico-chemical problems detectable during QC/A evaluation, with reformulation suggestions to resolve the problems (see Table 4).

If the softgel capsules are not to be finished immediately (due to scheduling conflicts, etc.) the capsules are transfered to deep (6-in.) trays for storage. The "deeps" are constructed in such as way that an airtight environment is created upon stacking. The tray interlock on all four sides, as compared to the "shallows," which interlock only at the corners. The "deeps" are held under optimum temperature and humidity conditions until further processing within the inspection/finishing area of the plant.

I. Finishing

Before proceding to the packaging area, softgel capsules are transported to a finishing area where special attributes may be incorporated. Capsules may be treated with 37% formalin or 10% acetone to make them easily fracturable (under finger pressure). Alternately, low-level (5%) solutions of formalin will render a softgel capsule enteric.

To maintain the high gloss or satin finish of softgels or to retard the development of stickiness, capsules may be coated (using conventional pan coaters) with substances such as stearic acid, acetylated monoglycerides, polyvinyl acetate, or high-molecular-weight polyethylene glycols. It should be noted that the effects of these coating materials on capsules is cosmetic and has no effect on the retention or loss of the equilibrium shell moisture. To ensure retention of the desired shell properties, suitable storage conditions and containers must be used.

Unique product identification is a desired attribute for any pharmaceutical dosage form. With softgel capsules, size, shape, and color aid in this critical factor. This unique dosage form is easily adaptable to direct markings with ink (roller or jetting) or "branding" [6]. This latter feature permits a permanent identification, even with additional printing. Softgels may be printed along either the long or the short axis (i.e., with or across the seam) to provide greater flexibility.

Table 4 Alphabetical List of Softgel Physicochemical Problems

Problem	Definition	Corrective action
Blooming	Visual crystallization of a solid on the shell resulting from substance migration from within. Frequently happens with Sorbitol.	Lower the thermodynamic activity of the crystallizing material.
Browning	Darkening of the shell due to the Maillard reaction, an interaction between proteins and polysaccharides. Color changes more noticeable in pastels than in darker colors.	Proper galatin selection, color selection, and rapid drying.
Color bleeding	Color transfer in two-tones. Blue colors especially prone to diffuse.	Selection of the gel formula, color system, and proper drying conditions.
Color change	Rapid change due to improper drying. FD&C Blue No. 2 is particularly unsuitable for use.	Proper drying and packaging.
Leakers	Seepage of fill material through shell. Polar leakage-corrosive incompatibility of materials. Seam leakers—poor sealing. Overfilling creates internal pressure. Slow drying weakens seal. Improper pump timing—entrapment of fill material in seal.	Reformulation of fill or shell, adjustment of encapsulation machine.

Table 4 (Continued).

Problem	Definition	Corrective action
Migration of components	Not a problem as long as it does not cause blooming, sweating, or brittle shells.	Reformualtion
Pellicle formation	Thin, fragile sac of gel left after most of shell has dissolved. May retain their contents and exhibit little or no dissolution. Known to develop in softgels containing lemon oil, perfumes, certain herbal extracts, creosote, and alkaline materials.	Little or no effect on bioavailability. May affect dissolution results.
Separation of fill	Suspensions solids precipitate	Add thickener or increase viscosity or density of the vehicle.

Final physical control processing and packaging may be accomplished by the following operations, conducted either in a batch mode or as a continuous in-line procedure.

1. A capsule diameter sorter (Fig. 32) allows passage to the next unit of any capsule within ±0.020 in. of the theoretical diameter of the particular capsules being tested. Overfills, underfills, and "foreign" capsules are discarded. The unit is fed from a hopper, and the capsules are passed through a final naphtha washing unit (Fig. 33) just prior to the sorter. The unit employs a syntron vibrator, which is a series of divergent wire lanes, and can be used for capsule diameters ranging from 0.200 to 0.500 in.
2. A capsule color sorter is the next unit in line. The capsules are fed to it automatically from the diameter sorter by a pneumatic conveyor. In this unit, any capsule whose color does not conform to the reference color standard for that particular product is discarded, while satisfactory capsules pass immediately to an electornic counting and packaging unit.

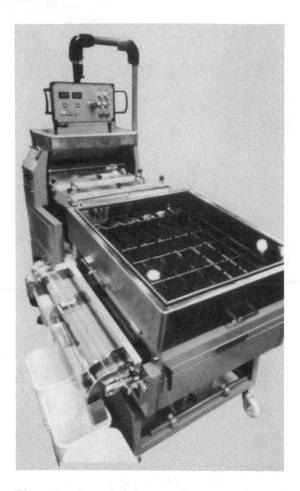

Fig. 32 Capsule-size quality control machine for evaluation the diameter of dried softgel capsules prior to packaging. (Courtesy of Pharmagel s.p.a., Italy.)

3. The electronic counting unit (Fig. 34) can count as many as 8000 capsules per minute (depending on size) directly into the bulk shipping carton, and a printout of the number of cartons is automatically produced and made part of the production record. Following this step, the cartons are labeled, sealed, and palletized and are then ready for shipment [9].

Since most softgel manufacturers are contract manufacturers, the primary packaging done is in bulk. This bulk package is only

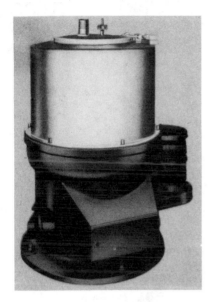

Fig. 33 Centrifuge for capsule washing. Bottom discharge of capsule onto in-line conveyor system. Capsules are provided a final
naphtha wash. (Courtesy of Pharmagel s.p.a., Italy.)

temporary protection from the normal changes in temperature and
humidity encountered during shipping. The industry standard bulk
package consists of a suitable moisture barrier (3-mil polyethylene
liner) in a standard corregated or fiberboard carton or drum. The
softgel capsules should be repackaged into suitable containers (bulk
trade bottles or unit-of-sale packages), which will provide a "permanent" vapor barrier, by the client as soon as possible to ensure
product integrity. This packaging operation and subsequent storage of bulk product, if repackaging cannot be done quickly, should
be done under the same temperature and humidity conditions maintained at the softgel manufacturer: that is, air-conditioned storage
at less than 45% RH and between 21°C and 24°C.

III. CONCLUSION

The softgel capsule dosage form is ideally suited to encapsulation of
materials that are impossible or difficult to produce in tablet or two-
piece hard-shell gelatin capsules [7]. The manufacturing process
for these one-piece, hermatically sealed (seamed) soft elastic gelatin
capsules has progressed from a one-at-a-time process with poor pre-

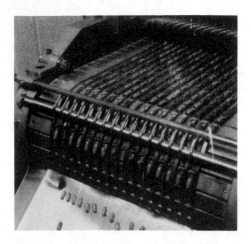

Fig. 34 Electronic capsule-counting machine capable of counting up to 8000 capsules per minute (depending on size) with automatic discharge into bulk packaging. (Courtesy of R. P. Scherer Corp., Troy, Mich.)

cision to one of several continuous processing methods, each with a high degree of precision. The reciprocating die method for powders (Accogel) or for "liquid" fill (Scherer method) is the worldwide standard of excellence in the specialized service industry of contract manufacturing. Machines of these types represent more than 90% of the machines used and manufactured around the world for the production of softgels.

IV. REFERENCES

1. F. S. Hom and R. J. Jimerson, in *Encyclopedia of Pharmaceutical Technology* (J. Swarbrick and J. C. Boylan, eds.), Marcel Dekker, New York, 1989.
2. Soft Elastic Capsule SEC Unicap Manufacturing Process, The Upjohn Company, Kalamazoo, Mich., 1988.
3. S. B. Amour, Personal communication, 1988.
4. R. P. Scherer Corporation, *Softgels—Pharmaceutical Applications,* a videotape, Scherer, Troy, Mich., 1988.
5. E. J. Rowe, in *Husa's Pharmaceutical Dispensing* (E. W. Martin, ed.), Mack, Easton, Pa., 1966.
6. J. P. Stanley, in *The Theory and Practice of Industrial Pharmacy* (L. Lachman, H. A. Leiberman, and J. L. Kanig, eds.), Lea & Febiger, Philadelphia, 1970.

7. W. R. Ebert, *Pharm. Technol.*, Oct. 1977.
8. J. P. Stanley, in *The Theory and Practice of Industrial Pharmacy* (L. Lachman, H. A. Leiberman, and J. L. Kanig, eds.), Lea & Febiger, Philadelphia, 1976.
9. J. P. Stanley, in *The Theory and Practice of Industrial Pharmacy* (L. Lachman, H. A. Leiberman, and J. L. Kanig, eds.), Lea & Febiger, Philadelphia, 1983.
10. A. G. Ward and A. Courts (eds.), *The Science and Technology of Gelatin*, Academic Press, New York, 1977.
11. A. Veis, *Macromolecular Chemistry of Gelatin*, Academic Press, New York, 1964.

Chapter 11

LARGE-SCALE PRODUCTION OF AEROSOL PRODUCTS

W. G. Gorman and Karl F. Popp*

Sterling Research Group, Rensselaer, New York

I. INTRODUCTION

Large-scale manufacture of aerosol production requires a practical understanding of chemistry, physics, and chemical and mechanical engineering, as well as Good Manufacturing Practices (GMPs). While at first somewhat overwhelming, many of the issues critical to the manufacture of this unique dosage form are similar to those encountered with other, more conventional, products such as solutions or suspensions.

On this basis, one may examine aerosol manufacture by reviewing those processes that are similar to other dosage forms, such as raw material handling, specifications, and manufacture of aerosol concentrates as extensions of the manufacturing of solutions or suspensions. Next, a look at those processes specific to aerosol products deserves attention.

Since aerosol manufacturing by its nature involves the coordination of multiple steps and variable processes, a look at the process in a general sense, followed by a definition of what aspects should be monitored and validated, should provide the reader with an understanding of aerosol product manufacturing.

Lastly, with an understanding of the technologies associated with the production of aerosol products, a discussion of the processes and issues encountered in commercial manufacturing may be comprehended.

This chapter has been assembled specifically to address issues relevant to large-scale aerosol production. In this content, it is assumed that the formulator has completed the prerequisite product development such as described in the Chemical Specialties Manufacturing Associations (CSMA) Premarketing Product Check List presented in Table 1 [1].

---

*Current affiliation: A. C. Stiefel Research Institute, Inc., Oak Hill, New York

Table 1 Premarketing Product Check

PREMARKETING CHECK LIST

The design of the check list assumes that various marketing questions have been answered and that the management of the company has decided to go ahead with the development and marketing of the product. This master check list, of necessity, refers to the broad base of all Aerosol and Aerated products and is meant to be applicable to all those currently produced and new products under development.

I. *Formulation Checks*
    1. Low temperature characteristics (stability, viscosity) of non-volatile concentrate
        a. 100°F
        b. 70°F
        c. 0°F
        d. −20°F
    2. Compatibility of non-volatile concentrate with propellant
        a. critical solubility range
        b. effect of ratio of propellant to concentrate on stability
        c. effect of temperature on stability of combination of propellant and non-volatile concentrate
            1. 100°F
            2. 70°F
            3. 0°F
            4. −20°F
    3. Specific heat of non-volatile concentrate
    4. Vapor pressure characteristics (curve below boiling point through 170°F)
    5. Specific heat of propellant (if product is cold filled)
    6. Co-efficient of expansion of completed formulation of non-volatile concentrate and propellant (giving head space requirements)
    7. Determination of flammability of product
    8. pH of product
    9. Density of product
    10. Determination of toxicity
    11. Effectiveness of product for purpose intended determined by commercially accepted techniques:
        a. Association test methods
        b. Federal specifications
        c. ASTM standards
        d. Bureau of Standards techniques
        e. FDA requirements
        f. USDA requirements

Table 1 (Continued).

II. *Container and Valve Components vs Formulation*
     Accelerated Aging at Loaboratory Level in Actual Container
     with Valve as Well as Individual Components Under Pressurized
     Glass
     1. Does product affect container?
         a. Effect on internal coating, lacquer or plate
         b. Effect on seam component
     2. Does product affect valve mechanism?
         a. Metal component
         b. Elastomeric seals
         c. Plastic components
     3. Performance of valve with formulated product
         a. Spray characteristics
         b. Spray Rate
         c. Valve action

III. *Valve and Container Selection*
     1. Suitability of container to formula (Sec II.2b)
     2. Bursting strength of container
     3. Effect of formulation on outside finish of container
     4. Susceptibility of valve to clogging
     5. Delivery rate of valve
     6. Spray characteristics of valve
     7. Valve attachment to dispenser
     8. Dip tube selection
     9. Valve testing prior to use
     10. Commercial history of containers and valves
     11. Sales appeal of container and valve
     12. Tamper-proof seal
     13. Packaging of empty dispensers (receiving cartons)
     14. Packaging of filled dispensers (shipping cartons)

IV. *Completed Products Use Test*
     1. Effectiveness of product (See Item I, II)
     2. Development of instructions and label (directions and
         cautions)
     3. Determination of odor
     4. Ease of operation
     5. Possible adverse effects on materials in home
     6. Flammability hazards
     7. Test pack for obtaining storage data at various tempera-
         tures and various positions of container during storage
         a. Effect on component parts of container and valve
         b. Changes in pressure characteristics of product

Table 1   (Continued).

IV.   *Completed Products Use Test*
      (Continued)
            c.   Changes in odor
            d.   Changes in color
            e.   Changes in pH
            f.   Effect on valve of intermittent spraying
            g.   Effect of tendency to leak
            h.   Effect on delivery rate
            i.   Possible crystallization in expansion chamber
      8.   Determination of products not exclusive of manufacturing
           cost

V.   *Manufacturing*
      1.   Bill of material
      2.   Filling processing procedure
      3.   Quality control procedure
            a.   Raw materials
            b.   Processing
            c.   Finished product
      4.   Manufacturing Cost

VI.   *Regulatory Considerations*
      1.   United States Department of Agriculture—Insecticide,
           Fungicide and Rodenticide Act. (Also State Acts)
      2.   Bureau of Explosives, Association of American Railroads,
           Interstate Commerce Commission, and Department of
           Transportation.
      3.   Food and Drug Administration—Federal Food, Drug and
           Cosmetic Act.   (Also State Acts)
      4.   Federal Hazardous Sub Labeling Act.
      5.   Child Protection Act.
      6.   State and Local Fire Regulation
      7.   State and Municipal Regulations

Thorough discussions of formulating for aerosol products for
cosmetics are available in the literature, such as the works of
Herzka [2] and Shepherd [3]. Cosmetic-class aerosols have also
been covered by Root [4], foams and emulsions by Sanders [5],
and inhalations aerosols by Gorman and Hall [6].

II. GENERAL PROCESSES OF AEROSOL MANUFACTURE

Aerosol products are recognized as specialized delivery systems and are produced by methods that, in many aspects, are similar to those for more conventional products, such as solutions or suspensions. The major difference is that aerosol manufacturing requires a propellant that generally involves a two-phase process. The first phase involves the manufacture of an aerosol concentrate such as a solution or suspension. The second phase involves combining the first phase with the necessary propellant at the time of filling. Since the manufacture of most aerosol product concentrates is accomplished using standard or generally accepted processes, as would normally be associated with the manufacture of solutions, emulsions, or suspensions, they present no truly unique manufacturing problems. The unique processes associated with aerosol manufacturing are those related to the handling and incorporation of the propellants and the handling and assembly of the container-dispensing system. Our discussion will focus on those aspects of processing that are somewhat specific to aerosol manufacturing.

In general, the issues addressed in the manufacture of an aerosol product are shown in Table 2. While the first three issues are common to many other dosage forms, several specific aspects are worthy of discussion.

A. Raw Material and Component Evaluation and Release

While the handling of material and component evaluations is generally universal, aerosol components require that special attention be given to physical dimensions and tolerances. This effort is particularly important for gaskets, moving parts, and orifices, as the failure to control any one of these specifications could result in product failure.

Care must be exercised in drawing specifications for individual components within the packaging system. Failures may result even though the integral parts meet their respective specifications, due to problems of assembly or use. This type of problem may not be obvious at first glance. However, as the assembled unit is used by the consumer and the parts wear from normal attrition, defects tend to become more obvious and accentuated.

B. Container and Packaging Component Cleaning

Cleaning of components must be accomplished so as not to alter the integrity of surfaces or gaskets. While container cleaning can be done by washing, blowing, vacuuming, etc., it is now standard practice to clean all containers before filling. Most container cleaning is done by inverting the container over a blast of dry, filtered air. Combination blowing and vacuum systems are also quite popular.

Table 2   Processes Associated with Aerosol Manufacture

A.   Raw material and Component evaluation and releases

B.   Container and packaging component cleaning

C.   Aerosol product concentrate manufacture

D.   Propellant blending or handling

E.   Aerosol product concentrate filling

F.   Propellant filling

G.   Headspace purging

H.   Valve crimping

I.   Leak testing and burst testing

J.   Spray and performance testing

K.   Actuator-Overcap Assembly

L.   Finished product evaluation and release

M.   Finishing operation, labeling, cartoner, etc.

The use of solvents should be avoided where possible, and if required, care should be taken to ensure that all solvent residues are
removed before putting the containers on the filling line.   Air-blow-
ing units must be carefully controlled, since they represent a major
potential source for introducing condensed moisture into the container
during cleaning.   Validation of any cleaning process to determine if
all detergent or solvent residues have been removed should be considered.

C.   Aerosol Product Concentrate Manufacture

Aerosol concentrates are generally solutions, suspensions, or emulsions, which are usually produced in conventional manners.   Parameters that may affect the manufacture or stability of the concentrate,
or the end product, must be identified and their tolerances established.   For example, manufacture of concentrates containing oxygen-
sensitive drugs, such as the adrenergic agent epinephrine, must be
prepared so as to remove any dissolved oxygen from the mixture
while protecting the solution or suspension from exposure to air
during handling.
      Temperature is another parameter to monitor during the manu-
facture of aerosol concentrates.   The solubility of a gas in any solvent increases dramatically as the solvent temperature decreases.

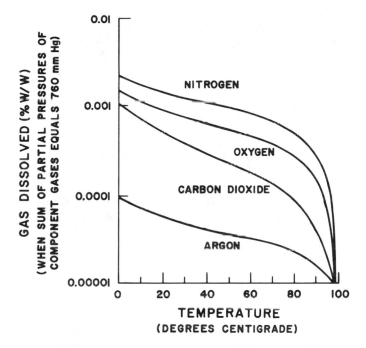

Fig. 1 Solubility of air gases in water as a function of temperature.

The concept that if a cold solution ($-10°C$) is good, then a colder solution ($-20°C$) is better is not necessarily true. Increases in the oxygen levels as a result of dissolving oxygen from the manufacturing tank headspace may occur. Figure 1 shows the effect of temperature on the amount of gas dissolved in water. Essentially, the same pattern is seen for most other solvents. Temperature may also affect the moisture content of an aerosol concentrate and the finished aerosol. Cold containers, solvents, tanks, nozzles, etc., will condense mositure from the air, possibly allowing it into product. If cold temperatures are involved in the manufacturing process, care must be taken to prevent excessive introduction of moisture. Suffice it to say that one must control and validate the processing of aerosol concentrates as one would any drug delivery system process.

III. PROCESSES SPECIFIC TO AEROSOL PRODUCTS

Successful large-scale manufacture of aerosol products results from careful attention to the details that make this specialized drug delivery system unique. Primary areas of interest involve the propellant

and the container-dispensing system. Since many of the processing
steps contain multiple variables, validation of processing parameters
is an essential element of producing high-quality aerosol products.
This discussion will focus on providing an understanding of the
various steps involved in aerosol manufacturing by examining those
process variables that may affect a product's integrity.

A. Propellant Handling

Purchased propellants are received, sampled, released, and stored
as raw materials. Quality control of propellants requires a system
for rigid and continuous inspection [7]. Storage containers, piping,
seals, pumps, etc., should all be of known composition and non-
reactive with the propellant. Safety and regulatory requirements
must, of course, be satisfied by the equipment installation.

Whether the propellants are compressed gases or volatile liquids,
several areas of concern need attention. Again, the variable elements of prime importance are discussed for each class separately.

B. Compressed-Gas Propellants

Compressed-gas propellants provide little chance for processing
variation (when used with a defined equipment assembly) other than
those resulting from temperature or pressure variations. Therefore,
pressure and temperature are measurable process variables in the
handling of compressed gases.

C. Liquefied Propellants

Processing variations could result with liquefied propellants as a
result of variations in temperature. Liquefied propellant blends
might also show in-processing variations as a result of fractionation,
especially as the storage container is depleted. Fractionation is
used here to describe a process where a mixture of volatile liquids
in equilibrium with their vapors changes in composition as a result
of differences between the vapor pressures of the liquid components.
In a mixture of volatile liquids, a more volatile liquid will vaporize
more readily than a less volatile liquid. Consequently, the vapor
phase above this liquid mixture will be richer in the more volatile
component than the underlying liquid. Thus, as vaporization occurs
during the emptying of a propellant or mixture tank, the composition of the propellant mixture may start to vary as it becomes less
concentrated in regard to the more volatile component. Figure 2
shows the composition of vapor in equilibrium with mixtures of di-
chlorodifluoromethane and trichlorofluoromethane [8]. The degree
of fractionation may be determined by direct assay of the liquid or

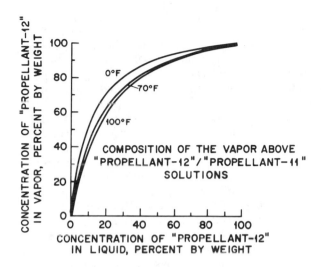

Fig. 2 Composition of vapor in equilibrium with mixtures of di-
chlorodifluoromethane (Propellant 12) and trichlorofluoromethane
(Propellant 11). (Adapted from Du Pont Freon Products Division
Technical Report FA-22, reproduced with permission of E. I.
Du Pont de Nemours and Company, Inc.)

estimated indirectly by vapor pressure. Therefore, temperature and
pressure are measurable process variables in the handling of liquefied
propellants.

D. Propellant Filling

Propellant filling is the process of adding propellant into the aerosol
product container. Propellant filling may be accomplished in several
ways, including (a) cold filling, (b) pressure filling, or (c) under-
to-cup filling.

E. Cold Filling

In cold filling, the propellant is refrigerated and added as a cold
liquid to an open aerosol product container, which is sealed after
product concentrate and propellant have been added. Whether the
propellant is added before the concentrate, after the concentrate,
or along with the concentrate, it is added as a cold liquid or slurry.
Once the procedure has been defined, processing variation can occur
as a result of weight or temperature variations. Weight variation
is readily monitored by routine checks of fill weights [9]. The effect

of temperature variation may be somewhat more subtle to assess.
Temperature variations may affect the dissolved gas (oxygen, etc.)
content in filled product. For example, gases such as oxygen are
more soluble in cold propellant than in hot propellant and, therefore, excessively cold propellant may transfer more oxygen to the
final package than warmer propellant. Excessively cold propellant
may not vaporize during filling and, therefore, not purge air from
the container headspace as might be done by a warmer propellant.
    For nonaqueous aerosol systems, the elimination of moisture
from the raw materials used to prepare the concentrate and the
finished product itself must be addressed, as the incorporation of
any moisture from any source, including condensation during processing, could cause corrosion or product instability.
    The effect of line speed may also indirectly affect cold filling.
Variations in line speed may alter container and processing temperatures. This may result in changes in fill weights and vapor
composition. Therefore, fill weights, moisture, temperature, and
line speed are measurable process variables associated with cold
filling. Figure 3 shows a typical filling line [10].

F. Pressure Filling

In pressure filling, the aerosol propellant is usually added to a sealed
aerosol product container, which previously had been filled with the
aerosol product concentrate, by forcing the propellant under pressure through the valve.
    Once the process is defined, the need for process validation
occurs as a result of variations in concentrate or propellant fill
weights. Since propellant is forced into a sealed container, residual
headspace gases may be undesirable. Headspace air may be compressed and, therefore, yield an increase in the apparent vapor
pressure of the product. The presence of oxygen in the headspace
air may also exert a detrimental effect on the product or the container. For these reasons, headspace purging is usually required
with pressure filling. While pressure measurements are definitely
desirable for an aerosol product, it is difficult to challenge or vaidate
pressure filling based on pressure measurements. Therefore, headspace purging and fill weights are measurable process variables involved in pressure filling.

G. Under-the-Cup Filling

In under-the-cup filling, the propellant is usually added to an open
aerosol product container by forcing propellant under the aerosol
valve cup just prior to sealing on the valve. The container is then
filled and sealed in the same unit operation. It is somewhat similar

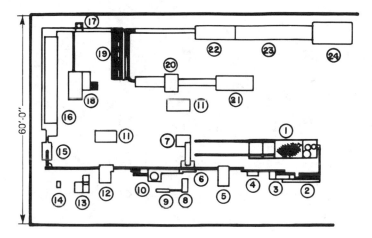

Fig. 3 Lehn and Fink hi-speed aerosol line.

1. Depalletizer.	12. Undercap Filler.
2. Unscrambler.	13. Propellent Pump.
3. Can Cleaner.	14. Heat Exchanger.
4. Can Bottom Coder.	15. Checkweigher.
5. Concentrate Filler	16. Water Bath.
6. Sorter Station of Valve Inserter.	17. Capper.
	18. Cap Sorter Station.
7. Hopper of Valve Inserter.	19. Accumulator Table.
	20. Case Packer.
8. Varidyne Motor.	21. Box Former.
9. Electrical Control Panel.	22. Case Sealer.
	23. Compression Unit and Case Coder Station.
10. Valve Inserter.	
11. Repair Benches.	24. Palletizer.

to pressure filling but is done before, rather than after, the valve is sealed onto the container. Process variables are similar to those of pressure filling.

H. Valve Crimping

Valve crimping (clinching, sealing, swaging) is the process of sealing the aerosol valve onto the container. It is usually accomplished by deforming the valve cup or ferrule so that it compresses a sealing gasket between the container rim and the valve cup or ferrule. While Budzilek [11, 12], Brinkley [13], and Sokol [14] have discussed various techniques of crimping aerosol units, parameters affecting processing will be addressed here.

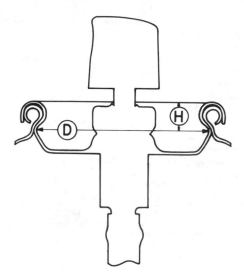

Fig. 4 Depth (H) and diameter (D) of a typical can valve crimp.

Can Valve Crimping

Can values are sealed onto cans by placing the valve inside the can
opening and then crimping or deforming the valve cap outward
beneath the can rim. Seal is accomplished by compressing a flowed-
in or fitted gasket between the valve cup and the can rim. Due to
the wide variety of can neck and curl configurations, crimping control can be a complicated situation. The CSMA Crimp Committee devised and approved a listing of 16 critical mechanical considerations
that affect the crimp. Table 3 represents this list [15]. The Crimp
Committee has not, however, developed any recommendations on
crimping specifications. Since it is difficult to measure gasket compression in such a system, crimping is usually controlled by controlling the depth and diameter of the valve crimp. Figure 4 illustrates the depth (H) and diameter (D) of a typical can valve crimp.
Since the dimensions of the valve cup, gasket, and can rim are
quite consistent, crimp measurements are usually adequate in assess-
ing can valve crimping. Therefore, crimp diameter and crimp depth
are measurable process variables in can valve crimping.

Bottle Valve Crimping

Bottle valves are sealed onto bottles (glass, plastic, or metal vials)
by placing the valve ferrule over the bottle rim and crimping or deforming the ferrule inward toward the bottle neck. The seal is accomplished by compressing a gasket between the valve ferrule and

Table 3 Critical Mechanical Considerations Affecting Valve Crimping

Critical dimensions of the can
1. Diameter of can opening   1.00 ± 0.004 in.
2. Can curl thickness: 0.130 ± 0.007 in.

Critical dimensions of the valve cup
These dimensions may be considered as "Proposed Tentative Standard Dimensions" provided through the CSMA. They apply only to tin-plate valve cups.
3. Outside cup diameter B_V
4. Inside skirt radius $R_V - T_V$
5. Tinplate thickness: T_V 0.011 ± 0.001
6. Flowed-in gasket thickness (dry) D_V
         0.023 ± 0.001 in.
7. Flowed in gasket length: E_V

Critical dimensions of the crimping collet
Applies only to six-segment, 3/64-in.-radius collets designed for standard 1-in. valves.
8. Collect foot radius: 0.047 ± 0.002
9. Check diametral integrity of collet in expanded position (ring gauge).
10. Check corner radius at each edge of all segments (radius gauge).

Critical dimensions of crimped valve cup
These dimensions apply only to 1-in. tinplate valve cups, crimped onto tinplate cans.
11. Measure crimp diameters across all segment impressions: 1.070 ± 0.005 in.
12. Measure crimp diameters across all segment gaps.[a]
13. Measure gap width between section of crimped impressions.[a]
14. Check for contact between can curl and valve cup at segment impression.[a]
     Check for contact between can curl and valve cup at gaps between segment impressions.[a]
15. Measure crimp depth at each collet: 0.185 ± (variable)
16. Measure mounting cup gasket compression at top of can curl, after Crimping.[a]
     a. Measure gasket thickness before crimping.
     b. Measure distance between top of can curl and inside surface of metal valve cup.

[a]Industry specifications not developed as of 1982.

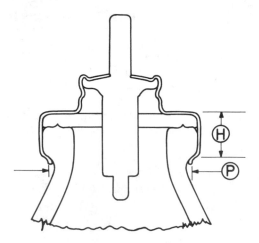

Fig. 5 Height (H) and pull-in (P) of a typical bottle valve crimp.

and the bottle neck. Budzilek [11] has suggested a method based
on crimp height and crimp diameter (pull-in). Gasket compression
is difficult to measure, and sealing is usually assessed by measuring
crimp height (H) and crimp pull-in (P). Figure 5 illustrates the
height (H) and pull-in (P) of a typical bottle valve crimp. For
bottle valve crimping, crimp height and crimp pull-in are measurable
process variables.

Rim Residues

Rim residues are films of powder, liquid, or semisolid usually in-
advertently left on the container rim. Regardless of whether the
residues occur on the container or valve, any residue between the
container rim and the valve gasket may adversely affect the container
seal even if all the crimping dimensions are controlled. Since it is
difficult to assess the presence and effect of rim residues, this is
best done by inspection of components, careful filling, and adequate
inspection during filling and crimping. Therefore, the presence or
absence of rim residues is a measurable process variable in the valve
crimping of can or bottle valves.

Leak Testing and Burst Testing

Leak and burst testing are the processes of ensuring that pressure-
tight seals have been made during valve crimping and that the con-
tainer-valve system is intact and can withstand the maximum of temperature and pressure that they are likely to encounter in commerce.
This testing is usually done by passing the filled and sealed aerosol

product containers through a heat tank or tunnel. While a hot-water tank is most commonly used, a heat tunnel has been successfully used with some products [16]. Containers should be heated to achieve their equilibrium pressure at 130°F (54.5°C) and observed for leakage or bursting. Adequate safety protection should be provided. In a hot-water tank, the submersion time necessary to warm filled units to this temperature may be many minutes and conceivably could slow production. So bath temperature above 130°F may be used. It is necessary to control the temperatures and pressures achieved during these procedures.

The detection of leakage or bursting is usually done by visual observation. Adequate safety precautions must be observed to protect workers inspecting units for leakage or bursting from fragment or chemical exposure from the product.

Once the general process of leak testing and burst testing has been established for a given product, bath temperature, product temperature, and batch submersion time will be considered as measurable processing variables.

I. Performance Testing

Performance testing is the process of checking and assuring the overall functionality of the filled aerosol unit. It is especially important in aerosol products, since lack of performance makes the product completely unavailable to the potential user.

Sampling

Since performance testing of filled units results in the loss of depletion of product, its use should be restricted or controlled. Sampling may be statistically controlled or done on a 100% basis. One hundred percent inspection is usually reserved for essential medicinal or metered valve products.

Product Depletion

As mentioned above, any product consumed in performance testing is not available to the purchaser. Samples used in performance testing must either be removed from those released for sale or must be tested in such a way as to assure the content and quality of the marketed product.

Valve or Nozzle Residues

When any aerosol product is sampled for performance testing, product residues are left in the valve and actuator. In any performance testing where tested product is to be marketed, care must be exercised to control valve or actuator residues.

Testing Methodology

When performance testing is done, it is important to make the testing
as definitive as possible. It may be necessary to devise special
testing methodology to meet special product performance requirements. Process variables in performance testing can only be identified once the performance testing itself has been established.

IV. PROCESS VALIDATION

As we have illustrated previously, there are a number of process
variables encountered in the manufacture of aerosol products. Many
of these variables are readily controlled with appropriate attention
to monitoring. Maintaining the process in control is not enough.
Determining the effect of variations in processing on the end
product's suitability is necessary, not only desirable. Every manufacturing process, whether large or small, exhibits some differences
on a batch-to-batch or day-to-day basis. This is normal in the
world of human involvement in dynamic processing. The ultimate
goal of validation is to establish the parameters of manufacture within
which a satisfactory product is produced. The following procedures
are suggested to facilitate the control and validation of the major
processes associated with the manufacture of aerosol products. Table
4 provides a listing of specific features of an aerosol filling line where
a process validation effort would be indicated [17].

A. Establish Process Variables

As discussed, process-variables can be difficult to determine. Only
by understanding and thoroughly analyzing the manufacturing process
can the variables be recognized and identified. A process cannot be
controlled until the variables have been identified.

B. Measurement Techniques

Once the processing variables have been identified, a method to measure or control those variables is needed. This could be very simple,
such as a temperature measurement, or quite difficult, such as the
analysis of vapor compositions. Regardless, it is necessary to measure the variable identified.

The *Annual Book of ASTM Standards*, Section 15, includes several
test monographs for aerosols [18]. Table 5 shows a listing of standardized test methods for aerosols. A wealth of information may also
be found in the publications of the Chemical Specialties Manufacturing
Associations (CSMA) [19].

Table 4 Specific Features of an Aerosol Filling Line Where Process Validation is Indicated

---

A. *Propellant handling*
  1. Compressed gas
     a. Pressure
     b. Temperature
  2. Liquefied propellants
     a. Temperature
     b. Fractionation

B. *Propellant filling*
  1. Cold filling
     a. Pressure
     b. Temperature
     c. Line speed
  2. Pressure filling
     a. Headspace purging
     b. Fill weights
  3. Under-cup filling
     a. Headspace purging
     b. Fill weights

C. *Valve crimping*
  1. Can valves
     a. Crimp diameter
     b. Crimp depth
     c. Rim residues
  2. Bottle valves
     a. Crimp height
     b. Crimp pull-in
     c. Rim residues

D. *Leak testing and burst testing*
  1. Bath temperature
  2. Submersion time
  3. Product temperature

E. *Performance testing*
  1. Sampling
  2. Product depletion
  3. Valve or nozzle residues
  4. Testing methodology

Table 5 Packaging Specifications, Test Methods, and Recommendations for Aerosol Products (ASTM Standards)

D 3057-72	Test for Moisture in Aerosol Products
D 3058-72	Spec. for Simple Can-Puncturing Device
D 3059-72	Test for Percent Product Retention in Pressurized Foods
D 3060-72	Test for Pressure Drop Rate of Compressed Gas-Propelled Products
D 3061-72	Spec. for Tin-Plate Fabricated Aerosol Cans
D 3062-72	Test for Solids Content of Aerosol Coatings
D 3063-72	Test for Pressure in Glass Aerosol Bottles
D 3064-72	Def. of Terms and Nomenclature Relating to Aerosol Products
D 3065-72	Test for Flammability of Aerosol Cans
D 3066-72	Rec. Practice for Labeling Aerosol Cans
D 3067-72	Rec. Practice of Reporting Laboratory Results When Checking Aerosol Containers
D 3068-72	Spec. for Safe Fill for Aerosol Containers
D 3069-72	Test for Delivery Rate of Aerosol Products
D 3070-72	Rapid Pressure Determination of Pressurized Products
D 3071-72	Drop Testing of Glass Aerosol Bottles
D 3072-72	Tests for Volatile Content of Aerosol Products
D 3073-72	Rec. Practice for Inspection of Glass Aerosol Containers
D 3074-72	Test for Pressure in Metal Aerosol Containers
D 3075-72	Test for Overrun of Food Aerosols
D 3076-72	Tests for Effective Crimping on Outside Crimped Valves of Aerosol Containers
D 3077-72	Rec. Practice for Comparison of Spray Patterns
D 3088-72	Test for Effectiveness of Aerosol and Pressurized Space Spray Insecticides Against Flying Insects
D 3089-72	Measurement of A-D Dimension of Aerosol Valve Dip Tubes
D 3090-72	Rec. Practice of Storage of Aerosol Products
D 3091-72	Rec. Practice for Safe Filling of Low-Pressure Pressurized Products

Table 5 (Continued).

D 3092-72	Test for Particle Size Distribution of Space Insecticide Aerosol
D 3093-72	Test for Pickup Efficiency of Residual Aerosol Insecticides
D 3094-72	Test for Seepage Rate of Aerosol Products
D 3095-72	Test for Effectiveness of Aerosol Insecticides Against Cockroaches
D 3096-72	Test for Liquid Densities of Pressurized Products
D 3097-72	Testing Aerosol Products for Delivered Mass

C. Challenge Testing

Challenge the process by altering and controlling the measurable variables. When methods have been established for measuring the identified processing variables, it is then necessary to measure the effects of variation of these variable on the product being manufactured. This may be done by subjecting the process to a series of controlled variations of these measurable variables. In the simplest case, each challenge could involve only a change on one variable to assess its effect on the overall process. To simplify the infinite variations possible, a challenge of each identified process variable could consist of testing each variable at some maximum and minimum value.

Alternatively, once the process variables have been identified and challenge ranges established, it may be more efficient to establish a program for statistically challenging the system. With this approach, it may be possible to device a challenge system that addresses more than one variable at a time and that also addresses variable interactions. It is desirable to obtain a statistical analysis early in the attempts to establish a process validation program to expedite the process validation with a minimum amount of effort.

As each variable is altered, its effect on the process and the resulting product should be carefully assessed. Records must be kept of each challenge and the results of the variable challenges evaluated individually and collectively. It is desirable to retain records as long as possible, since they may be useful in aspects of future validation based on a review of these records as historical data.

D. Establishment of Validated Process Criteria

Once the process variables have been challenged and the results of
these challenges evaluated, a proposed validated process should be
defined. Target ranges or specifications based on the validation
data should be selected for each identified measurable processing
variable. Since each variable has been challenged and controlled,
the overall process should be in control.

Monitor the proposed validated process for its continued suitability. Records should be kept of each lot of product made using
the proposed validated process. These records should include the
values of each measurable processing variable, and, if necessary,
the proposed validated process can be further modified to allow for
other manufacturing conditions from which a suitable product would
be realized.

V. COMMERCIAL PRODUCTION

Large-scale manufacturing of aerosols requires an understanding of
various aspects of chemical and mechanical engineering. The handling
of volatile liquids such as liquefied gases may be accomplished under
pressure, extremely low temperatures, or a combination of both. In
many instances, the loss of propellant on a filling line due to a leak
would go unnoticed until someone realized the yields were down or a
vapor-pressure check on a container indicated a problem.

Construction of an aerosol filling line requires the installation of
special storage tanks, manufacturing kettles and rooms, customized
filling equipment, in addition to the variety of usual apparatus found
in manufacturing plants. The materials of construction are critical
to the line's integrity and generally add to the cost of installation.
Pressure-rated, sealable, glass-lined or stainless steel tanks are
commonly used for preparing aerosol concentrates. The necessary
refrigeration, environment, and safety equipment for the aerosol
processing area requires significant floor space, and energy resources
and must be given due consideration. A detailed discussion of aerosol production equipment and plant design can be found in *The Aerosol Handbook* [20].

VI. CONCLUSION

This chapter has addressed aspects affecting the large-scale manufacture of aerosol products. Our goal has been to provide a discussion that covers those issues encountered with aerosol manufacturing
with an emphasis on topics specific to the pharmaceutical industry.
With an understanding of the manufacturing and control processes

involved in the production of aerosols, successful commercialization of this specialized drug delivery system can be attained.

VII. REFERENCES

1. M. A. Johnson (ed.), *The Aerosol Handbook*, 1st ed., Wayne Dorland Company, N.J., 1972, pp. 391–392.
2. A. Herzka (ed.), *International Encyclopedia of Pressurized Packaging (Aerosols)*, Pergamon Press, Elmsford, N.Y., 1966.
3. H. R. Shepherd (ed.), *Aerosols: Science and Technology*, Interscience, New York, 1961.
4. M. Root, *Cosmetics, Science and Technology*, Vol. 2, 2nd ed., John Wiley, New York, 1972, pp. 417–485.
5. P. A. Sanders, *Principles of Aerosol Technology*, Van Nostrand Reinhold, New York, 1970.
6. W. G. Gorman and G. D. Hall, "Inhalation Aerosols," Current Concepts: Dosage Form Design and Bioavailability," Lea & Febinger, Philadelphis, 1974, pp. 97–148.
7. D. E. Dean, Quality control of propellants and propellant systems, *CSMA Proc.*, Part 47-1:59–60 (1960).
8. E. I. du Pont de Nemours, Vapor Pressure and Liquid Density of "Freon" Propellants, Freon Aerosol Report FA-22, E. I. du Pont de Nemours & Co., Wilmington, Del., 1957.
9. T. Frost, Application of in-line check weighing, *Manufacturing Chemist*, June 1982, pp. 38, 39, 41, 43.
10. M. A. Johnson (ed.), *The Aerosol Handbook*, 2nd ed., Wayne Dorland Company, N.J., 1982, p. 384.
11. E. Budzilek, Crimping aerosol bottles, *Drug and Cosmetic Industry*, December 1968, p. 45.
12. E. Budzilek, Checking the crimp of glass aerosols, *Aerosol Age*, *12*(4):34 (1967).
13. E. Brinkley, Crimping aerosol cans, *Aerosol Age*, *12*(2):25 (1967).
14. H. Z. Sokol, The fine points of closing miniature aerosol containers, *Packaging Eng.*, May 1967, p. 88.
15. M. A. Johnson (ed.), *The Aerosol Handbook*, 2nd ed., Wayne Dorland Company, N.J., 1982, p. 287.
16. R. B. Holmgren, Schering-Plough crosses the Atlantic; brings back aerosol line, *Packaging Eng.*, November 1981, pp. 41–45.
17. W. G. Gorman, K. F. Popp, W. A. Hunke, and E. P. Mariani, Process validation of aerosol products, *Aerosol Age*, *32*(3): 24–28 (1987).
18. American Society for Testing and Materials, *Annual Book of ASTM Standards*, Section 15, Vol. 1509, American Society for Testing and Materials, Philadelphia, 1984.

19. Chemical Specialties Manufacturing Associations, New York.
20. M. A. Johnson (ed.), *The Aerosol Handbook*, 2nd ed., Wayne
     Dorland Company, N.J., 1982, pp. 373–409.

INDEX